Obsessive-Compulsive Symptoms in Schizophrenia

Lieuwe De Haan
Frederike Schirmbeck
Mathias Zink
Editors

Obsessive-Compulsive Symptoms in Schizophrenia

Springer

Editors
Lieuwe De Haan
Department of Psychiatry
University of Amsterdam
Academic Medical Centre
Amsterdam
The Netherlands

Mathias Zink
Psychiatry and Psychotherapy
Central Institute of Mental Health
Mannheim
Germany

Frederike Schirmbeck
Department of Psychiatry
University of Amsterdam
Academic Medical Centre
Amsterdam
The Netherlands

ISBN 978-3-319-34958-9 ISBN 978-3-319-12952-5 (eBook)
DOI 10.1007/978-3-319-12952-5

Springer Cham Heidelberg New York Dordrecht London

Softcover reprint of the hardcover 1st edition 2015

Printed on acid-free paper

Springer is part of Springer Science+Business Media (www.springer.com)

Preface

The aim of this book is to summarize the current advances in our understanding of obsessive-compulsive symptoms (OCS) in schizophrenia.

It all starts with our patients, for example Anna who is convinced that others are able to read her thoughts. Therefore she tries to think as superficial as possible and to stop thinking about emotional matters. Because this is difficult to do and makes her tense and tired, she prefers to stay at home alone. She always has been excessively clean and is preoccupied with the thought that she needs to wash her hands 7 times after she touches something that might have been touched by others. She knows that it is a silly thing to do but she cannot stop it.

Or Thomas, who was diagnosed with a first psychotic episode, when he was 20 years old, and reported to fear that others could read his thoughts and that he was hearing commanding voices. He was further convinced that his neighbors and the police were spying on him and that they were able to control everything that happened to him. He was admitted to the hospital several times and was then treated with clozapine. He reported subsequent remission of psychotic symptoms, but when the medication was at the highest level, he developed obsessions related to contamination and fire, which led to the checking of electronic devices and excessive hand washing about 30 times per day. He further avoided specific objects and public places and needed constant reassurance from his mother.

Obsessive-compulsive disorder (OCD) or OCS occur far more frequent in schizophrenia patients when compared to the general population. A recent meta-analysis reported prevalence rates of OCS, defined as any obsession or compulsion, in 30.3% of patients with psychotic disorders. Co-morbid OCD according to international criteria was found in 13.6% with an even higher prevalence in chronic populations (see Chap. 4). Schizophrenia patients with co-morbid OCD often display a reduced quality of life, a poor treatment response, worse long-term outcome, and greater functional impairments.

As shown in the cases of Anna and Thomas, the clinical presentation of OCS in patients with schizophrenia is diverse and can emerge before, concurrent with, or after the first onset of psychotic symptoms, and it may be related to treatment with antipsychotic medication (see Chap. 3).

Over the past decades, several research groups investigated this co-morbidity and accumulated evidence regarding epidemiology, clinical characteristics, and etiological explanations and provided suggestions for pharmacological treatment interventions and cognitive behavioural therapy (see Chaps. 11 and 12).

Schizophrenia is a heterogeneous disorder. Differences between patients and longitudinal courses over time within patients are substantial. These differences and changes are important to consider in staging and profiling of the disorder. Ultimately the goal is to deliver individualized treatment options dedicated to the stage and individual profile of patients in order to achieve recovery and improve quality of live. Comorbid psychiatric syndromes, like OCS, interfere with successful treatment and must be integrated into an individualized concept of therapeutic interventions.

We asked world leading researchers and clinicians to contribute, in order to provide a 'state of the art book' concerning OCS as a clinical relevant profile in schizophrenia and related disorders.

In Part I, comorbidities of schizophrenia and OCD will be described along the lines of multidimensional concepts in psychiatry leading to clinical relevant profiles. In Part II, the phenomenology of OCS in patients with psychotic disorders will be reviewed: clinical presentation; epidemiology; dimensional overlap; associations with other symptoms, general functioning; and neurocognitive impairment. In Part III, gene-environment interactions, neurophysiological and neuroimaging findings, and effects of antipsychotic treatment on OCS will be reviewed. In Part IV, medication strategies and cognitive behavioural therapy will be extensively discussed. Finally, the editors will provide a summary of a possible future research agenda.

We are very fortunate in having gathered a talented group of authors and thank them for their enthusiastic participation. We are confident that this book will provide a comprehensive summary of the current scientific knowledge. We hope to increase the awareness and stimulate the improvement of effective treatment strategies for schizophrenia patients with comorbid OCS.

Amsterdam, The Netherlands	Lieuwe De Haan
Amsterdam, The Netherlands	Frederike Schirmbeck
Mannheim, Germany	Mathias Zink

Contents

Part I

From Diagnostic Categories to Multidimensional Concepts in Psychiatry

Comorbid Psychiatric Disorders in Schizophrenia: More than Just a Chance Co-occurrence

1

Peter F. Buckley and Michael Y. Hwang

1.1 Are Comorbidities Chance Co-occurrences?

Psychiatric symptoms that aggregate as comorbid conditions are more the rule than the exception among people with schizophrenia. Foremost among these are depression, anxiety, obsessive-compulsive (OC) symptoms, and substance abuse (Buckley et al. 2009). In a meta-analysis of 52 studies of psychiatric comorbidities in schizophrenia, Achim and colleagues (2011) reported a prevalence rate for OCD of 12.1 %, 9.8 % for panic disorders, 12.4 % for PTSD, and 14.9 % for social phobia. While the pathogeneses and even the prevalence of each among people with schizophrenia are widely debated, their existence is not disputed, and such comorbidities substantially complicate the management of schizophrenia, a condition which alone is already challenging enough to understand and treat (Kim et al. 2013; Opler et al. 2013). This book focuses on one symptom constellation – namely, obsessive-compulsive symptoms – and it carefully teases out the biological significant and clinical implications of the OC comorbidity in schizophrenia from several complementary vantage points. The purpose of this brief chapter is to illuminate the prevailing themes and set the stage concerning the vexing question of psychiatric comorbidities and schizophrenia.

Robert Kendall, the British phenomenologist and famed student of psychiatric nosology, ascribed an intuitive hierarchy to mental health diagnoses (Surtees and

P.F. Buckley, MD (✉)
Medical College of Georgia, Georgia Regents University,
1120 15th Street, AA-1002, Augusta, GA 30912, USA
e-mail: pbuckley@gru.edu

M.Y. Hwang, MD
Department of Psychiatry (116A),
New York Medical College, F.D.R VAMC, Montrose,
New York, NY 10548, USA
e-mail: michael.hawng@va.gov

L. De Haan et al. (eds.), *Obsessive-Compulsive Symptoms in Schizophrenia*,
DOI 10.1007/978-3-319-12952-5_1

Table 1.1 Prevalence estimates of co-occurrence of psychiatric condition in patients with schizophrenia

Condition	% of patients
Depression	50
Anxiety disorders	30
PTSD[a]	12
Obsessive compulsive symptoms[a]	12[b]
Substance abuse	50

[a]Derived from meta-analysis of studies by Achim et al. (2011)
[b]In another meta-analysis and meta-regression by Swets et al. (2014), obsessive-compulsive disorder prevalence was recorded as 12.3 % (rising to 13.6 % by meta-regression); any OC symptoms were recorded in 30 % of patients

Kendell 1979). He eloquently espoused that schizophrenia was foremost in this hierarchy and that, in essence, if you were diagnosed with schizophrenia, then you couldn't simultaneously be diagnosed with other "lower-order" conditions such as anxiety disorders or depression.

While such early diagnostic concept has guided the research approaches and clinical management for over a century, time and systematic epidemiological, clinical, and biological studies have variously chipped away at this notion, and there is now compelling evidence that some of these psychiatric comorbidities – with clinical features analogous to their presentation in nonpsychotic patients – occur at greater prevalence and may have biopsychosocial pathogeneses. Consequently, the current evidence suggests that patients with comorbid disorders in schizophrenia require specific diagnostic assessment and appropriate treatment interventions to achieve an optimal outcome (Hwang et al. 2009; Swendsen et al. 2010; Opler et al. 2013; Buckley et al. 2009; Reynolds et al. 2013).

A summary of prevalence rates is given in Table 1.1.

1.2 Clinical Case Illustrations

Case 1 A 45-year-old white male presented with a 27-year history of chronic undifferentiated schizophrenia, including 16 years of institutionalization. On his last hospital admission 4 years previously, he was agitated, psychotic, and engaged in a number of bizarre, stereotyped behaviors such as repeated face and hand washing and touching door frames in a ritualistic manner before walking through them. He remained unchanged or worsened during the next year, despite trials of various neuroleptics, both alone and in combination with lithium, carbamazepine, propranolol, and lorazepam. A neurological work-up, including EEG, brain CT scan, and skull series, was unremarkable. Treatment with chlorpromazine (CPZ) 1,000 mg bid resulted in only partial improvement of psychosis, and he benefited mainly from its sedating effects. The bizarre rituals persisted and a clinical trial of fluoxetine was started. After 2 weeks of treatment on 40 mg/day, his rituals became less frequent and intense. His self-care skills improved, and he became more responsive toward routines and to staff attempts to engage him in therapeutic activities. After a year of treatment, when fluoxetine was reduced to 20 mg/day, frequency and intensity of his rituals increased. A subsequent increase to 60 mg/day of fluoxetine for 6 weeks brought about marked symptom relief and improvement. The patient remained improved and stable during 2 years of follow-up with combined CPZ and fluoxetine treatment.

Case 2 A 35-year-old white male with hallucinations and paranoia was diagnosed at age 12 as with undifferentiated schizophrenia. Several acute psychotic episodes had been well controlled with neuroleptic treatment. However, during his most recent hospitalization, in which he presented with acute paranoid delusions, auditory/visual hallucinations, and catatonic behavior, he responded poorly to a variety of antipsychotic and adjunctive medications. Unlike previous episodes, he remained markedly psychotic and dysfunctional despite treatment. In addition, he began to exhibit bizarre, compulsive rituals including repetitive touching of objects, opening and closing of doors, drinking water, and forcefully rubbing and injuring his own eyes. His neurologic examination, including brain CT scan, was unremarkable. CMI was added to the ongoing fluphenazine decanoate and lithium carbonate (1,200 mg/day) treatment regimen, starting at 25 mg/day increased to 50 mg/day over a 2 week period. After 4 weeks on 50 mg/day of CMI, rituals became less frequent and intense, with improved engagement in the treatment milieu. However, when CMI was further increased to 150 mg/day, he became restless, hyperactive, impulsive, and agitated. Subsequent dose reduction to 50 mg/day resulted in symptom relief and functional improvement. He was discharged and followed as an outpatient, and for over 2 years he has remained stable.

Case 3 Ms. L. is a 32-year-old Asian female, diagnosed with paranoid schizophrenia 13 months prior to our encounter with the patient. Although her psychosis was well controlled with risperidone treatment, 5 months after initial diagnosis, she exhibited compulsive counting and checking behaviors. Due to the parkinsonian adverse effects, her treatment regimen was subsequently changed to clomipramine 175 mg, risperidone 0.5 mg, diazepam 15 mg, and propranolol 30 mg/day with good control of psychotic symptoms without medication side effects. However, her OC symptoms persisted, and she was transferred to our facility with a Y-BOCS score of 33 (16 for obsessions/17 for compulsions). Clomipramine was increased to 450 mg/day for 6 weeks but resulted in intolerable anticholinergic side effects and severe tremor. Clomipramine was then changed to fluoxetine 80 mg/day, and risperidone was titrated up to 6 mg/day. After 2 weeks of hospitalization, the patient had only partial improvements in rituals and was discharged to initiate cognitive-behavioral therapy as outpatient. After 6 month of combination treatment of psychotherapy and pharmacotherapy, OC symptoms were in remission with continued remission of other psychotic symptoms. Ms. L. is currently maintained symptom-free on risperidone 1 mg, fluoxetine 60 mg, and clonazepam 1 mg.

1.3 Well...Maybe These Features Are All Just Part of Schizophrenia Anyway?

The development of psychiatric nosology after Kendell and in subsequent iterations of the Diagnostic and Statistical Manuel (DSM) and International Classification of Diseases (ICD) has sought to refine and characterize the essence of this enigmatic condition termed schizophrenia (Tandon 2012). Conceptualizations have variously highlighted positive symptoms, negative symptoms, cognitive deficits, and illness course. Additionally, the boundaries of schizophrenia have been blurred by substantial overlap of the clinical manifestations between psychotic disorders and mood (neurotic) disorders (Waddington and Buckley 2013), between psychotic (paranoid and delusional) states, and between even broader developmental spectrum disorders (Tandon 2012). Many have asserted that DSM-5 rather than clarifying these issues has added further complexity, including the recognition of attenuated psychosis syndrome ("schizophrenia lite," just like a "head cold" might resemble and presage a "flu") (Tandon 2012; Frances and Nardo 2013; Regier et al. 2013). Zink and colleagues (2014) observed more similarities than differences [although higher positive symptoms overall] in individuals with at-risk mental states who had OC symptoms compared to those individuals who did not.

It was hoped that DSM-5 would afford, based upon fundamental advances in the neurobiology of psychiatric conditions, the opportunity to advance beyond approaches that are overly reliant on aggregations of symptoms and move to a higher understanding based on the basic neurobiological constructs that may underlie the protean expressions of specific symptom or group of psychiatric conditions ("spectrum disorder") (Regier et al. 2013). The Research Domain Criteria (RDOC) represents the latest effort – firmly at a research rather than clinical level – to understand the neurobiology of mental illnesses (Cuthbert and Insel 2013).

Given such sustained and uncertain technetronic shifts in nosology, it is hardly surprising that psychiatric comorbidities in schizophrenia remain a nosological conundrum and are inadequately studied to date. There is, of course, still the hope that by further exploration of comorbid psychiatric conditions may provide better insight whether they are intricate to the illness, define some distinct subgroup, or speak to some other etiological process or vulnerability that results in the high co-occurrence of distinct psychiatric comorbidities in patients with schizophrenia (Kim et al. 2013; Opler et al. 2013; Buckley et al. 2009).

1.4 Psychiatric Comorbidities and Schizophrenia: Pathobiological Speculations and Avenues for Inquiry

There is now emergent evidence that people with schizophrenia are at greater risk of childhood physical and psychological trauma, effects that might also lead to comorbidities like anxiety and substance abuse as a result of shared epidemiological risk factors (Clarke et al. 2013). Another plausible explanation for co-occurrence is that there is some shared genetic vulnerability. There is now ample evidence of substantial overlap of genetic aberrancies between schizophrenia and other psychiatric and neurodevelopmental disorders (Cross-Disorder Group 2013). There may also be fundamental biological perturbations that represented a shared "final common pathway" for psychosis and for a specific psychiatric comorbidity. As just one example, extant neuroscience literature now points to a similar neurobiological end point of dopamine receptor "supersensitivity" both in psychosis and in craving among addiction disorders (Wang et al. 2010). Reynolds, Mehta, and Nasrallah point to the overlap between depression and schizophrenia with respect to perturbations in brain-derived neurotrophic factor (BDNF). Another, often-cited reason for comorbidities is the effects of stress. As one example, it is proposed that people with schizophrenia will self-medicate their stress and symptoms like hallucinations by using alcohol or drugs like marijuana (Buckley et al. 2009). At the other end of this range of multiple plausible explanations for psychiatric comorbidities, there is also evidence that our medications may also be contributory. For example, the expression of OC symptoms as a side effect of clozapine (and, to a lesser extent, also with other second-generation antipsychotic medications) is now well appreciated (Table 1.2) (Doyle et al. 2014).

While further work is clearly needed, current evidence suggests a biopsychosocial multifactorial pathogeneses for the OC phenomena in patients with schizophrenia, and we propose a preliminary outline for the pathogeneses of OC schizophrenia below.

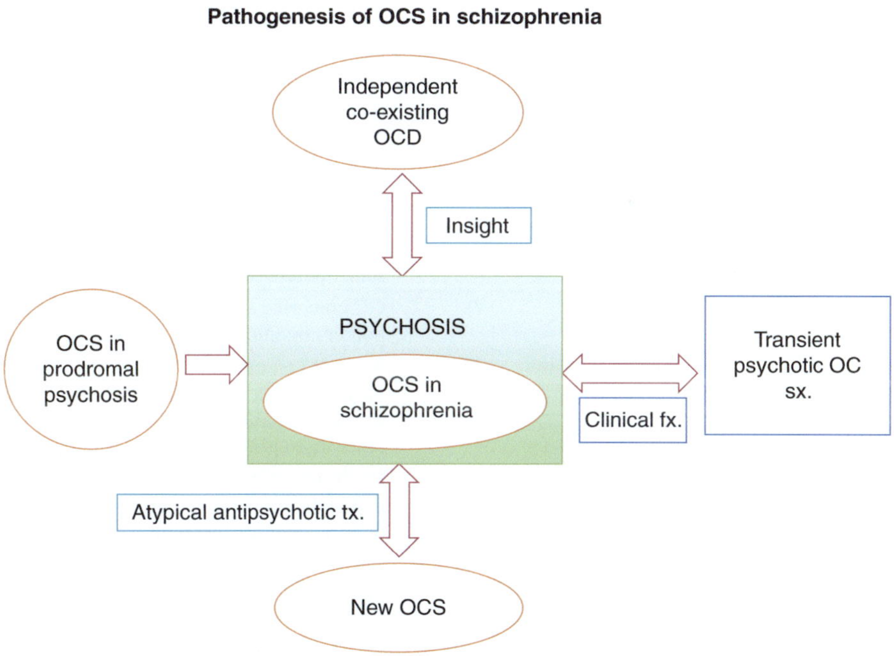

Table 1.2 Recent (2013–2014) studies of psychiatric comorbidities in schizophrenia

Authors	Comorbidity focus	Patients	Findings/conclusions
Doyle et al. (2014)	OC symptoms	97	Compared OC symptoms and characteristics in 62 clozapine-treated schizophrenia patients and 35 OCD without schizophrenia. Most patients developed OC symptoms de novo on clozapine – more cognitive OC than behavioral OC in primary OCD patients
Eryilmaz et al. (2013)	OCS	4	Aripiprazole added to clozapine reduced OC symptoms
Frias et al. (2014)	OC symptoms	67	More similarities than differences between "OCD" schizophrenia patients and patients without OCD
Frommann et al. (2013)	Violence	38	Poor facial recognition in violent/ forensic patients compared with nonviolent schizophrenia patients
Jones and Steel (2014)	PTSD		More intrusive memories in high PTSD symptom patients
Landgraf et al. (2013)	Psychiatric comorbidities	70	Female forensic patients have more psychiatric comorbidities than female patients with schizophrenia in general
Michalopoulou et al. (2014)	OC symptoms	40	No differences apart from minor processing skill deficit in patients with "OCD" and schizophrenia
Pope et al. (2013)	Substance use, mood, anxiety disorders	214	Persistence of comorbidities at 1-year reevaluation in first-episode psychosis patients
Swets et al. (2014)	OC symptoms	3,978	Meta-analysis and meta-regression; mean prevalence of OCD at 12.3 %, although any OC symptoms observed in 30.7 %
Tsai and Rosenheck (2013)	Psychiatric comorbidities	1,446	Separation on latent class analysis between addiction comorbidity, anxiety/ depressive disorders comorbidity, and schizophrenia alone
Whitton and Henry (2013)	OCS	78	OC comorbid symptoms associated with poorer cognition and social performance
Wobrock et al. 2013	Substance abuse	323	31 % of first-episode psychosis patients have substance use comorbidity, mostly cannabis; similar clinical features to other first-episode psychosis patients
Zink et al. (2014)	OC symptoms	233	Prodromal subjects with OC symptoms had higher positive symptoms and poorer cognitive function

1.5 Concluding Remarks

Among the several psychiatric comorbidities that are commonly observed in patients with schizophrenia, OC symptoms in schizophrenia are noteworthy for both their enduring nature and disabling clinical effects as well as an opportunity to explore the biopsychosocial effects on the etiopathogeneses of the OC phenomena in patients with schizophrenia (Hwang et al. 2009; Kim et al. 2013; Opler et al. 2013; Frias et al. 2014; Zink et al. 2014). The expression, potential neurobiological and treatment attributes of OC exemplify many of the considerations highlighted above in this brief review.

References

Achim AM, Maziade M, Raymond E, Olivier D, Mérette C, Roy MA (2011) How prevalent are anxiety disorders in schizophrenia? A meta-analysis and critical review on a significant association. Schizophr Bull 37(4):811–821

Buckley PF, Miller B, Lehrer D, Castle D (2009) Psychiatric comorbidities and schizophrenia. Schizophr Bull 35(2):383–402

Clarke MC, Tanskanen A, Huttunen MO, Cannon M (2013) Sudden death of father or sibling in early childhood increases risk for psychotic disorder. Schizophr Res 143(2–3):363–366

Cross-Disorder Group of the Psychiatric Genomics Consortium; Genetic Risk outcome of Psychosis (GROUP) Consortium (2013) Identification of risk loci with shared effects on five major psychiatric disorders: a genome-wide analysis. Lancet 381(9875):1371–1379

Cuthbert BN, Insel TR (2013) Toward the future of psychiatric diagnosis: the seven pillars of RDoC. BMC Med 11:125

Doyle M, Chorcorain AN, Griffith E, Trimble T, O'Callaghan E (2014) Obsessive compulsive symptoms in patients with Schizophrenia on Clozapine and with Obsessive Compulsive disorder: a comparison study. Compr Psychiatry 55(1):130–136

Eryilmaz G, Hizli Sayar G, Ozten E, Gogcegoz Gul I, Karamustafalioglu O (2013) Aripirazole augmentation in clozapine-associated obsessive-compulsive symptoms in schizophrenia. Ann Gen Psychiatry 12(1):40

Frances AJ, Nardo JM (2013) ICD-11 should not repeat the mistakes made by DSM-5. Br J Psychiatry 203(1):1–2

Frias A, Palma C, Farrols N, Salvador A, Bonet J, Bernáldez I (2014) Psychopathology and quality of live among patients with comorbidity between schizophrenia spectrum disorder and obsessive-compulsive disorder: no evidence for a "schizo-obsessive" subtype. Compr Psychiatry 55(5):1165–1173

Frommann N, Stroth S, Brinkmeyer J, Wolwer W, Luckhaus C (2013) Facial affect recognition performance and event-related potentials in violent and non-violent schizophrenia patients. Neuropsychobiology 68(3):139–145

Hwang MY, Kim SW, Yum SY, Opler LA (2009) Management of schizophrenia with obsessive-compulsive features. In: Hwang MY, Nasrallah HA (eds) Psychiatric and physical comorbidity in schizophrenia. Psychiatr Clin North Am 32(4):835–851

Jones V, Steel C (2014) Examining vulnerability to intrusive memories in schizophrenia comorbid with post traumatic stress disorder. Schizophr Res 15(2):487–489

Kim SW, Lindenmayer J-P, Hwang MY (2013) Schizophrenia with obsessive-compulsive symptoms: clinical and conceptual issues. Psychiatr Ann 43(10):442–445

Landgraf S, Blumenauer K, Osterheider M, Eisenbarth H (2013) A clinical and demographic comparison between a forensic and a general sample of female patients with schizophrenia. Psychiatry Res 210(3):1176–1183

Michalopoulou PG, Konstantakopoulos G, Typaldou M, Papageorgiou C, Christodoulou GN, Lykouras L, Oulis P (2014) Can cognitive deficits differentiate between schizophrenia with and without obsessive-compulsive symptoms? Compr Psychiatry 55(4):1015–1021

Opler LA, Hwang MY, Opler MG (2013) Comorbidities in schizophrenia: challenges for researchers and clinicians. Psychiatr Ann 43(10):438–441

Pope MA, Joober A, Malla AK (2013) Diagnostic stability of first-episode psychotic disorders and persistence of comorbid psychiatric disorders over one year. Can J Psychiatry 58(10): 588–594

Regier DA, Kuhl EA, Kupfer DJ (2013) The DSM-5: classification and criteria changes. World Psychiatry 12(2):92–98

Reynolds D, Mehta P, Nasrallah HA (2013) Evaluation and treatment strategies in patients with schizophrenia and comorbid depression. Psychiatr Ann 43(10):446–453

Surtees PG, Kendell RE (1979) The hierarchy model of psychiatric symptomatology: an investigation based on present state examination ratings. Br J Psychiatry 135:438–443

Swendsen J, Conway KP, Degenhardt L, Glantz M, Jin R, Merikangas KR, Sampson N, Kessler RC (2010) Mental disorders as risk factors for substance use, abuse and dependence: results from the 10-year follow-up of the National Comorbidity Survey. Addiction 105(6):1117–1128

Swets M, Dekker J, Van Emmerik-van Oortmerssen K, Smid GE, Smit F, de Haan L, Schoevers RA (2014) The obsessive compulsive spectrum in schizophrenia, a meta-analysis and meta-regression exploring prevalence rates. Schizophr Res 152(2–3):458–468

Tandon R (2012) The nosology of schizophrenia: toward DSM-5 and ICD-11. Psychiatr Clin North Am 35(3):557–569

Tsai J, Rosenheck RA (2013) Psychiatric comorbidity among adults with schizophrenia: a latent class analysis. Psychiatry Res 210(1):16–20

Waddington JL, Buckley PF (2013) Psychotic depression: an underappreciated window to explore the dimensionality and pathobiology of psychosis. Schizophr Bull 39(4):754–755

Wang M, Pei L, Fletcher PJ, Kapur S, Seeman P, Liu F (2010) Schizophrenia, amphetamine-induced sensitized state and acute amphetamine exposure all show a common alteration: increased dopamine D2 receptor dimerization. Mol Brain 3:25

Whitton AE, Henry JD (2013) The relationship between sub-clinical obsessive-compulsive symptoms and social cognition in chronic schizophrenia. Br J Clin Psychol 52(2):115–128

Wobrock T, Falkai P, Schneider-Axmann T, Hasan A, Galderisi S, Davidson M, Kahn RS, Derks EM, Boter H, Rybakowski JK, Libiger J, Dollfus S, Lopez-Ibor JJ, Peuskens J, Hranov LG, Gaebel W, Fleischhacker WW, EUFES study group (2013) Comorbid substance abuse in first-episode schizophrenia: Effects on cognition and psychopathology in the EUFEST study. Schizophr Res 147(1):132–139

Zink M, Schirmbeck F, Rausch F, Eifler S, Elkin H, Solojenkina X, Englisch S, Wagner M, Maier W, Lautenschlager M, Heinz A, Gudlowski Y, Janssen B, Gaebel W, Michel TM, Schneider F, Lambert M, Naber D, juckel G, Krueger-Oezguerdal S, Wobrock T, Hasan A, Riedel M, Müller H, Klosterkötter J, Bechdolf A (2014) Obsessive-compulsive symptoms in at –risk mental states for psychosis: associates with clinical impairment and cognitive function. Acta Psychiatr Scand 130(3):214–226

Comorbid Psychiatric Disorders in Obsessive-Compulsive Disorder: The Spectrum Concept

2

Anne Katrin Külz and Ulrich Voderholzer

OCD is a multifaceted and heterogeneous disorder comprising various subtypes with different phenomenology. Several other disorders share similarities with OCD in their behavioral features and underlying pathophysiology. The DSM-5 concept for OCD/OC spectrum disorders tries to accommodate these common characteristics by grouping similar diagnostic constructs into a new category of "obsessive–compulsive and related disorders" (OCRDs). Since pure OCD without comorbidities is rather an exception than the rule, it seems extremely important to take potential comorbidities into account. This chapter provides an overview of subtypes of OC symptoms and also presents related disorders and disorders comorbid with OCD.

2.1 Introduction

With a 12-month prevalence of 0.6 % and lifetime prevalence rates of about 2–3 %, obsessive–compulsive disorder (OCD) is one of the most common psychiatric disorders (Crino et al. 2005). This makes it more than twice as frequent as, for example, schizophrenia or panic disorder. In the age group between 15 and 44, OCD was identified among the 20 leading causes for years of life lived with disability (YLD; World Health Organization 2001). The disease pattern is accompanied by substantial impairment in the quality of life and often causes problems in social or family

A.K. Külz (✉)
OCD Outpatient Unit, University Medical Center Freiburg, Clinic of Psychiatry and Psychotherapy, Hauptstraße 5, Freiburg D-79104, Germany
e-mail: anne.katrin.kuelz@uniklinik-freiburg.de

U. Voderholzer
Schoen Clinic Roseneck, am Roseneck 6, Prien am Chiemsee D-83209, Germany
e-mail: UVoderholzer@Schoen-Kliniken.de

L. De Haan et al. (eds.), *Obsessive-Compulsive Symptoms in Schizophrenia*,
DOI 10.1007/978-3-319-12952-5_2

life while also affecting work and the career options. If left untreated, obsessive–compulsive disorder usually takes a relapsing course and becomes chronic (Abramowitz et al. 2009; Visser et al. 2014).

Patients with OCD suffer from recurrent and intrusive thoughts, impulses, or images and/or repetitive behaviors (compulsions) like washing, ordering, or checking. Compulsions are aimed at reducing distress, fear, uneasiness, or worry caused by obsessions or serve to prevent a dreaded event. Typically, they are excessive or not reasonably connected to what they are supposed to prevent. Common compulsions include rituals such as repeatedly checking whether the stove has been turned off or the door is locked to alleviate fears about harm. Another example is excessive hand washing and household cleaning, which often counters an exaggerated fear of contamination. Some patients, however, show only mental rituals (e.g., repetitive praying or counting), which they feel compelled to do in response to an obsession, whereas others experience only obsessions (e.g., intrusive thoughts of hurting one's own baby) without compulsions or subject themselves to rituals that must be performed according to strict rules.

2.2 Subtypes of OCD

Obsessive–compulsive disorder itself represents a phenotypically heterogeneous, multidimensional condition. Although massive research efforts have been undertaken to identify distinct OCD subtypes, attempts to dissect the disorder into homogeneous categories have been limited by the large diversity of identified subgroups stemming from a wide range of criteria, data sources, and applied statistical methods. However, regarding the *symptoms* of OCD, there is growing agreement to classify OCD into three to five symptom dimensions to reduce the complexity of this multifaceted disorder (Abramowitz et al. 2010):

- Obsessions about being responsible for causing or failing to prevent harm with checking compulsions and reassurance seeking
- Contamination obsessions with washing and cleaning rituals
- Symmetry obsessions with ordering, arranging, and counting rituals
- Obsessions without visible compulsions or the so-called "pure" obsessions
- Hoarding obsessions and compulsions

Family studies (Hasler et al. 2007) indicate that a small but statistically significant preferential sharing of symptom dimensions runs in families and that it shows some gender dependence. As stated by van den Heuvel et al. (2009), both distinct and overlapping neural substrates such as specific gray matter and white matter volumes in several brain regions exist between different subtypes. Moreover, there is growing evidence suggesting that specific subtypes of OCD are associated with different treatment responses. Obsessions about overinflated responsibility for harm, for example, were associated with a significantly better diagnosis, whereas remission in patients with hoarding symptoms was significantly less likely (Eisen et al. 2013).

Some investigators have suggested an OCD *subclassification based on comorbid disorders* (e.g., Nestadt et al. 2009). According to their analysis on 706 patients with OCD, the authors found three classes of syndromes in OCD: first, an OCD simplex class, which is characterized by major depression as the most frequent additional disorder; second, OCD classes with tic-related comorbidity, in which affective syndromes are markedly rarer; and third, a comorbid affective-related class in which panic disorder and affective syndromes are predominant (Nestadt et al. 2009). Members of the class with tic-related comorbidity are more likely to be male and to show a high conscientiousness. Class 3 members, in contrast, more frequently are of female gender and have a young age at onset, obsessive–compulsive personality disorder (OCPD) features, high scores on the "taboo" factor of OCD symptoms, and low conscientiousness.

Other authors prefer placing obsessive–compulsive and related disorders on a crosscutting *spectrum between compulsivity and impulsivity* (Robbins et al. 2012; Berlin and Hollander 2014). In addition, several attempts have been undertaken to classify OCD patients according to other *phenomenological characteristics* or *clinical correlates*. Some studies suggest that OCD patients with *early onset of symptoms* are more likely to develop certain comorbidities such as tic disorder and Tourette syndrome than patients where OCD emerges in adulthood (Janowitz et al. 2009). A systematic review suggests that two distinguishable groups exists, one characterized by a mean onset of 11 years and the other by a mean onset of 23 years (Taylor 2011). Based on this classification, about three quarters of OCD patients fall into the category of early onset.

A further aspect that has been brought into play is that OCD patients differ on the basis of their *insight* into the senselessness of their obsessions and compulsive rituals. DSM-IV did not specify whether a patient with poor insight should be diagnosed with OCD or a psychotic disorder. DSM-5 introduced the insight specifier, which allows the determination of the degree of insight within a broader range of several options. This seems especially relevant from a clinical perspective as patients with poor insight may especially benefit from motivational interview techniques used in conjunction with CBT (Meyer et al. 2010). Recent results by Phillips et al. (2012) support the introduction of an insight specifier. They found that the level of insight spans a broad range from absent to excellent in OCD but also in body dysmorphic disorder.

Finally, an interesting approach focuses on the *motivational core dimensions* of OCD symptoms. Whereas, for a long time, OC symptoms have mainly been considered as motivated by harm avoidance, more recent research focuses on sensations of "not just right" or of things being incomplete which may also underlie symptoms. While obsessional thoughts seem to be predominantly related to harm avoidance, symptoms regarding symmetry and ordering seem to be mainly motivated by a sense of incompleteness (Ecker and Gönner 2008).

2.3 OCD Spectrum Disorders

2.3.1 Overview

Whereas DSM-IV grouped OCD with the anxiety disorders, the DSM Working Group felt that a wide range of differences between anxiety disorders and OCD as well as OC spectrum disorders justified the conceptualization of a new Obsessive–Compulsive and Related Disorders chapter. In DSM-5, the new category "OCD and related disorders" (OCRDs) is introduced as a nosologically distinct spectrum including several disorders with common features such as obsessive preoccupation and impulsive, repetitive behaviors. In addition to phenomenological characteristics, preliminary data converge on an etiological, psychobiological, or treatment overlap of OCRDs with OCD (Ameringen et al. 2014). In addition to obsessive–compulsive disorder, trichotillomania (hair-pulling disorder) and body dysmorphic disorder as well as two new disorders, namely, hoarding disorder and excoriation (skin-picking) disorder, are included in this new chapter of DSM-5 (see Fig. 2.1).

The following paragraph describes the OCD spectrum disorders according to DSM-5.

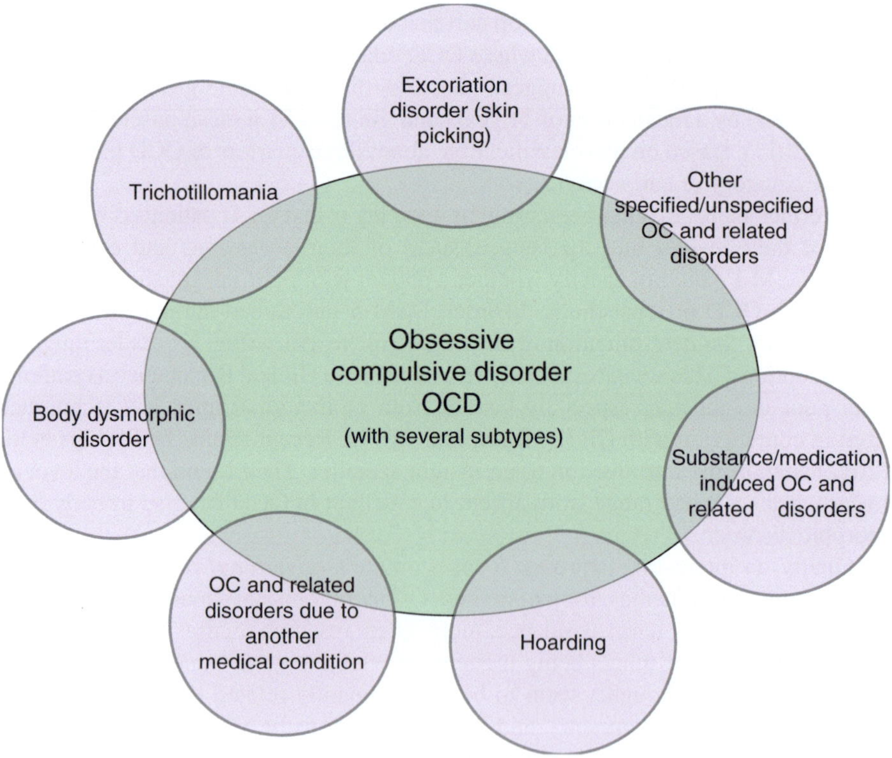

Fig. 2.1 OCD and related disorders

2.3.2 Trichotillomania

Trichotillomania (repeatedly pulling one's hair) is a condition formerly found in the "impulse control disorder not elsewhere classified" section. The diagnostics in DSM-5 involve visible hair loss, a feeling of tension immediately prior to pulling, and a sense of relief or pleasure when pulling out hair. According to DSM-5, individuals have to repeatedly attempt to stop hair pulling. This requirement was not part of the diagnostic criteria in DSM-IV and brings the hair-pulling disorder more in line with the repetitive and ritualized behavior and urges in OCD (Ameringen et al. 2014).

Recent results confirm evidence for the genetic transmission of hair pulling and suggest a familial subtype of hair pulling with comorbid OCD. However, there was no evidence for an etiologic relationship between hair pulling and skin picking (Keuthen et al. 2014).

Rogers et al. (2014) propose a stepped care model with a Web-based self-help program as step 1 followed by the opportunity to engage in an in-person habit reversal training for 8 weeks (step 2). The model was tested in 60 patients and proved to be highly accepted. On top of that, participants showed significant reduction of symptoms and increased quality of life.

2.3.3 Excoriation Disorder (Skin Picking)

As for trichotillomania, excoriation disorder was previously classified under impulse control disorders. Even with a lifetime prevalence estimate of between 2 and 4 % (Grohol 2013), excoriation disorder is new to DSM-5. Patients with this disorder have to suffer from a recurrent urge to pick at one's own skin resulting in skin lesions. The disorder is further characterized by repeated attempts to decrease or stop the skin picking. Excoriation disorder can be very time consuming as individuals sometimes spend up to 8 h per day picking their skin.

Unlike OCD, skin picking is not preceded by obsessions but a high level of tension and an urge to scratch, pick, or squeeze otherwise healthy skin. Several studies suggest that symptom severity tends to fluctuate with stress levels but typically has a chronic course associated with substantial emotional distress and functional impairments (e.g., Odlaug et al. 2010).

Recent data support the conceptualization of excoriation disorders as a valid diagnostic entity (Snorrason et al. 2013). First, skin picking is characterized by a distinct constellation of symptoms, phenomenology, and course. Second, recent data suggest an underlying dysfunction and familiarity that cannot be completely explained by comorbid disorders. Third, skin picking is associated with certain characteristic environmental and temperamental factors such as stress and emotional reactivity.

SSRIs seem to be less effective in the treatment of skin picking, in contrast to OCD, whereas the opioid agonist naltrexone, for example, has demonstrated efficacy in this disorder. Similarly, exposure treatment, the method of first choice in

OCD, seems to be ineffective, whereas patients with skin picking, like patients with trichotillomania, benefit from habit reversal training (Grant et al. 2012). Here, patients are instructed to develop awareness of the picking behavior and, in a next step, to replace it with a harmless habit that makes it impossible.

2.3.4 Hoarding Disorder

Hoarding disorder is a chronic and very debilitating condition characterized by a difficulty in discarding and/or excessive acquiring of things, gathering of clutter, and subsequent distress and impairment due to the hoarding behavior. Often, functional impairment also extends to relatives who live with the patient, so involving family members in the treatment is crucially important.

There is mounting evidence that hoarding pathology is associated with worse treatment outcome compared to other OC symptoms (e.g., Knopp et al. 2013). A large body of research suggests that hoarding disorder is clinically and neurobiologically distinct from OCD and necessitates a somewhat different kind of treatment. In line with this, hoarders seem to have a different pattern of cerebral glucose metabolism than non-hoarding patients with OCD (Saxena et al. 2004).

Though OCD symptoms and hoarding symptoms occasionally co-occur, many patients with hoarding disorder do not suffer from OCD. Recent results, however, suggest that individuals with only hoarding disorder show similar deficits on measures of executive functions as patients with both OCD and severe hoarding. This points toward a similar underlying neuropsychological dysfunction. The authors interpret their results as an argument for the inclusion of hoarding disorder within the new Obsessive–Compulsive and Related Disorders chapter (Morein-Zamir et al. 2014).

2.3.5 Body Dysmorphic Disorder

DSM-5 moved body dysmorphic disorder (BDD) from the somatoform disorders to the obsessive–compulsive spectrum disorders. Recent research on BDD yields a prevalence rate of about 1.8 % (Buhlmann et al. 2010).

Patients with BDD are constantly haunted by feelings of ugliness or an imagined defect in their looks despite a normal appearance or only a slight and trivial abnormality in appearance. Physical features that commonly raise concerns about perceived imperfections or flaws involve the skin, nose, ears, mouth, genitals, or hair. Some subjects, for example, focus their concern on perceived excessive facial hair or a disfigured shape of the nose. The preoccupation must cause clinically significant distress or impaired social or occupational functioning, clearly differentiating the disorder from normal concerns about one's appearance. Many subjects tend to constantly ask for reassurance from others, are engaged in ritualistic checking behaviors, and make time-consuming attempts to improve the perceived imperfection. Others show avoidance behavior, for example, social withdrawal and avoiding mirrors; alternating between excessive checking and avoidance is also not unusual.

Insight in BDD is generally poorer than in OCD. Phillips et al. (2006), for example, investigated the two variants of BDD, namely, delusional and non-delusional. Their study found that about one third (36 %) of BDD subjects were delusional. The proportion of delusional BDD was higher in adolescents than in adults. A recent comparison of insight in BDD and OCD revealed that in both disorders insight can range from excellent to absent. Most OCD patients, however, showed excellent or good insight on the Brown Assessment of Beliefs Scale (BABS), and only 2 % of OCD patients had delusional beliefs. In contrast, the majority of BDD patients scored within the range of poor or absent insight (Phillips et al. 2012), and 32 % showed delusional beliefs.

Buhlmann and Winter (2011) point to several similarities between OCD and BDD. These include checking rituals, similar age of onset and course of illness as well as tendencies to hide the disorder from others due to excessive shame or embarrassment, and a high comorbidity. Major depression and anxiety disorders, however, are also very often comorbid with BDD, and the disorder is frequently associated with suicidal ideation (31 %) and suicide attempts (22 %) (Buhlmann et al. 2010).

So far, serotonin reuptake inhibitors and cognitive behavioral treatment are considered the treatment of choice. A recently evaluated manualized modular cognitive behavioral therapy for BDD over 24 weeks was well received by patients and proved very effective in reducing BDD symptoms (Wilhelm et al. 2014).

2.3.6 Other OCRD Conditions

Substance-/medication-induced OCRD must occur immediately after or during substance intoxication or withdrawal or develop as a consequence of a specific medication. For example, obsessions or compulsive rituals can be caused by certain stimulating drugs containing amphetamines or by corticosteroid therapy (Bhangle et al. 2013).

As OCD can also be caused by certain *medical conditions*, a medical evaluation is always required to rule out that a medical factor is causing obsessions or compulsions. Pediatric autoimmune neuropsychiatric disorders associated with streptococcal infections (PANDAS), for example, can lead to a sudden onset of severe OCD symptoms in children. There is evidence that patients with this type of OCD may benefit from antibiotics in addition to CBT or medication with antidepressants (Murphy et al. 2012). Another example is certain neurodegenerative diseases of the basal ganglia such as Huntington's or Wilson's disease, which can be associated with OC symptoms. New onset of OCD has also been reported secondary to other neurological disorders such as brain tumors, stroke lesions, postencephalopathic disorders, or traumatic brain injury.

Finally, there are *other specified and unspecified obsessive–compulsive and related disorders* for individuals who fulfill some but not all the diagnostic criteria for one of the disorders described above. One example is body dysmorphic-like disorder with actual flaws, which command excessive preoccupation. Another example is obsessional jealousy, which is characterized by non-delusional preoccupation with a partner's perceived infidelity and repetitive behaviors or mental acts concerning the perceived infidelity. Also Jikoshu-kyofu or olfactory reference syndrome – a strong fear of having bad body odor – falls into this category.

2.4 Common Comorbidities

2.4.1 Comorbidity in OCD

A recent study on 955 patients with obsessive–compulsive disorder revealed that only 7.7 % showed no lifetime prevalence of any comorbid DSM-IV Axis I disorder (Torres et al. 2013). In line with this, Murphy et al. (2013) report that comorbidities with psychiatric disorders are two- to eightfold higher in individuals with OCD than the rates of neuropsychiatric disorders in the general US population. The most common psychiatric comorbidities in OCD as determined by several studies are presented in Fig. 2.2 (for a review, see Zaudig 2011). It shows depression as the most frequent comorbid disorder followed by personality disorders and anxiety disorders. Table 2.1 provides a more detailed overview by listing results from studies on comorbidities with large samples of OCD patients ($n>300$). In the following section, the most frequent psychiatric comorbidities of OCD are described.

2.4.2 Affective Disorders

Depression is the most frequent comorbidity in OCD. A large body of research suggests that about two thirds of patients with OCD fulfill criteria for major depression during their lifetime and one third of OCD patients experience a depressive episode at the time of evaluation (Tükel et al. 2002; Timpano et al. 2012).

Depression mostly occurs after the onset of OCD (Bartz and Hollander 2006). This may indicate that patients with OCD develop depressive symptoms mainly due to the functional impairment or the loss of positive reinforcement and of self-esteem

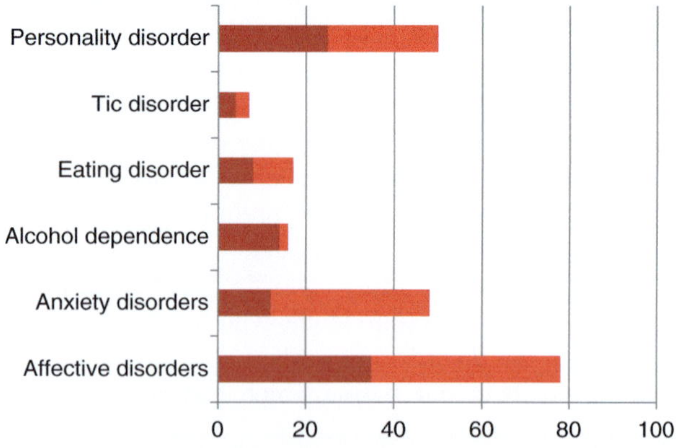

Fig. 2.2 Comorbidities of obsessive–compulsive disorders (%). According to various studies, lower and upper numbers in studies

Table 2.1 Lifetime comorbidity rates of patients with obsessive–compulsive disorder in large studies ($n > 300$)

Comorbid disorder	LaSalle et al. (2004)[a] $N=334$[a]	Hasler et al. (2007)[a] $N=418$	Miguel et al. (2008)[a] $N=630$	Ruscio et al. (2010)[b] $N=2073$	Gomes de Alvarenga et al. (2012)[a] $N=813$	Torres et al. (2014)[a] $N=1,001$
Affective disorders					70.7	60.8
Major depression	66	69	69.7	40.7		56.4
Dysthymia	24	14.1	10.6	13.1		11.9
Bipolar disorder	13	7.0	10.0	23.4		8.2
Social phobia	23	42.6	36.8	43.5	35.2	34.6
Specific phobia	12	38.9	32.4	42.7	33	31.4
Panic disorder with or without agoraphobia	23	21.0	6.2	20.0	5.7	15.3
Agoraphobia without history of panic disorder	18	16.3	5.7	7.8	5	4.9
Generalized anxiety disorder	18	45.8	35.4	8.3	33.8	34.3
Bulimia nervosa	10	5.0	2.9		11.3	
Anorexia nervosa	9	6.2	2.7			
Somatization disorder			3.5		Somatoform disorder 2.8	2.3
Hypochondriasis		7.7				3.4
Alcohol abuse/dependence	23		7.5	38.6		7.9

[a]The Structured Clinical Interview for DSM-IV/Clinical Version (SCID-I/CV) was used to diagnose the Axis I disorders
[b]The Composite International Diagnostic Interview was used to diagnose the Axis I disorder

that OC symptoms cause. In many cases, this leads to a vicious circle that involves depressive mood, growing inactivity, lowered self-esteem, an increase in OC symptoms, and, consequently, worsening of depressive symptoms. There is evidence that OCD patients with comorbid depression benefit less from cognitive behavioral or pharmacological treatment (Overbeek et al. 2002). Moreover, depressive symptoms seem to occur more frequently in response to excessive obsessions than compulsions.

A recently published review on comorbid *bipolar disorder* and OCD (Amerio et al 2014) stated that 11–21 % of patients suffering from bipolar disorder experience obsessive–compulsive disorder in their lifetime, whereas the lifetime prevalence rate of bipolar disorder is about 6–10 % in patients with current OCD. Interestingly, in patients who fulfill both diagnoses, OC symptomatology takes a more episodic course. As might be expected, patients typically show improvement of symptoms during manic or hypomanic episodes and exacerbation of symptoms during depressive episode.

Whereas cognitive behavioral therapy has been established as highly efficacious in OCD, patients with comorbid depression seem to be slightly less responsive to behavioral-based treatment alone (Hohagen et al. 1998). Therefore, in the case of comorbid depression, CBT should be combined with selective serotonin reuptake inhibitors.

2.4.3 Anxiety Disorders

As mentioned above, OCD was formally classified as anxiety disorder in DSM-IV. While individuals with anxiety disorders often try to help themselves by avoiding feared situations or stimuli such as closed places or spiders in certain specific phobias, individuals with OCD predominantly engage in rigid rituals or repetitive behavior to achieve temporary relief from their distressing thoughts. In contrast to general anxiety disorder, obsessions mostly go beyond daily worries and focus on one or only a few underlying themes (e.g., "I could have killed someone unintentionally," "there may be germs that make me sick"). As already mentioned, OCD is often accompanied by anxiety, but some patients experience other emotional qualities such as disgust, for example.

A large cross-sectional study with 1,001 OCD patients by Torres et al. (2014) revealed that about 20 % had a lifetime diagnosis of panic disorder and/or agoraphobia. Patients in this subgroup were also more likely to have other Axis I diagnoses, especially other anxiety disorders, hypochondriasis, or mood disorders.

Sometimes patients with severe OCD experience social anxiety resulting from low self-esteem and deficits in social skills due to their longtime social isolation. Moreover, OC symptoms frequently also serve to keep distance from others or to shun social demands (Külz et al. 2010). As noticed by Jakubovski et al. (2013), avoidance tendencies in patients with comorbid anxiety disorder can compromise adherence to exposure treatment. On the other hand, experiencing the mechanisms of stimulus confrontation and habituation can effect relief regarding both OC symptoms and comorbid anxiety disorder.

2.4.4 Substance Use Disorder and Alcohol Dependency

Some individuals with OCD suffer from secondary alcohol dependency or drug addiction. In the study of Mancebo et al. (2008), 27 % of OCD patients had a lifetime diagnosis of substance use disorder. The majority of individuals reported that OCD preceded substance use disorder by at least 1 year; the median was 8 years.

In the study by Gentil et al. (2009), 7.5 % of OCD patients showed alcohol-use disorder comorbidity. These patients were more likely to be men and had a higher rate of suicidal thoughts and suicide attempts. Other comorbidities such as generalized anxiety and somatization disorders were also more common in this group of OCD patients. It is remarkable, however, that the rates of alcohol-use disorder in OCD patients do not seem to differ strongly from community prevalence rates (Wakefield and Schmitz 2014).

Clinical experience generated the hypothesis that some individuals turn to overconsumption of alcohol or to drug use in order to cope with OCD symptoms. For some patients, the intake of alcoholic beverages can easily become a fixed element of the daily routine when social relationships and positive activities fall by the wayside because rituals and absorbing thoughts are highly time-consuming. Unfortunately, this makes it even more difficult to resist the obsessive impulses in the medium term. It seems essential to treat alcoholism or drug addiction first before exposure therapy can be administered effectively.

2.4.5 Personality Disorders

There is a constant interest in possible relations between OCD and obsessive–compulsive personality disorder (OCPD). In a recent study by Starcevic et al. (2013), almost half of the OCD patients (47.3 %) fulfilled the criteria of an obsessive–compulsive personality disorder (OCPD). However, individuals diagnosed with both OCD and OCPD did not differ from other OCD patients regarding demographic variables, mean age of onset of OC symptoms, clinician-rated severity of OCD, or levels of disability. Other authors, however, found an association between comorbid obsessive–compulsive personality disorder and early onset of OC symptoms (e.g., Maina et al. 2008).

In contrast to OCD, OCPD is characterized by an enduring pattern of preoccupation with perfectionism, doubt, excessive consciousness, orderliness, and interpersonal control in all or almost all aspects of daily life. Rigid adherence to rules and an excessive devotion to work, which impairs family activities and social relationships, are frequent. While patients with OCD feel tortured by their unwanted thoughts and impulses and consider them unreasonable, patients with OCPD usually believe that their rigid system of rules makes sense. Subjective suffering often results from interpersonal conflicts, for example, when family members do not comply with the patients' high standards or feel neglected when work and achievement take up too much time.

Interestingly, OCPD seems to be as frequent in anxiety disorders (Pena-Garijo et al. 2013), which argues against a continuum between OCPD and OCD.

Apart from OCPD, cluster C personality disorders in general are common in OCD (Pena-Garijo et al. 2013). Nevertheless, it is important to bear in mind that patients with OCD can present various different personality traits. In some patients, for example, OC symptoms can have a compensatory function, for example, to deal with impulsivity, feeling fragmented, or lacking identity.

Concerning comorbidity with schizotypal personality disorder, there is some evidence for higher rates of OC symptoms on symmetry, ordering/arranging, and checking in patients with a high level of schizotypy (Brakoulias et al. 2014). Besides, comorbidity with major depression, posttraumatic stress disorder, substance abuse, and general psychopathology seems to be more common than in patients with a low level of schizotypy.

With regard to treatment response, cluster A personality disorders, especially schizotypal personality disorder, narcissistic personality disorder, and the presence of two or more comorbid personality disorders, were found to be associated with poorer treatment outcomes. For other clusters, the results are inconsistent (Thiel et al. 2013).

2.4.6 Schizophrenia

The comorbidity between OCD and schizophrenia will be discussed in more detail in the following chapters. Contrary to earlier reports, the risk of developing schizophrenia is not significantly elevated in primary OCD. Roughly one quarter of patients with schizophrenia, however, will experience OC symptoms during their lifetime, and about 12 % meet the criteria for OCD (e.g., Braga et al. 2013). The high prevalence of OC symptoms in schizophrenia might be an indication of shared neurobiological characteristics.

Moreover, in a recent study (Zink et al. 2014), about 11 % of patients with at-risk mental states for psychosis had OC symptoms and 5 % fulfilled the criteria for OCD. In this study, comorbid OC symptoms were associated with higher impairment of psychosocial functioning. Remarkably, the presence of OC symptoms was related to less impairment in verbal working memory and verbal immediate, suggesting that OC symptoms serve as a protective factor. Other studies on OC symptoms in schizophrenia, however, found that patients without comorbid obsessions or compulsions showed better cognitive performance (e.g., Schirmbeck et al. 2013). One important point is that second-generation antipsychotics, especially clozapine, may aggravate or even induce OC symptoms (Schirmbeck and Zink 2013).

One essential criterion for differentiating between psychotic symptoms and OC symptoms is that OC patients realize that their intrusive thoughts or impulses are a product of their own thinking mind. Another criterion is that OC patients have – at least from time to time – some insight into the irrationality of their obsessions and rituals. However, as mentioned above, while most OC patients have excellent or very good insight into the senselessness of their obsessions and compulsions, a minority of patients possess low insight. Finally, resistance against psychotic symptoms such as delusions and hallucinations is typically not very strong, while patients with OC symptoms usually try to distance themselves via a certain degree of resistance against their obsessions and compulsions.

2.4.7 Eating Disorders

Eating disorders and OCD have similar phenomenological features such as recurrent intrusive thoughts and a compulsive urge to perform rituals in order to reduce anxiety and to prevent feared consequences.

Concerning comorbidity between eating disorders and obsessive–compulsive disorders, Sallet et al. (2010) conducted a large cross-sectional study and found a lifetime comorbidity rate of 11.3 % with binge eating disorder being most frequent

(7.2 %). Only 2 % of OCD patients experienced bulimia nervosa or anorexia nervosa. Studies on eating disorder individuals show different results: Whereas a comorbid OCD uncommonly co-occurs with bulimia nervosa or binge eating disorder, it is more frequent in anorexia nervosa (lifetime prevalence 15–69 %) (Serpell et al. 2002). Comorbid OCD patients were more likely to be women with higher anxiety and depression scores and a higher prevalence of previous psychiatric treatment. The comorbidity leads to an increased severity of the eating disorder symptoms, a longer length of hospital stay (Weltzin et al. 2007), and longer duration of illness (AWMF 2010). Therefore, it should be important to develop special therapeutic programs to improve and enhance the therapeutic outcome in these patients.

In a previous study, Hasler et al. (2005) reported that eating disorder was mainly related to contamination obsessions and cleaning compulsions.

Recently, Pollack and Forbush (2013) aimed at evaluating why obsessive–compulsive disorder and eating disorder frequently co-occur. The authors used a transdiagnostic approach, which postulates that shared maintaining factors contribute to risk for various disorders. Their results suggest that neuroticism and perfectionism are underlying mediating variables for the comorbidity between eating disorders characterized by binge eating and dietary restraint and obsessive–compulsive disorder. Perfectionism seems a developmental risk factor for OCD (Obsessive Compulsive Cognitions Working Group 1997), and it shows higher scores in individuals with anorexia nervosa and bulimia nervosa than in individuals with anxiety disorders, depression, or controls (Bulik et al. 2003).

2.4.8 Autism Spectrum Disorders

Individuals with autism spectrum disorders (ASD) often show repeating, hoarding, or touching rituals and tend toward self-injuring behavior or excessive rigidity, which is not driven by harm avoidance as in OCD. Nevertheless, OCD symptoms can also frequently be found in autism spectrum disorders. In a sample of patients with Asperger syndrome and high-functioning autism, about one quarter also met formal diagnostic criteria of OCD (Russell et al. 2008).

Similarly, autistic personality traits such as restricted patterns of behavior and interests are rather common in OCD patients. As pointed out by Bejerot et al. (2014), ASD and OCD share a wide spectrum of commonalities such as neurological soft signs, mild neuropsychological dysfunction, and personality disorders within the obsessive–compulsive, avoidant, and schizotypal/schizoid domains. Especially in patients with both autism spectrum disorder and tic disorder, comorbidity including "just right" feeling and problems with impulse control are very common.

2.4.9 Tic Disorder and Tourette Syndrome

OCD comorbid with chronic tic disorders including Tourette syndrome (TS) is associated with a high prevalence of early onset and also sensory experiences such as "just right" feeling. With regard to symptom dimensions, patients with tic-related

OCD most frequently report symptoms concerning symmetry, but symptoms on the aggression dimension are also common and typically persist for several years.

To account for the differences between OCD patients with and without comorbid tics, a tic-related specifier was added to DSM-5.

Although it is sometimes difficult to differentiate between tics and OC symptoms, tics are typically preceded by uncomfortable somatic sensations in certain body parts or a diffuse tension, but not by anxiety. Moreover, a behavior is more likely an OC ritual than a tic if it is performed in a certain order or a certain number of times, especially when it occurs in response to obsessional thinking. Nevertheless, the differentiation between a tic-like compulsion and a tic behavior can be tricky, particularly in the case of complex behaviors such as touching an object.

Roughly 7 % of OCD patients meet the diagnostic criteria of Tourette syndrome, which is characterized by multiple vocal and motor tics. On the other hand, about one third to one half of children with Tourette syndrome or multiple tics will also suffer from OC symptoms at some point during their lifetime (Bloch et al. 2006). OCD patients with comorbid tic disorder are more likely to be males, to report an early onset of OC symptoms, and to suffer from aggressive obsessions, cleaning compulsions, and trichotillomania (Jaisoorya et al. 2008): Interestingly, preliminary evidence indicates that children and adolescents both with OCD and with Tourette syndrome show a higher prevalence of allergic diseases (Yuce et al. 2014).

2.5 Discussion

Despite significant advances in the understanding of OCD, there are still many different, partially diverging approaches to evaluating the structure and relevant comorbidities of this disabling disorder.

Concerning OCD symptom dimensions, the various conditions share similarities regarding clinical symptomatology, comorbidity, and neurobiological mechanisms such as alterations in the frontobasal pathways including the orbitofrontal cortex and the anterior cingulate cortex. On the other hand, there is evidence for a more widespread network of cerebral changes than previously thought. This possibly explains the heterogeneous clinical dimensions of OCD (for a review, see Piras et al. 2013). In line with this, recent research suggests that certain cognitive deficits are mediated by several subtypes of OCD. While it has long been known that OCD patients show mild neuropsychological deficits regarding visuospatial organization and nonverbal memory (Külz et al. 2004; Vandborg et al. 2014), deficits in nonverbal memory and organizational strategy are reported to be related to the symmetry/ordering dimension and the obsessions/checking dimension, respectively (Jang et al. 2010).

Current data on OC spectrum disorders suggest a number of promising avenues for exploration. One future question will be how related genes are involved in the comorbidity of OC spectrum disorders and other psychiatric disorders. One recent study (Monzani et al. 2014), for example, suggests that OCD, body dysmorphic disorder, and hoarding disorder share a common genetic factor, but are also influenced by unique disorder-specific factors, whereas trichotillomania and skin picking are mainly determined by the same latent genetic factor.

As Murphy et al. (2013) point out, there is also considerable overlap in some genetic variants identified in OCD and the whole spectrum of affective and anxiety disorders, including the serotonin transporter gene or the brain-derived neurotrophic factor.

Regarding the various attempts at subtyping OCD and related disorders, the situation is somewhat similar to the story of the six blind men palpitating an elephant, who were asked what an elephant looked like and gave six different answers due to feeling different parts of the elephant's body (see Gardner 1995): Only combining information from different perspectives will give the overall picture of OCD. With regard to treatment and future research, however, comparing and potentially integrating the subtyping categories and comorbidities of OCD could prove very valuable. OCD with early onset, for example, may be largely compatible with tic-related OCD and a sense of incompleteness or "just right" feeling. Nestadt et al. (2009) argue that reducing the heterogeneity would be helpful both in identifying which treatment strategies are most effective for which patients and in investigating characteristics of distinct OCD subpopulations. On the other hand, many patients show symptoms from various areas, though some obsessions might be more intrusive than others or one comorbid disorder might be more prominent than another.

Bearing in mind these limitations, the development of specialized therapeutic approaches for different subgroups seems essential, but cognitive behavioral treatment with or without selective serotonin reuptake inhibitors remains the first choice in treating OCD. As shame often prevents OCD patients from seeking help, comorbidities such as mood disorders often become the initial reason for patients to consult a medical professional. With this knowledge in the back of the mind, one should also consider screening patients with major depression, anxiety disorders, or other common comorbidities for potential symptoms of OCD.

The treatment of OC individuals with accompanying comorbidities can be demanding. For example, triggered obsessions (e.g., the fear of having done something completely wrong) can trigger comorbid emotions (e.g., feelings of worthlessness in avoidant personality disorder or guilt in comorbid depression), resulting in processes that amplify each other. In view of the fact that comorbidity is associated with worse long-term treatment outcome in OCD (Jakubovski et al. 2013), the development of effective therapeutic approaches tailored to individuals with comorbidities seems to be crucial. To address the comorbidity aspect more fully and appropriately, additional research will have to establish more detailed and specific relationships between various subtypes, spectrum disorders, and other psychiatric comorbidities of OCD.

References

Abramowitz JS, Taylor S, McKay D (2009) Obsessive-compulsive disorder. Lancet 374(9688): 491–499

Abramowitz JS, Deacon BJ, Olatunji BO et al (2010) Assessment of obsessive-compulsive symptom dimensions: development and evaluation of the Dimensional Obsessive-Compulsive Scale. Psychol Assess 22:180–198

Ameringen MV, Patterson B, Simpson W (2014) DSM-5 obsessive compulsive and related disorders. Clinical implications of the new criteria. Depress Anxiety 31:487–493

Amerio A, Odone A, Liapis CC, Ghaemi SN (2014) Diagnostic validity of comorbid bipolar disorder and obsessive-compulsive disorder: a systematic review. Acta Psychiatr Scand 129:343–358
AWMF (2010) S-3 Leitlinie "Diagnostik und Therapie bei Essstörungen". Arbeitsgemeinschaft der Wissenschaftlichen Medizinischen Fachgesellschaften. AWMF online: 051/026
Bartz JA, Hollander E (2006) Is obsessive-compulsive disorder an anxiety disorder? Prog Neuropsychopharmacol Biol Psychiatry 30:338–352
Bejerot S, Weizmann A, Gross-Isseroff R (2014) Communality between obsessive compulsive disorder and autism spectrum disorder. In: Vinood BP, Patel RP, Martin CR (eds) Comprehensive guide to autism. Springer, New York, pp 671–692
Berlin GS, Hollander E (2014) Compulsivity, impulsivity, and the DSM-5 process. CNS Spectr 19(1):62–68
Bhangle SD, Kramer N, Rosenstein ED (2013) Corticosteroid-induced neuropsychiatric disorders: review and contrast with neuropsychiatric lupus. Rheumatol Int 33(8):1923–1932
Bloch MH, Peterson CH, Scahill L, Otka J, Katsovich L, Zhang H, Leckman JF (2006) Adulthood outcome of tic and obsessive-compulsive symptom severity in children with Tourette syndrome. Arch Pediatr Adolesc Med 160:65–69
Braga RJ, Reynolds GP, Siris SG (2013) Anxiety comorbidity in schizophrenia. Psychiatry Res 210:1–7
Brakoulias V, Starcevic V, Berle D et al (2014) The clinical characteristics of obsessive compulsive disorder associated with high levels of schizotypy. Aust N Z J Psychiatry 48:852–860
Buhlmann U, Winter A (2011) Perceived ugliness: an update on treatment-relevant aspects of body dysmorphic disorder. Curr Psychiatry Rep 13(4):283–288
Buhlmann U, Glaesmer H, Mewes R et al (2010) Updates on the prevalence of body dysmorphic disorder: a population-based survey. Psychiatry Res 178:171–175
Bulik C, Tozzi F, Anderson CH, Mazzeo S, Aggen S, Sullivan P (2003) The relation between eating disorders and components of perfectionism. Am J Psychiatr 160:366–368
Crino R, Slade T, Andrews G (2005) The changing prevalence and severity of obsessive compulsive disorder criteria from DSM-III to DSM-IV. Am J Psychiatr 162(5):876–882
Ecker W, Gönner S (2008) Incompleteness and harm avoidance in OCD symptom dimensions. Behav Res Ther 46:895–904
Eisen JL, Sibrava NJ, Boisseau CL et al (2013) Five-year course of obsessive-compulsive disorder: predictors of remission and relapse. J Clin Psychiatry 74:233–239
Gardner M (1995) Famous poems from bygone days. Courier Dover Publications, New York, p 124
Gentil AF, de Mathis MA, Torresan RC, Diniz JB et al (2009) Alcohol use disorders in patients with obsessive-compulsive disorder: the importance of appropriate dual-diagnosis. Drug Alcohol Depend 100:173–177
Gomes de Alvarenga P, de Mathis MA, Dominguez Alves AC et al (2012) Clinical features often-related obsessive-compulsive disorder: results from a large multicenter study. CNS Spectr 17:87–93
Grant JE, Odlaug BL, Chamberlain SR et al (2012) Skin picking disorder. Am J Psychiatry 169: 1143–1149
Grohol JN (2013) Psych Central. Available at: http://pro.psychcentral.com/2013/dsm-5-changes-obsessive-compulsive-and-related-disorders/004404.html
Hasler G, LaSalle-Ricci VH, Ronquillo JG et al (2005) Obsessive-compulsive disorder symptom dimensions show specific relationships to psychiatric comorbidity. Psychiatry Res 135:121–132
Hasler G, Pinto A, Greenberg BD et al; OCD Collaborative Genetics Study (2007) Familiality of factor analysis-derived YBOCS dimensions in OCD-affected sibling pairs from the OCD Collaborative Genetics Study. Biol Psychiatry 61:617–625
Hohagen F, Winkelmann G, Rasche-Räuchle H et al (1998) Combination of behaviour therapy with fluvoxamine in comparison with behaviour therapy and placebo. Results of a multicentre study. Br J Psychiatry Suppl 35:71–78

Jaisoorya TS, Reddy YC, Srinath S, Thennarasu K (2008) Obsessive-compulsive disorder with and without tic disorder: a comparative study from India. CNS Spectr 13:705–711

Jakubovski E, Diniz JB, Valerio C et al (2013) Clinical predictors of long-term outcome in obsessive-compulsive disorder. Depress Anxiety 30(8):763–772

Jang JH, Kim HS, Ha TH et al (2010) Nonverbal memory and organizational dysfunctions are related with distinct symptom dimensions in obsessive-compulsive disorder. Psychiatry Res 180(2–3):93–98

Janowitz D, Grabe HJ, Ruhrmann S et al (2009) Early onset of obsessive-compulsive disorder and associated comorbidity. Depress Anxiety 26:1012–1017

Keuthen NJ, Altenburger EM, Pauls D (2014) A family study of trichotillomania and chronic hair pulling. Am J Med Genet B Neuropsychiatr Genet 165(2):167–174

Knopp J, Knowles S, Bee P, Lovell K, Bower P (2013) A systematic review of predictors and moderators of response to psychological therapies in OCD: do we have enough empirical evidence to target treatment? Clin Psychol Rev 33:1067–1081

Külz AK, Hohagen F, Voderholzer U (2004) Neuropsychological performance in obsessive-compulsive disorder: a critical review. Biol Psychol 65:185–236

Külz AK, Lumpp A, Herbst N et al (2010) Functions of obsessive-compulsive symptoms: results of an In-Patient Study. Verhaltenstherapie 20:101–109

LaSalle VH, Cromer KR, Nelson KN et al (2004) Diagnostic interview assessed neuropsychiatric disorder comorbidity in 334 individuals with obsessive-compulsive disorder. Depress Anxiety 19:163–173

Maina G, Albert U, Salvi V et al (2008) Early-onset obsessive-compulsive disorder and personality disorders in adulthood. Psychiatry Res 15:217–225

Mancebo MC, Grant JE, Pinto A et al (2008) Substance use disorders in an obsessive compulsive disorder clinical sample. J Anxiety Disord 23:429–435

Meyer E, Shavitt RG, Leukefeld C et al (2010) Adding motivational interviewing and thought mapping to cognitive-behavioral group therapy; results from a randomized clinical trial. Rev Bras Psiquiatr 32:20–29

Miguel EC, Ferrão YA, Rosário MC et al; Brazilian Research Consortium on Obsessive-Compulsive Spectrum Disorders (2008) The Brazilian Research Consortium on Obsessive-Compulsive Spectrum Disorders: recruitment, assessment instruments, methods for the development of multicenter collaborative studies and preliminary results. Rev Bras Psiquiatr 30:185–196

Monzani B, Rijsdijk F, Harris J, Mataix-Cols D (2014) The structure of genetic and environmental risk factors for dimensional representations of DSM-5 obsessive-compulsive spectrum disorders. JAMA Psychiatry 7:182–189

Morein-Zamir S, Papmeyer M, Pertusa A et al (2014) The profile of executive function in OCD hoarders and hoarding disorder. Psychiatry Res 215:659–667

Murphy TK, Storch EA, Lewin AB et al (2012) Clinical factors associated with pediatric autoimmune neuropsychiatric disorders associated with streptococcal infections. J Pediatr 160(2):314–319

Murphy DL, Moya PR, Fox MA et al (2013) Anxiety and affective disorder comorbidity related to serotonin and other neurotransmitter systems: obsessive-compulsive disorder as an example of overlapping clinical and genetic heterogeneity. Philos Trans R Soc Lond B Biol Sci 368(1615):20120435. doi:10.1098/rstb.2012.0435

Nestadt G, Di CZ, Riddle MA et al (2009) Obsessive-compulsive disorder: subclassification based on co-morbidity. Psychol Med 39:1491–1501

Obsessive Compulsive Cognitions Working Group (1997) Cognitive assessment of obsessive-compulsive disorder. Behav Res Ther 35(7):667–681

Odlaug BL, Kim SW, Grant JE (2010) Quality of life and clinical severity in pathological skin picking and trichotillomania. J Anxiety Disord 27:611–626

Overbeek T, Schruers K, Vermetten E, Griez E (2002) Comorbidity of obsessive-compulsive disorder and depression: prevalence, symptom severity, and treatment effect. J Clin Psychiatry 63:1106–1112

Pena-Garijo J, Edo Villamón S, Meliá de Alba A, Ruipérez MA (2013) Personality disorders in obsessive-compulsive disorder: a comparative study versus other anxiety disorders. Scientific World Journal 2013:856846. doi:10.1155/2013/856846
Phillips KA, Menard W, Pagano ME et al (2006) Delusional versus nondelusional body dysmorphic disorder: clinical features and course of illness. J Psychiatr Res 40:95–104
Phillips KA, Pinto A, Hart AS et al (2012) A comparison of insight in body dysmorphic disorder and obsessive-compulsive disorder. J Psychiatr Res 46(10):1293–1299
Piras F, Piras F, Chiapponi C et al (2013) Widespread structural brain changes in OCD: a systematic review of voxel-based morphometry studies. Cortex pii: S0010-9452(13)00046-4. doi:10.1016/j.cortex.2013.01.016
Pollack LO, Forbush KT (2013) Why do eating disorders and obsessive-compulsive disorder co-occur? Eat Behav 14:211–215
Robbins TW, Gillan CM, Smith DG et al (2012) Neurocognitive endophenotypes of impulsivity and compulsivity: towards dimensional psychiatry. Trends Cogn Sci 16(1):81–91
Rogers K, Banis M, Falkenstein MJ et al (2014) Stepped care in the treatment of trichotillomania. J Consult Clin Psychol 82:361–367
Ruscio AM, Stein DJ, Chiu WT, Kessler RC (2010) The epidemiology of obsessive-compulsive disorder in the National Comorbidity Survey Replication. Mol Psychiatry 15:53–63
Russell AJ, Mataix-Cols D, Anson M, Murphy DG (2008) Obsessions and compulsions in Asperger syndrome and high-functioning autism. Br J Psychiatry 186:525–528
Sallet PC, de Alvarenga PG, Ferrão Y et al (2010) Eating disorders in patients with obsessive–compulsive disorder: prevalence and clinical correlates. Int J Eat Disord 43:315–325
Saxena S, Brody AL, Maidment KM, Smith EC, Zohrabi N, Katz E, Baker SK, Baxter LR Jr (2004) Cerebral glucose metabolism in obsessive-compulsive hoarding. Am J Psychiatry 161:1038–1048
Schirmbeck F, Zink M (2013) Comorbid obsessive-compulsive symptoms in schizophrenia: contributions of pharmacological and genetic factors. Front Pharmacol 4:99
Schirmbeck F, Rausch F, Englisch S et al (2013) Stable cognitive deficits in schizophrenia patients with comorbid obsessive-compulsive symptoms: a 12-month longitudinal study. Schizophr Bull 6:1261–1271
Serpell L, Livingstone A, Neiderman M, Lask B (2002) Anorexia nervosa: obsessive-compulsive disorder, obsessive-compulsive personality disorder, or neither? Clin Psychol Rev 22(5):647–669
Snorrason I, Stein DJ, Woods DW (2013) Classification of excoriation (skin picking) disorder: current status and future directions. Acta Psychiatr Scand 128:406–407
Starcevic V, Berle D, Brakoulias V (2013) Obsessive-compulsive personality disorder co-occurring with obsessive-compulsive disorder: conceptual and clinical implications. Aust N Z J Psychiatry 47:65–73
Taylor S (2011) Early versus late onset obsessive-compulsive disorder: evidence for distinct subtypes. Clin Psychol Rev 31:1083–1100
Thiel N, Hertenstein E, Nissen C et al (2013) The effect of personality disorders on treatment outcomes in patients with obsessive-compulsive disorders. J Pers Disord 27:697–715
Timpano KR, Rubenstein LM, Murphy DL (2012) Phenomenological features and clinical impact of affective disorders in OCD: a focus on the bipolar disorder and OCD connection. Depress Anxiety 29:226–233
Torres AR, Shavitt RG, Torresan RC et al (2013) Clinical features of pure obsessive-compulsive disorder. Compr Psychiatry 54(7):1042–1052
Torres R, Ferrão YA, Shavitt RG, Diniz JB et al (2014) Panic Disorder and Agoraphobia in OCD patients: clinical profile and possible treatment implications. Compr Psychiatry 55:588–597
Tükel R, Polat A, Ozdemir O, Aksüt D, Türksoy N (2002) Comorbid conditions in obsessive-compulsive disorder. Compr Psychiatry 43:204–209
van den Heuvel OA, Remijnse PL, Mataix-Cols D et al (2009) The major symptom dimensions of obsessive-compulsive disorder are mediated by partially distinct neural systems. Brain 132:853–868

Vandborg SK, Hartmann TB, Bennedsen BE, Pedersen AD, Thomsen PH (2014) Memory and executive functions in patients with obsessive-compulsive disorder. Cogn Behav Neurol 27:8–16
Visser HA, van Oppen P, van Megen HJ et al (2014) Obsessive-compulsive disorder; chronic versus non-chronic symptoms. J Affect Disord 152–154:169–174
Wakefield JC, Schmitz MF (2014) How many people have alcohol use disorders? Using the harmful dysfunction analysis to reconcile prevalence estimates in two community surveys. Front Psychiatry 5:10. doi:10.3389/fpsyt.2014.00010
Weltzin T, Cormella-Carlson T, Weisensel N, Timmel P, Hallinan P, Bean P (2007) The combined presence of obsessive compulsive behaviors in males and females with eating disorders account for longer length of stay and more severe eating disorder symptoms. Eat Weight Disord 2:176–182
Wilhelm S, Phillips KA, Didie E et al (2014) Modular cognitive-behavioral therapy for body dysmorphic disorder: a randomized controlled trial. Behav Ther 45:314–327
World Health Organization (2001) The world health report 2001. Mental health: new understanding – new hope
Yuce M, Guner SN, Karabekiroglu K et al (2014) Association of Tourette syndrome and obsessive-compulsive disorder with allergic diseases in children and adolescents: a preliminary study. Eur Rev Med Pharmacol Sci 18:303–310
Zaudig M (2011) Heterogeneity and comorbidity of obsessive-compulsive disorder. Nervenarzt 82:290, 292, 294–296
Zink M, Schirmbeck F, Rausch F et al (2014) Obsessive-compulsive symptoms in at-risk mental states for psychosis: associations with clinical impairment and cognitive function. Acta Psychiatr Scand 130:214–226. doi:10.1111/acps.12258, PubMed PMID:24571191

Part II

Phenomenology

Clinical Presentation of Obsessive-Compulsive Symptoms in Patients with Psychotic Disorders Psychopathological Concepts, Differential Diagnosis, and Symptom Presentation

3

Lieuwe de Haan and Mathias Zink

Abbreviations

OCD	Obsessive-compulsive disorder
OCS	Obsessive-compulsive symptoms
Y-BOCS	Yale-Brown Obsessive-Compulsive Scale

3.1 Case Presentation

A first-person account from a website called PsychCentral describes the story of a 20-year-old woman with both obsessive-compulsive and psychotic symptoms:

> For as long as I can remember I have always been a shy and quiet girl. When I was twelve I became less active and preferred to stay in my room all day. I began to develop a habit of needing to keep things clean and organized. I would alphabetize my books and cds, and I would color code all of my clothing. If anything was untidy or disorganized, I would begin to feel hopeless and overwhelmed. At this point I began procrastinating, putting things off until I was in the mood to do it, which sometimes never came.
>
> Things got worse and new problems developed throughout my years in middle school and high school. It got so bad that I ended up dropping out of high school at the beginning of my senior year. I have pretty much cut all contact with my friends and whenever they

L. de Haan (✉)
Department of Psychiatry, University of Amsterdam Academic Medical Centre, Amsterdam, The Netherlands
e-mail: l.dehaan@amc.uva.nl

M. Zink, MD
Department of Psychiatry and Psychotherapy, Medical Faculty Mannheim, Central Institute of Mental Health, Heidelberg University, 12 21 20, Mannheim D-68072, Germany

L. De Haan et al. (eds.), *Obsessive-Compulsive Symptoms in Schizophrenia*,
DOI 10.1007/978-3-319-12952-5_3

would try to call me, I would ignore them, not wanting to talk to them or to go anywhere. I hardly ever left home, hardly left my room for months on end.

Now at the age of twenty I am still living at home with my parents with no job, spending my days in my room. I just feel too stressed, too depressed to do anything, even the things I once enjoyed dearly.

Now I have become extremely paranoid and it has gotten so bad that I am afraid to go to sleep at night. I also have these intrusive, morbid, tormenting thoughts, most revolving around death, disasters and violence. I cannot control these thoughts nor can I make them go away. Moreover, I need to wash my hands every time I touch something outside my room. The thoughts make me feel so helpless and make want to cry my eyes out. But the truth is I have not been able to cry since… I don't know when. I mean I could not even bring myself to cry when my grandfather died five years or so ago, which made me feel completely guilty.

Aside from the intrusive thoughts, I hear voices a lot, sometimes they sound as if they are just in my mind, and then other times they sound as if they are right behind me or next to me, like someone else is there. I have such difficult time thinking and focusing on things and my short term memory is deteriorating rather rapidly.

This patient suffers from OCS, psychosis, and depression and her social functioning is severely disturbed. The dimensions of her psychopathology interact with each other. She might be paradigmatic for several other patients, but in other patients the order of events and the courses over time markedly differ. These aspects refer to the aims of this chapter.

In this chapter, we will present a concise overview of the history of psychopathological concepts of OCS comorbidity, the differential diagnosis between OCS and psychosis, and the clinical presentation of OCS in patients with psychotic disorders.

3.2 Historical Perspective on Concepts of OCS Psychopathology in Psychotic Disorders and Their Differentiation

Psychopathological descriptions and concepts of obsessions and compulsions underwent substantial changes during history. Here, we will present a concise overview concerning different historical approaches.

French and German pioneers of psychiatry published very divergent theories in the nineteenth and twentieth century. Based on single-case analyses or small case series, authors like Esquirol and Morel proposed that OCS were driven by emotional factors (Berrios 1989). Later Westphal (1878) proposed a more cognitive view, assuming primary cognitive dysfunctions. He was the first to distinguish OCS from psychosis. From his long-term clinical observations, he concluded that OCS never evolved to psychotic syndromes. Therefore, he proposed a clear-cut distinction of both syndromes concerning clinical presentation, treatment, prognosis, and outcome. This stimulated the view that OCS might indicate an internal defense strategy against psychosis, which could prevent the development or progression of schizophrenia. In line with this, Stengel (1945) observed a tendency toward remission in patients with comorbid OCS. Based on 14 cases suffering from both OCS and psychosis, he suggested that catatonic or hebephrenic syndromes did not occur while OCS were present and that psychotic patients with OCS comorbidity frequently realized the irrationality of their psychotic cognitions. In those days, it was generally assumed that "psychosis resulted in a release of primitive impulses which had previously been kept under control with the aid of obsessional symptoms" (Stengel 1945). In 1957, Rosen hypothesized that OCS might delay psychosis-caused "personality disorganization" by preventing the development of "malignant schizophrenia." He also observed that none of his patients developed obsessive symptoms after the onset of schizophrenia (Rosen 1957).

These thoughts resulted into the view that OCS and psychosis should be categorized as antagonistic disorders, in which OCS was considered as partially preventive and indicative of a favorable prognosis. Later on this view changed dramatically.

An important issue, the difficulty to differentiate OCS from psychosis, is already apparent in the publications of abovementioned clinicians. Below we will give an overview of the thoughts of influential clinicians showing the different conceptualizations of obsessions and compulsions in relation to psychosis and reality distortion. In earlier editions of his psychiatric textbook, Kraepelin subsumed delusion within obsessive-compulsive disorder and made no distinction between delusional ideas, obsessive thoughts, and overvalued ideas (Kraepelin 1896). Kronfeld (1924) conceptualized obsession as a state in which the feeling of activity as such is lost, and the obsessive reaction is immediate, without interference of reflexive consciousness. Westphal underscores the self-reflexive distance to own contents of consciousness in obsessions; he described that it seems as if the ego faces itself. Because the obsessive image "feels" as no longer under the person's control, it seems abnormal (even alien) and lacks an affective bond. In later work, Kraepelin (1915) differentiated obsessions from delusions, and he agreed with Westphal that obsessions are reflexive in character. In trying to describe the relationship between obsessions and "the ego," Jaspers (1973) made a distinction between obsessions in the broader sense and obsessions in the strict sense. In obsessions in the broader sense, there is an inner struggle. Jaspers describes that in an obsession in the broader sense, the person is facing himself and has an image which is his own and which he nevertheless does not want to have. The patient has an impulse which he wants to follow and at the same time against which he is fighting. The ego is no longer in control when it comes to making a choice and the contents of consciousness persist against one's own will. In obsessions in the strict sense, there is more distance between the content of the obsession and the ego. The content of obsessions is assessed as being unfounded, nonsensical, and incomprehensible, and therefore, the ego defends itself against them. The difference between obsessions in the strict sense and obsessions in the broad sense is gradual, depending on the feeling a person has that obsessions are strange, unwanted, mental phenomena he does not want to have.

Schneider (1939) emphasized that contents of obsessions cannot be repressed although the person assesses them as being nonsensical or as dominating without reason. However, as also is pointed out in the ICD-10, persisting obsessive thoughts and compulsive acts can be accompanied by minimal resistance. According to the DSM-IV criteria for the diagnosis OCD, patients need to realize at some point in the course of the disorder that the obsessive thoughts and compulsive acts are exaggerated. Bürgy (2007) points out that persisting obsessions may increasingly be integrated into one's own experiencing and thereby can acquire an ego-syntonic character. Burgy (2007) also emphasized the importance of evaluating "obsession in the strict sense" to differentiate between obsessions and delusions in schizophrenia. In obsessions in the strict sense, the patient is always able to reflect upon himself and to evaluate his own thoughts as nonsensical, whereas in the case of delusional ideas, self-reflexivity collapses. The deluded patient is no longer able to keep an evaluating distance from the contents of consciousness, but is completely seized by them. Only retrospectively, when the delusional idea subsides, the person regains the ability to take a reflexive stance and to evaluate the contents of the delusions. In the case of obsession in the strict sense, simultaneous reflexivity and evaluation of the nonsensical nature of the obsessive images is possible. It is clear that in obsessions in the strict sense, insight is preserved.

The recently published DSM-5 introduced changes compared to the DSM-IV that are relevant for the issue of co-occurrence of OCS and severe psychotic disorders. The old DSM-IV specifier "with poor insight" has been modified from being an all or nothing specifier to a specifier that allows three degrees on a spectrum of insight in accordance to the levels used by clinical rating scales such as the Y-BOCS. These degrees of insight are defined as "good or fair insight," "poor insight," or "absent insight/delusional OCD beliefs (complete conviction that OCD beliefs are true)." This change emphasizes that absent insight/delusional beliefs may be compatible with a diagnosis of OCD or related disorder, rather than with a schizophrenia spectrum disorder. Catapano et al. performed a 3-year prospective study focusing on the prognosis of OCD with poor insight. Compared to their good insight counterparts, the OCD patients with poor insight showed a greater severity of obsessive-compulsive and depressive symptomatology, an earlier age at onset, a higher rate of schizophrenia spectrum disorder in their first-degree relatives, and a higher comorbidity with schizotypal personality disorder (for a comprehensive discussion concerning the OCD and schizotypal personality disorder, we would like to refer to Chap. 5). During the follow-up period, poor insight OCD patients were less likely to achieve at least a partial remission of OCS, required a significantly greater number of therapeutic trials, and received more frequently augmentation with antipsychotics (Catapano et al. 2010). These findings suggest that the specifier "poor insight" helps to identify a subgroup of patients at the more severe end of OCD spectrum, characterized by a more complex clinical presentation, a diminished response to standard pharmacological interventions, and a poorer prognosis, and importantly a stronger association with the spectrum of psychosis vulnerability. On the other hand, it also seems an acknowledgment of our inability to make a sharp distinction between OCS and psychosis in some cases. Another change in the DSM-5 is that the delusional variant of body dysmorphic disorder (which identifies individuals who are completely convinced that their perceived defects are truly abnormal appearing) is no longer classified as both delusional disorder, somatic type, and body dysmorphic disorder. Instead, it gets a "delusional belief" specifier to the classification of body dysmorphic disorder.

3.3 The Differential Diagnosis Between OCS and Psychosis and the Classification of These Disorders

The abovementioned historic and current clinical experience underscores the major challenge we face: the identification of OCS in schizophrenia or related disorders and the differentiation of obsessions from delusions and of compulsions from schizophrenic mannerisms and stereotypical behavior. Here we will describe several aspects that may be evaluated in clinical practice in describing obsessions or compulsions and in differentiating them from psychotic phenomena.

The aspects to consider are attribution and insight, uncertainty, content, association with schizophrenia symptoms, timing of onset, and remission (course).

3.3.1 Attribution and Insight

Attribution, insight, and resistance can be distinguished, although they are also related to each other. Patients suffering from OCD typically attribute the obsessions, impulsive symptoms, and compulsions to their own thinking, declare with insight their unreasonableness, and show some degree of resistance against them. These patients would have been classified by Jaspers as having obsessions in the strict sense. Concerning insight, the differentiation of obsessions from delusions is guided by the fact that obsessions are characterized as recurrent, intrusive, ego-dystonic thoughts, accompanied by the insight that they are senseless, whereas a psychotic patient typically lacks insight in the distorted quality of their thoughts. Delusions of a psychotic patient cannot be influenced by rational arguments or evidence to the contrary; they are held with strength in the face of evidence or social pressure (Zink et al. 2008). On the other hand, patients with obsessions typically try to resist these thoughts; they feel as unwanted and not belonging to their personal characteristics.

3.3.2 Uncertainty

Another way of evaluating the differences between psychosis and OCS is the phenomenological aspects of the "feelings of uncertainty." As discussed, most patients with OCD recognize that their obsessive thoughts are "a product of their own mind" and that the content of these thoughts is unreasonable. They view these thoughts as not in line with what they really value and want; their obsessions are so-called ego-dystonic. As mentioned this is in sharp contrast with delusions in which patients are convinced that their ideas are true, important, and held with vigor. Delusions are ego-syntonic; the delusion feels as an important insight and is held with conviction.

In other words, obsessions and delusions differ in the level of certainty patients attach to their thoughts. Moreover, people with obsessive thoughts are in doubt, they do not know for sure. In fact, they are searching for relief for their feeling of uncertainty accompanied with feelings of insecurity. They would like to know for sure that the situation is safe for themselves or for the people they love. But they cannot reach this feeling of safety. Szechtman and Woody (2006) propose that disturbances in the so-called security motivation system may underlie OCS and OCD. The security motivation system represents a fundamental biologically primitive motivational system that is activated by potential danger to self or intimate others and engages a set of behaviors (such as checking and washing) to handle potential danger. Because the task of the security motivation system is open ended, in the sense that no stimuli can exist in the real world to indicate the absence of any potential danger, the shutdown of security motivation is produced by a self-generated feeling of knowing, a feeling that "the situation is good enough and that it is safe." In this elegant theory, OCS and OCD result from a failure to generate this feeling of safety. Therefore the patient persists in a strong motivational state having to do with basic threats to existence. This leads to prolonged engagement in security-related behaviors, such as repetitive thoughts, checking and washing, characteristic of the symptoms of OCD: compulsions and obsessions. Recently, Hinds et al. (2012) found support for this theory in humans. Compared to controls, OCD patients with washing compulsions did not differ significantly in their levels of initial activation to the threat of contamination; however, they were significantly less able to reduce this activation by engaging in the corrective behavior of hand washing. They conclude that OCD is characterized by a reduced ability of security-related behavior to terminate motivation evoked by potential danger, rather than a heightened initial sensitivity to potential threat.

How different is the situation in people who have delusions? These people are not in doubt; they even show the metacognitive bias of hasty decision making (jumping to conclusion) due to an overestimation of the reliability of information. During delusional thinking, they are convinced that their idea is correct. Their belief in the content of their delusion is robust. Delusions are defined by the characteristics of certainty, incorrigibility, and impossibility to falsify their content. The subjects believe them with absolute conviction, despite compelling counterarguments or even proof of the contrary. Thus, delusions describe implausible, bizarre, or patently untrue "facts." Hallucinations are perceived with the character of sensory information originating from an external source. The subject classically attributes the content of the hallucination not to his own thinking but to an external source. In contrast, as earlier mentioned, obsessions and compulsions are intrusive thoughts/actions that originate from the subjects' own thinking. The patients report insight into the unreasonable nature and try to resist or ignore them. Lincoln (2007) found that the distress associated with delusions as well as beliefs involving persecution and loss of control to be the most relevant aspects in distinguishing persons with schizophrenia from persons without schizophrenia. Moritz and Van Quaquebeke (2013) found that a higher degree of belief conviction aggravates the behavioral consequences of persecutory beliefs in a linear fashion. Jacobsen et al. investigated whether the abovementioned reasoning bias ("jumping to conclusions") is also associated with high-conviction beliefs in obsessive-compulsive disorder (OCD). They compared high-conviction OCD patients with people with low-conviction OCD and with people with delusions and nonclinical controls. They found that "jumping to conclusions" is associated with delusions but not with high- nor low-conviction beliefs in OCD. This is consistent with the view that high-conviction OCD should not be classified as a psychotic disorder. Although, high-conviction OCD shares features with psychotic disorders concerning symptoms and outcome.

3.3.3 Content

Besides the level of insight, there are other characteristics that may help to differentiate obsessions from delusions. Usually, obsessions have a typical content which distinguishes them from delusions. Obsessions frequently have, as theme contamination, aggressive or sexual themes or symmetry, while delusions frequently have as theme persecution, ideas of reference, diminishing barriers between the person and the surrounding, or grandiosity. Another aspect that may help in differentiation of obsessions or compulsions from delusions or psychosis-related behavior is the relationship between the content of OCS and the content of psychosis. We propose that ruminations or stereotypic ego-dystonic cognitions with direct relation with the content of psychotic thoughts should not be diagnosed as obsessions.

Particularly catatonic symptoms in schizophrenia (Fink 2013) confer several problems to psychopathological assessment in daily clinical practice. Even the established psychometric instruments such as the catatonia rating scale (Bräunig et al. 2000) and the Yale-Brown Obsessive-Compulsive Scale (de Haan et al. 2006; Woody et al. 1995) share many symptomatic dimensions. They facilitate the assessment of severity, but do not allow a clear-cut differentiation. Historically, a more precise characterization and differentiation of symptoms was achieved by an undisguised view on the natural long-term course of schizophrenia. The work of Karl Leonhard (Beckmann et al. 2000) contains case descriptions that allowed a clear discrimination between OCS and catatonic symptoms most importantly in patients with the so-called manieristic catatonia. At present, most patients are evaluated during antipsychotic treatment and present with attenuated symptoms. We propose to differentiate catatonic or compulsive behavioral phenomena according the general clinical context and the criterion of the subject's attribution as ego-dystonic.

3.3.4 Association with Schizophrenia Symptoms

In studies of patients with schizophrenia and comorbid OCD, a lack of association between the major OCD symptom categories and schizophrenia symptom dimensions is found.

As mentioned above, ruminations or stereotypic ego-dystonic cognitions with direct relation to the contents to psychotic thinking should not be diagnosed as obsessions.

3.3.5 Timing of Onset and Remission (Course)

Last but not least, a final issue in differentiating OCS from psychosis is the relation in time between these phenomena. This association may point to differences in etiology between these phenomena. We will describe issues concerning onset in the following paragraph. The diagnosis depends, among others, on the relationship in time between OCS and psychosis. In general, the final decision whether the patient really suffers from a valid comorbid OCD should be postponed until the remission of psychotic symptoms, in order to evaluate OCS independently from the content of the psychotic thinking. However, this may introduce a false appearance of diagnostic certainty, since OCS may also fluctuate during the course of the illness. Having said this, a complete remission of OCS, together with a remission of psychotic symptoms, shows most likely that there is no alone-standing comorbid OCD.

Clinical aspects to consider when differentiating between psychotic symptoms and OCS are summarized in Table 3.1.

Recently, Oulis et al. (2013) also listed the phenomenological features of typical obsessions/compulsions and delusions/repetitive delusional behaviors, respectively, and proposed a list of features that should be evaluated in differential diagnosis. This list can be kept in mind in evaluating the differential classification of these symptoms. They mention seven features concerning obsessions/delusions that may be of importance in differentiating these symptoms: (1) source or origin and sense of ownership of the thought, (2) conviction, (3) consistency with one's belief system, (4) awareness of its inaccuracy, (5) awareness of its symptomatic nature, (6) resistance, and (7) emotional impact. They also propose five features of repetitive behaviors that are important in differentiating symptoms: (1) aim of repetitive behaviors, (2) awareness of their inappropriateness, (3) awareness of their symptomatic nature, (4) their immediate effect on underlying thought, and (5) their emotional impact. These clinical features may help to discriminate obsessions and compulsive rituals from delusions and delusional repetitive behaviors in patients with schizophrenia or related disorders. Throughout Oulis et al. stress the importance of the feature of mental reflexivity for understanding the nature of insight and the ambiguous diagnostic status of poor insight in OCD which may be either a marker of the chronicity of obsessions or a marker of their delusionality. With these notions we return to earlier-mentioned thoughts concerning "obsessions in the strict sense" and "obsessions in the broader sense" according to Jaspers (1973).

With the abovementioned aspects in mind, psychotic symptoms and OCS can often be clearly distinguished; however, relatively frequent there is a marked overlap between psychotic symptoms and obsessive-compulsive symptoms. Sometimes it is not possible to make a robust unequivocal distinction between OCS and psychosis. Given the similarities in neurobiology, pathophysiology, prognosis, and therapeutic response of "psychotic OCS" or "obsessive-compulsive psychosis," this may not come as a surprise.

Taken together, a comprehensive assessment of the abovementioned aspects of OCS or psychotic symptoms helps to differentiate them, or at least, in cases were a robust unequivocal distinction between OCS and psychosis is not possible, they help to place them on a dimensional line between those classifications.

Table 3.1 Differential diagnostic identification of obsessive-compulsive symptoms in schizophrenia

Attribution and insight	Insight criterion	Patients suffering from OCD typically fulfill three symptom characteristics: (1) they attribute obsessions, impulsive symptoms, and compulsions to their own thinking, (2) declare with insight their unreasonableness, and (3) show some degree of resistance against them. In particular, the first two properties allow a differentiation from hallucinations and delusions
Uncertainty	Doubt	Typically OCD patients are in doubt, whereas deluded patients know for sure
Content	OCS not solely related to the psychotic content	For instance, cleaning or checking behavior should be diagnosed as compulsions only if it is accompanied by typical obsessions and not if the patient currently suffers from delusions of contamination, intoxication, or infection
	Theme	Typical themes of obsessions are contamination, aggressive or sexual topics, or symmetry
		Typical themes of delusions are persecution, ideas of reference, diminishing barriers between the person and surrounding, or grandiosity
	Catatonic symptoms	Repetitive behavior or stereotypic actions should be discriminated from catatonic symptoms most importantly in patients with the so-called manieristic catatonia
	Obsessions presented as pseudohallucinations	A subgroup of OCS patients who experience their obsessions as extremely aversive and burdening and use expressions such as "voices" or "foreign thought content," but in most cases these phenomena can be characterized as pseudohallucinations
Association with schizophrenia symptoms	No association with schizophrenia symptoms: comorbid OCD	In most studies of patients with schizophrenia and comorbid OCD, a lack of association between the major OCD symptom categories and schizophrenia symptom dimensions is found
	Association with schizophrenia symptoms: no comorbid OCD	Ruminations or stereotypic ego-dystonic cognitions with direct relation to the contents to psychotic thinking should not be diagnosed as obsessions
Time of occurrence	Antipsychotic-induced OCS	Patients without a previous history of OCS might develop these phenomena during antipsychotic treatment
Course	Reevaluation of OCS after remission of psychotic symptoms	If the first manifestation of OCS occurs simultaneously with the first psychotic exacerbation, the final decision whether there is a valid comorbid condition should be postponed until the remission of psychotic symptoms

Clinical aspects to consider when differentiating between psychotic symptoms and OCS

3.4 Clinical Presentation of OCS in Patients with Psychotic Disorders

Throughout this book, details will be given concerning the clinical presentation of OCS in patients with psychotic disorders. Here we will give a concise overview concerning the following aspects: (a) time of occurrence, (b) symptom structure, (c) course of comorbid OCS, and (d) association with schizophrenia symptoms. For more details concerning these aspects, we will refer to the relevant chapters.

3.4.1 Time of Occurrence

OCS may occur in schizophrenia patients as (1) *preceding prodromal symptoms*: (1.1) before the development of psychosis as an independent, coexisting syndrome that can be diagnosed as OCD; (1.2) before the occurrence of the first psychotic episode as part of the at-risk mental state (ARMS) in subjects with mild psychotic complaints; or as (2) *comorbid condition*, during a psychotic episode or during recovery form psychosis: (2.1) together with psychotic symptoms during the first psychotic episode; (2.2) during the course of chronic schizophrenia as a waxing and waning condition; (2.3) simultaneously with the first psychotic exacerbation; (2.4) during the course of chronic schizophrenia as a persistent morbidity; or (3) *de novo associated with antipsychotic treatment*, as markedly aggravated or de novo occurring after initiation of specific antipsychotic treatment (Hwang et al. 2009; Schirmbeck and Zink 2012, 2013).

For prevalence estimations for different stages of the psychotic disorder, and for differences in symptom presentation in these subgroups, we would like to refer to Chaps. 4, 8, and 10.

3.4.2 Symptom Structure

Several researchers evaluated whether the symptom structure of well-described OCS in patients with schizophrenia is comparable to the symptom structure of OCS in patients with OCD.

Faragian et al. (2009) studied 110 patients who met DSM-IV criteria for both schizophrenia and OCD. They performed an exploratory factor analysis of the Yale-Brown Obsessive-Compulsive Scale (Y-BOCS) checklist. They found a five-factor solution that accounted for 58.7 % of the total variance:

1. Aggressive, sexual, and religious obsessions and counting
2. Symmetry and ordering/hoarding compulsions
3. Contamination and cleaning
4. Somatic obsession and repeating compulsion
5. Hoarding obsession and checking/repeating compulsions

Moreover, they evaluated the interrelationship between the resulting factors and schizophrenia symptom dimensions. Here they found no significant correlation between the Y-BOCS symptom dimensions and schizophrenia symptom dimensions. The five symptom dimensions are comparable to those revealed in "pure" OCD. The first three symptom dimensions identified in their study, namely, aggressive, sexual, and religious obsession and counting compulsion, symmetry/ordering, and cleanliness/washing, are remarkably similar to the OCD factors that emerged from a meta-analysis of the symptom structure in "pure" OCD and designated as forbidden thought factor, symmetry factor, and cleaning factor (Bloch et al. 2008). These findings are supported by a recent study in which Kim et al. (2012) found a high level of similarity between the nature of symptoms and dimensions identified in patients with antipsychotic medication-induced OCS and those revealed in OCD patients. Taken together, these similarities suggest the involvement of universal mechanisms in the pathogenesis of OCD regardless of the presence of schizophrenia. Moreover, the lack of intercorrelation between the major OCD symptom categories and schizophrenia symptom dimensions lends additional support to the independent nature of OCD in these patients suffering from schizophrenia and OCD. For more details concerning OCD subtypes and spectrum disorders, we refer the reader to Chap. 2.

3.4.3 Course of Comorbid OCS

Course patterns may be important in distinguishing clinical relevant differences in etiology, prognosis, and therapeutic opportunities. Therefore, a precise estimate of occurrence and persistence of OCS/OCD in schizophrenia is needed. The few studies so far that prospectively evaluated the course of comorbid OCS/OCD in general showed considerable fluctuation in the course of OCS (Craig et al. 2002; de Haan et al. 2012). Regarding the subgroup of schizophrenia patients treated with clozapine or olanzapine, OCS may be remarkable persistent (Schirmbeck et al. 2013).

For differences in pattern of onset and clinical course, we would like to refer to Chaps. 4 and 10.

3.4.4 Association with Schizophrenia Symptoms

Several studies evaluated the association between OCS and symptoms of schizophrenia. Although patients with schizophrenia with OCS tend to have more severe depressive symptoms and overall poorer functional capacities, no consistent pattern of association with positive and negative symptoms has emerged. However, Guillem et al. (2009) found a strong positive relationship between delusions and obsessions and between auditory hallucinations and compulsions. These findings are interpreted that they are consistent with the view that psychosis and OCS reflect manifestations of similar mechanisms. On the other hand, they found inverse relationships between somatic obsessions and disorganization and between hoarding and delusions or auditory hallucinations. These inconsistencies may be explained by methodological issues. However, an alternative explanation may be that two (or more) subgroups in patients with schizophrenia and OCS can be identified: those with "pure" OCD independent of schizophrenia symptoms and those with the so-called "schizotypal" OCD because symptoms partially overlap with positive symptoms (Poyurovsky et al. 2003) (see Chap. 5).

For a more comprehensive discussion concerning associations between OCS and schizophrenia symptoms, we would like to refer to Chap. 5.

In conclusion, precise psychopathological investigation allows in most cases the attribution of cognitive and behavioral symptoms to the spectrum of OCS or to psychosis. Frequently, retrospective data, information from family members or caregivers, and longitudinal observations turn out to be very helpful. The precise classification of symptoms in individual patients facilitates specific therapeutic interventions that are described in Chaps. 11 and 12.

References

Beckmann H, Bartsch AJ, Neumärker K-J, Pfuhlmann B, Verdaguer MF, Franzek E (2000) Schizophrenia in the Wernicke-Kleist-Leonhard School. Am J Psychiatry 157:1024–1025

Berrios GE (1989) Obsessive-compulsive disorder: its conceptual history in France during the 19th century. Compr Psychiatry 30:283–295

Bloch MH, Landeros-Weisenberger A, Rosario MC, Pittenger C, Leckman JF (2008) Meta-analysis of the symptom structure of obsessive-compulsive disorder. Am J Psychiatry 165:1532–1542

Bräunig P, Krüger S, Shugar G, Höffler J, Börner I (2000) The catatonia rating scale I–development, reliability, and use. Compr Psychiatry 41:147–158

Bürgy M (2007) Obsession in the strict sense: a helpful psychopathological phenomenon in the differential diagnosis between obsessive-compulsive disorder and schizophrenia. Psychopathology 40:102–110

Catapano F, Perris F, Fabrazzo M, Cioffi V, Giacco D, De Santis V, Maj M (2010) Obsessive-compulsive disorder with poor insight: a three-year prospective study. Prog Neuropsychopharmacol Biol Psychiatry 34:323–330

Craig T, Hwang MY, Bromet EJ (2002) Obsessive-compulsive and panic symptoms in patients with first-admission psychosis. Am J Psychiatry 159:592–598

de Haan L, Hoogeboom B, Beuk N, Wouters L, Dingemans PM, Linszen DH (2006) Reliability and validity of the Yale-Brown Obsessive-Compulsive Scale in schizophrenia patients. Psychopharmacol Bull 39:25–30

de Haan L, Sterk B, Wouters L, Linszen DH (2012) The 5-year course of obsessive-compulsive symptoms and obsessive-compulsive disorder in first-episode schizophrenia and related disorders. Schizophr Bull 39:151–160

Faragian S, Pashinian A, Fuchs C, Poyurovsky M (2009) Obsessive-compulsive symptom dimensions in schizophrenia patients with comorbid obsessive-compulsive disorder. Prog Neuropsychopharmacol Biol Psychiatry 33:1009–1012

Fink M (2013) Rediscovering catatonia: the biography of a treatable syndrome. Acta Psychiatr Scand Suppl 127:1–47

Guillem F, Satterthwaite J, Pampoulova T, Stip E (2009) Relationship between psychotic and obsessive compulsive symptoms in schizophrenia. Schizophr Res 115:358–362

Hinds AL, Woody EZ, Van Ameringen M, Schmidt LA, Szechtman H (2012) When too much is not enough: obsessive-compulsive disorder as a pathology of stopping, rather than starting. PLoS One 7:e30586

Hwang MY, Kim SW, Yum SY, Opler LA (2009) Management of schizophrenia with obsessive-compulsive features. Psychiatr Clin North Am 32:835–851
Jaspers K (1973) Allgemeine psychopathologie, 9th edn. Springer, Berlin
Kim JH, Ryu S, Nam HJ, Lim M, Baek JH, Joo YH, Kwon JS, Ha TH, Hong KS (2012) Symptom structure of antipsychotic-induced obsessive compulsive symptoms in schizophrenia patients. Prog Neuropsychopharmacol Biol Psychiatry 39:75–79
Kraepelin E (1896) Psychiatrie, 5th edn. Barth, Leipzig
Kraepelin E (1915) Psychiatrie, 8th edn. Barth, Leipzig
Kronfeld A (1924) Zur Phänomenologie des Triebhaften. Zeitschrift für die gesamte Neurologie und Psychiatrie 92:379–395
Lincoln TM (2007) Relevant dimensions of delusions: continuing the continuum versus category debate. Schizophr Res 93:211–220
Moritz S, Van Quaquebeke N (2013) Are you sure? Delusion conviction moderates the behavioural and emotional consequences of paranoid ideas. Cogn Neuropsychiatry 19:164–180
Oulis P, Konstantakopoulos G, Lykouras L, Michalopoulou PG (2013) Differential diagnosis of obsessive-compulsive symptoms from delusions in schizophrenia: a phenomenological approach. World J Psychiatry 22:50–56
Poyurovsky M, Kriss V, Weisman G, Faragian S, Kurs R, Schneidman M, Fuchs C, Weizman A, Weizman R (2003) Comparison of clinical characteristics and comorbidity in schizophrenia patients with and without obsessive-compulsive disorder: schizophrenic and OC symptoms in schizophrenia. J Clin Psychiatry 64:1300–1307
Rosen I (1957) The clinical significance of obsessions in schizophrenia. J Ment Sci 103:773–785
Schirmbeck F, Zink M (2012) Clozapine-induced obsessive-compulsive symptoms in schizophrenia: a critical review. Curr Neuropharmacol 10:88–95
Schirmbeck F, Zink M (2013) Comorbid obsessive-compulsive symptoms in schizophrenia: contributions of pharmacological and genetic factors. Front Pharmacol 4:99
Schirmbeck F, Rausch F, Englisch S, Eifler S, Esslinger C, Meyer-Lindenberg A, Zink M (2013) Differential effects of antipsychotic agents on obsessive-compulsive symptoms in schizophrenia: a longitudinal study. J Psychopharmacol 27:349–357
Schneider K (1939) Begriffliche Untersuchung über den Zwang. Allgemeine Zeitschrift Psychiatrie und ihre Grenzgebiete 112:17–24
Stengel E (1945) A study on some clinical aspects of the relationship between obsessional neurosis and psychotic reaction types. J Ment Sci 91:166–187
Szechtman H, Woody E (2006) Obsessive-compulsive disorder as a disturbance of security motivation: constraints on comorbidity. Neurotox Res 10:103–112
Westphal K (1878) Ueber Zwangsvorstellungen. Arch Psychiatr Nervenkr 8:734–750
Woody SR, Steketee G, Chambless DL (1995) Reliability and validity of the Yale-Brown Obsessive-Compulsive Scale. Behav Res Ther 33:597–605
Zink M, Englisch S, Dressing H (2008) Neurobiology confirms psychopathology: on the antagonism of psychosis and obsessive-compulsive syndromes. Psychopathology 41:279–285

4 Epidemiology: Prevalence and Clinical Characteristics of Obsessive-Compulsive Disorder and Obsessive-Compulsive Symptoms in Patients with Psychotic Disorders

Frederike Schirmbeck, Marije Swets, and Lieuwe de Haan

4.1 Obsessive-Compulsive Symptoms in Schizophrenia: Epidemiological Perspective

The associations between psychotic disorders and obsessive-compulsive symptoms have interested scientists since Carl Friedrich Otto Westphal in the nineteenth century (Westphal 1878). But it was not before the later decades of the twentieth century that notable concern and an increased research interest about this problem arose. Since then, several epidemiological studies have investigated the occurrence of obsessions and compulsions in patients with psychotic disorders. Subsequently, data of these primary investigations have been evaluated and summarized in recent reviews and meta-analysis (Achim et al. 2011; Braga et al. 2013; Buckley et al. 2009; Swets et al. 2014).

Within their meta-analyses, Achim et al. included 34 studies with a total of 3,007 patients, which reported data on co-morbid obsessive-compulsive disorder (OCD) in schizophrenia. Their estimation of a sample size weighted mean prevalence rate revealed that 12.1 % (95 % CI, 7.0–17.1) of patients with schizophrenia also fulfil the

F. Schirmbeck, PhD (✉)
Department of Psychiatry, Academic Medical Centre, University of Amsterdam, Meibergdreef 5, Amsterdam 1105 AZ, The Netherlands
e-mail: n.f.schirmbeck@amc.nl

M. Swets
Arkin Mental Health and Addiction Treatment Centre, Amsterdam, The Netherlands
e-mail: marijeswets@upcmail.nl

L. de Haan
Department of Psychiatry, Academic Medical Centre, University of Amsterdam, Amsterdam, The Netherlands
e-mail: l.dehaan@amc.uva.nl

L. De Haan et al. (eds.), *Obsessive-Compulsive Symptoms in Schizophrenia*,
DOI 10.1007/978-3-319-12952-5_4

criteria for OCD (Achim et al. 2011). This number largely exceeds prevalence rates of OCD in the general population where the lifetime prevalence for OCD is 2–3 % (Angst et al. 2004; Fineberg et al. 2013). In contrast to this high lifetime risk for patients with schizophrenia to suffer from co-morbid OCD, primary OCD patients most frequently present with co-morbid affective or anxiety disorders. However, two recent epidemiological case register studies from Denmark and Sweden concluded that a diagnosis of OCD was also associated with higher rates of schizophrenia and schizophrenia spectrum disorders (Cederlof et al. 2014; Meier et al. 2014).

In line with earlier reports, Achim et al. point out that the variability of reported OCD prevalence rates in patients with schizophrenia is considerably high, ranging from as low as 0.6 % to as high as 55.0 % (Achim et al. 2011). Previously this heterogeneity led other authors to conclude that the exact prevalence rates of co-morbid OCD in schizophrenia remain unclear (Mukhopadhaya et al. 2009). To identify the variables that are responsible for this heterogeneity, Achim et al. considered the effect of several moderator variables related to sampling and methodological aspects. Whereas gender or the primary diagnosis of schizophrenia vs. schizoaffective disorder did not have an effect, results revealed a significant moderating effect of the stage of illness, with higher prevalence rates in later disease stages, when compared to first-episode patients. Furthermore, differences in the applied diagnostic instruments had a significant effect. Studies applying the more recent version of the Diagnostic and Statistical Manual of Mental Disorders (DSM-IV) and those supplementing the Structured Clinical Interview for DSM Disorders (SCID) with additional instruments (e.g. the Yale-Brown Obsessive Compulsive Scale (YBOCS)) reported significantly higher prevalence rates. However, adjusting analyses for these moderating variables still left considerable residual heterogeneity within the strata of studies unexplained (Achim et al. 2011).

4.1.1 Prevalence Estimations Accounting for Different Levels of Symptom Severity

Swets et al. recently conducted a second meta-analysis, suggesting that the inclusion of studies with different diagnostic thresholds used to define OCD may have added to the observed variability. Their study therefore specifically focused on the whole spectrum of obsessive-compulsive symptoms (OCS), aiming to provide best estimate of both OCS and OCD prevalence in schizophrenia patients. Overall, 36 studies with a total of 3,308 subjects provided data on a clinical OCD diagnosis (see Fig. 4.1). Furthermore, prevalence estimations for subthreshold OCS not fulfilling diagnostic criteria and rates for different YBOCS subcategories were calculated. Closely in line with the finding reported by Achim et al., the pooled prevalence rate for OCD was 12.3 % (95 % CI, 9.7–15.4 %) (Swets et al. 2014).

The pooled prevalence rate of 30.7 % (95 % CI, 23.0–39.6 %) for the OCS category was considerably higher, suggesting that almost every third patient with a psychotic disorder reported subclinical obsessive, distressing, intrusive thoughts and/or compulsions (e.g. repeated handwashing, checking behaviour, counting or

OCD prevalence

Study name	Statistics for each study				
	Event rate	Lower limit	Upper limit	Z-Value	p- Value
Bermanzohn 2000	0,135	0,057	0,286	-3,861	0,000
Braga 2005	0,151	0,077	0,274	-4,501	0,000
Byerly 2005	0,230	0,158	0,322	-5,085	0,000
Cassano 1998	0,290	0,158	0,470	-2,262	0,024
Ciapparelli, 2007	0,238	0,133	0,389	-3,212	0,001
Cosoff 1998	0,138	0,078	0,232	-5,652	0,000
Craig 2002	0,040	0,021	0,075	-9,321	0,000
Eisen 1997	0,078	0,035	0,163	-5,812	0,000
Fabisch 2001	0,003	0,000	0,053	-3,889	0,000
Farrelly 2007	0,016	0,005	0,049	-6,973	0,000
Goodwin 2001	0,117	0,071	0,188	-7,116	0,000
Goodwin 2003	0,054	0,029	0,098	-8,778	0,000
Huppert 2002	0,375	0,227	0,551	-1,399	0,162
Haan, de 2002	0,150	0,095	0,228	-6,584	0,000
Koen 2003A scid	0,042	0,006	0,244	-3,073	0,002
Koen 2003B digs	0,008	0,001	0,114	-3,408	0,001
Kruger 2000	0,158	0,092	0,258	-5,320	0,000
Lee 2009	0,370	0,212	0,562	-1,335	0,182
Lysaker 2002	0,175	0,100	0,289	-4,676	0,000
Niehaus 2005	0,006	0,002	0,018	-8,903	0,000
Nimwegen, van 2008	0,148	0,095	0,223	-6,865	0,000
Ohta 2003	0,183	0,109	0,290	-4,875	0,000
Öngür 2005	0,085	0,046	0,151	-7,199	0,000
Pallanti 2004	0,225	0,147	0,329	-4,619	0,000
Porto 1997	0,260	0,157	0,398	-3,244	0,001
Poyurovsky 1999	0,140	0,068	0,266	-4,454	0,000
Poyurovsky 2006	0,160	0,082	0,289	-4,299	0,000
Sa 2009	0,167	0,092	0,283	-4,643	0,000
Seedat 2007a	0,108	0,081	0,142	13,106	0,000
Seedat 2007b	0,043	0,014	0,125	-5,266	0,000
Sim 2006	0,063	0,033	0,117	-7,816	0,000
Strakowski 1993	0,074	0,019	0,252	-3,437	0,001
Strakowski 1995	0,111	0,028	0,352	-2,773	0,006
Tibbo 2000	0,250	0,151	0,384	-3,430	0,001
Ücok 2006	0,096	0,046	0,188	-5,644	0,000
Kessler 2005	0,041	0,013	0,120	-5,341	0,000
Sevincok 2004	0,283	0,178	0,418	-3,049	0,002
Overall prevalence	**0,123**	**0,097**	**0,154**	**14,529**	**0,000**

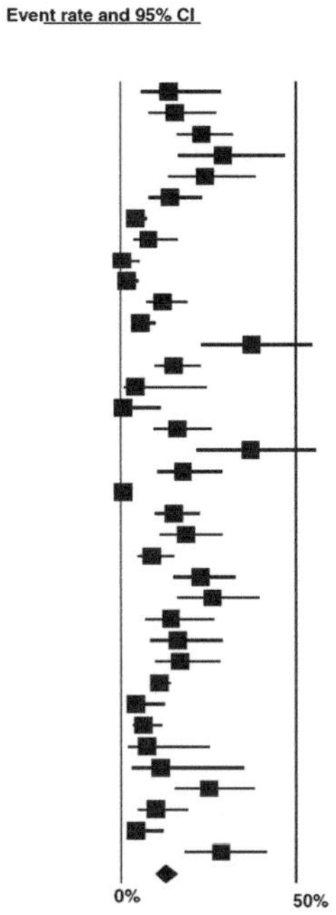

Fig. 4.1 Results of studies on obsessive-compulsive disorder and their 95 % confidence intervals included in the meta-analysis by Swets et al. (Figure reprint with permission Swets et al. (2014))

cleaning). Accordingly, mean prevalence estimations depended on different diagnostic thresholds used to define OCS: YBOCS threshold 1–5, mean prevalence of 35.3 % (95 % CI, 20.9–53.1 %); threshold 6–9, mean prevalence of 30.3 % (95 % CI, 23.9–37.6 %); threshold 10–13, mean prevalence of 20.5 % (95 % CI, 12.9–30.9 %); and threshold 14–17, mean prevalence of 14.8 % (95 % CI, 11.9–18.2 %) (see Fig. 4.2) (Swets et al. 2014).

In addition to the meta-analytical review of previous studies, Swets et al. recently evaluated the occurrence of OCS/OCD in the large multicentre Genetic Risk and Outcome of Psychosis (GROUP) study, a prospective investigation of a representative cohort of patients, their nonpsychotic siblings and healthy controls in the Netherlands. Overall, 2,526 subjects were included in one or more analyses (987 patients and 973 siblings, coming from 978 families, and 566 controls). In concordance with the mentioned pooled prevalence rates resulting from meta-analysis, they found clinically relevant OCS (YBOCS > 9) in 19.0 % of patients. This number highly exceeded the occurrence of clinically relevant OCS in siblings (4.3 %) and healthy controls (1.6 %) (M. Swets et al. unpublished data).

Although distinguishing between OCD and OCS and addressing different severity thresholds partly explain the heterogeneity of previous results, the variability of prevalence rates within the OCD and OCS categories was still significantly high

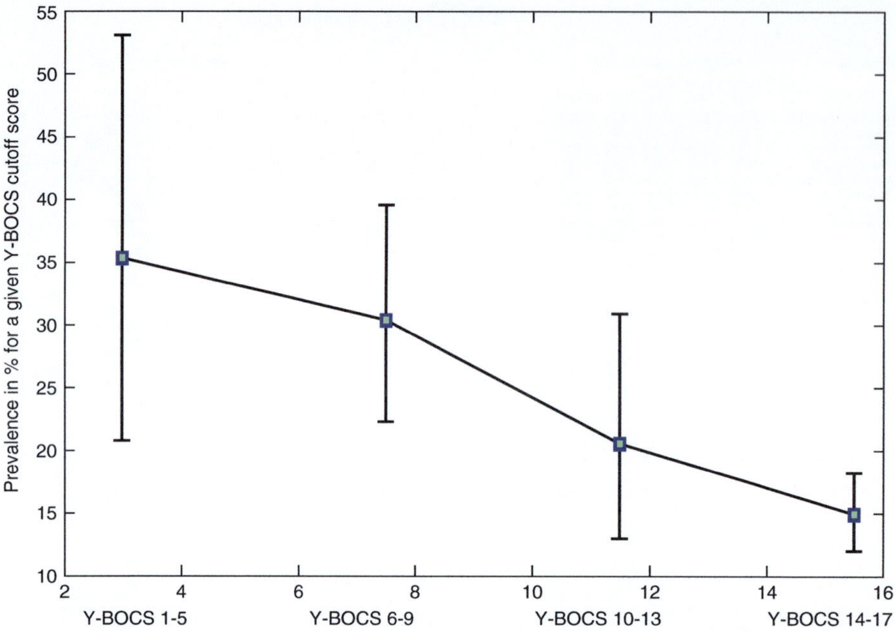

Fig. 4.2 Prevalence (in %) for different YBOCS threshold severity scores. The figure indicates the average prevalence and error bars (±1.96 SD) (Figure reprint with permission Swets et al. (2014))

(see Fig. 4.2). Therefore, Swets et al. conducted additional meta-regression analyses to identify potential moderators. In line with findings by Achim et al., again stage of illness, the applied DSM version (DSM-III vs. DSM-IV), used diagnostic instrument (DIGS vs. SCID) and application of supplement assessments specifically addressing OCS (e.g. the YBOCS) were associated with the level of reported OCD rates. These variables explained almost 60.0 % of the heterogeneity across studies. After adjustment, the overall OCD prevalence changed from 12.3 to 13.6 %. The confidence interval narrowed accordingly, now ranging from 11.8 to 15.8 %. With respect to the OCS prevalence estimates, only the additional assessment with symptom-specific instruments retained a statistically significant association. This variable explained 27.1 % of the heterogeneity, leading to an adjusted overall OCS prevalence in 30.3 %, with a narrower confidence interval ranging from 24.2 to 37.3 % (Swets et al. 2014).

4.1.2 Prevalence Estimations for Different Stages of the Psychotic Disorder

Both meta-analytical studies mentioned illness duration as a significant moderator with prevalence rates in later disease stages being significantly higher than in the early course of psychotic illness. Consequently, separate analyses of prevalence

Table 4.1 OCS/OCD prevalence rates in ARMS and FEP patients

	Cohort size (*n*)	OCD (%)	OCS (%)
ARMS			
Lencz et al. (2004)	82	11	
Rosen et al. (2006)	29	4	
Shioiri et al. (2007)	219	1.5	2.7
Rubino et al. (2009)	197	8.1	
Niendam et al. (2009)	64	14	20
Sterk et al. (2011)	29	3.4	20.7
Fontenelle et al. (2011)	396	8.1	
Bechdolf et al. (2011)	156	3.8	11.1
Hur et al. (2012)	65		36.9
De Vylder et al. (2012)	20	30	60
Fusar-Poli et al. (2012)	509	2	
Zink et al. (2014)	233	5.2	11.2
FEP			
Poyurovsky et al. (1999)	50	14	
Strakowski et al. (1993)	27	7.4	
Strakowski et al. (1995)	18	11.0	
Craig et al. (2002)	225	4.0	16.9
De Haan et al. (2002, 2005)	106	15.0	29.2
De Haan et al. (2004)	200	7	
Sterk et al. (2011)	270	1.5	10.7
De Haan et al. (2013)	198		11.6
De Haan et al. (2013)	186	11.8	31.2

Abbreviations: *ARMS* at-risk mental state, *FEP* first-episode patients, *OCD* obsessive-compulsive disorder, *OCS* obsessive-compulsive symptoms

estimations in different stages of the psychotic illness could be a useful approach in further explaining heterogeneity of reported results.

In a recent study, Zink et al. published data on OCS and OCD occurrence in an at-risk mental state (ARMS) sample and reviewed existing data of prevalence rates in the early course of psychotic illness (see Table 4.1). Including their findings in the calculation of sample size weighted mean prevalence rates, 13.0 % (95 % CI, 10.8–15.5) of ARMS patients report OCS, while 5.4 % (95 % CI, 4.5–6.5) fulfil the criteria for OCD. Slightly higher averaged rates for OCS (17.1 %, 95 % CI, 14.6–19.8) and OCD (7.0 %, 95 % CI, 5.7–8.6) were found in first-episode patients (see Fig. 4.3). Thus, in comparison to the general population, a remarkably large subgroup of patients already reports OCS during the early course of psychotic illness (Zink et al. 2014). Again, variability of epidemiological data between studies can be explained by methodological aspects, including differences in the definition of ARMS criteria and differences in the psychometric assessment of OCS or OCD.

In comparison to OCD prevalence rates in early stages of the disease, the mentioned co-morbidity rates in mixed and later disease stages are considerably higher,

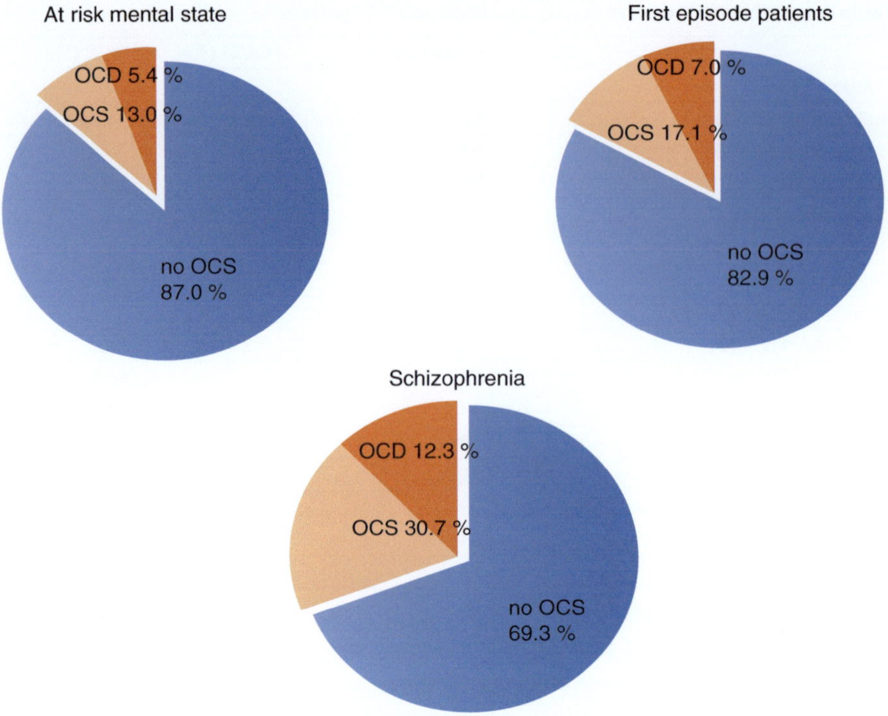

Fig. 4.3 Prevalence rates for different stages of psychosis

frequently exceeding estimations of more than 30 % (Lysaker and Whitney 2009; Sevincok et al. 2006). This finding is in line with the general assumption that more severe psychopathology is characterized by higher levels of co-morbidity. Furthermore, several case reports, cases series and systematic evaluations reported the de novo development or marked aggravation of OCS during treatment with atypical antipsychotics, in particular clozapine (Mukhopadhaya et al. 2009) (see Chap. 10). High prevalence rates of up to 70 % in groups treated with clozapine markedly contrast with lower prevalence and severity of OCS, for example, in patients treated with haloperidol or other second-generation antipsychotics (de Haan et al. 1999; Schirmbeck et al. 2011, 2013; for a review, see Schirmbeck and Zink 2013). The fact that chronic patients are more likely to use clozapine may partly explain the higher co-morbidity rates in later disease stages. Another explanation may be that the propensity to develop antipsychotic-resistant psychotic symptoms is associated with the risk to develop OCS.

In summary, meta-analyses highlight the fact that obsessions and compulsions are highly prevalent in patients with psychotic disorders and require specific attention. The noticeable heterogeneity in prevalence rates throughout cross-sectional studies can be attributed to several factors such as the levels of symptom severity, stage of the psychotic illness or methodological differences. Taking symptom severity into account, Swets et al. concluded that around 30 % of patients with a psychotic disorder experienced broadly defined OCS, 20 % experience at least mild OCS and 12 % fulfil the criteria for a co-morbid OCD. The evaluation of prevalence estimations at different stages of psychotic illness reveals an increase in co-occurring OCS/OCD with longer illness duration.

4.2 Differences in Pattern of Onset and Clinical Course

Apart from differences in first manifestation of co-occurring OCS/OCD, little is known about the longitudinal course of symptoms over time. Prevalence estimations based on the presence of OCS/OCD at one cross-sectional assessment or based on short-term retrospective assessments do not account for the fact that OCS may appear as fluctuating symptoms that they may remit, relapse or worsen over time. To provide a more realistic lifetime estimate of occurrence and persistence of OCS/OCD in schizophrenia, detailed longitudinal assessments are needed. This data will further aid to provide information on the course and possible interactions of symptoms.

To date, only few studies prospectively assessed the course of co-morbid OCS/OCD over time. Craig et al. reassessed schizophrenia/schizoaffective patients 24 months after inclusion and found remission of baseline OCS/OCD in two-thirds of their investigated sample. Concomitantly, during follow-up, there was an incidence of newly reported OCS and OCD roughly equal to about one-third of the lifetime prevalence rate found at baseline (Craig et al. 2002). In line with these findings, a recent study of a large sample of first-episode patients ($n = 172$) showed considerable fluctuation in co-morbid OCS/OCD over a period of 5 years. The point prevalence for OCS at admission was 32.2 %; the 5-year prevalence rate for OCS was 51.1 %, with only 13.4 % reporting OCS at all four assessments (de Haan et al. 2012). Similarly, the vast majority of co-morbid patients of the earlier mentioned GROUP study reported symptom changes either as remitting, de novo development or intermittent OCS over the first 3 years of prospective investigation (see Fig. 4.4) (F. Schirmbeck et al. unpublished data). In contrast, a 1-year observational investigation of a subgroup of schizophrenia patients treated with clozapine or olanzapine found remarkable persistence in reported OCS over time (Schirmbeck et al. 2013).

As a result of reported findings, different types of OCS onset and development over time have been proposed (see Fig. 4.5).

The reason for the variation in course of co-occurring OCS and substantial fluctuation in a large subgroup of co-morbid patients is not clear. Analyses within the GROUP sample revealed that changes in OCS were significantly associated with changes in psychotic symptoms, general psychopathological symptoms and emotional distress, not only in patients but also in unaffected siblings (F. Schirmbeck et al. unpublished data). These findings hint towards dynamic interactions between symptoms, but they are limited by infrequent assessments, with a large interval of 3 years in-between. Changes of affective or psychotic symptoms, transient OCS or

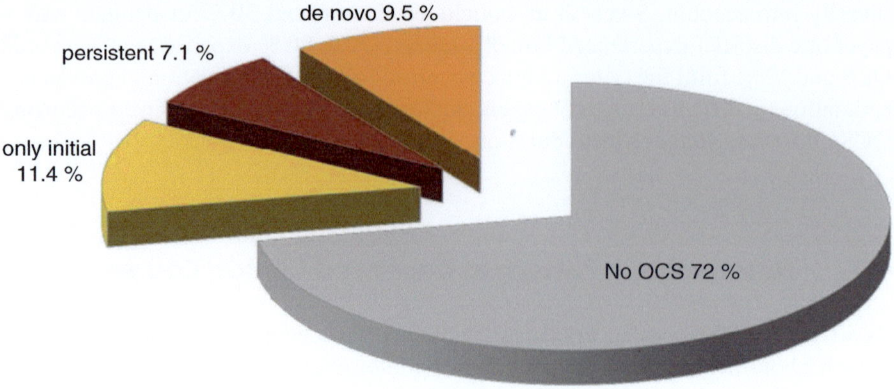

Fig. 4.4 Course of obsessive-compulsive symptoms over 3 years

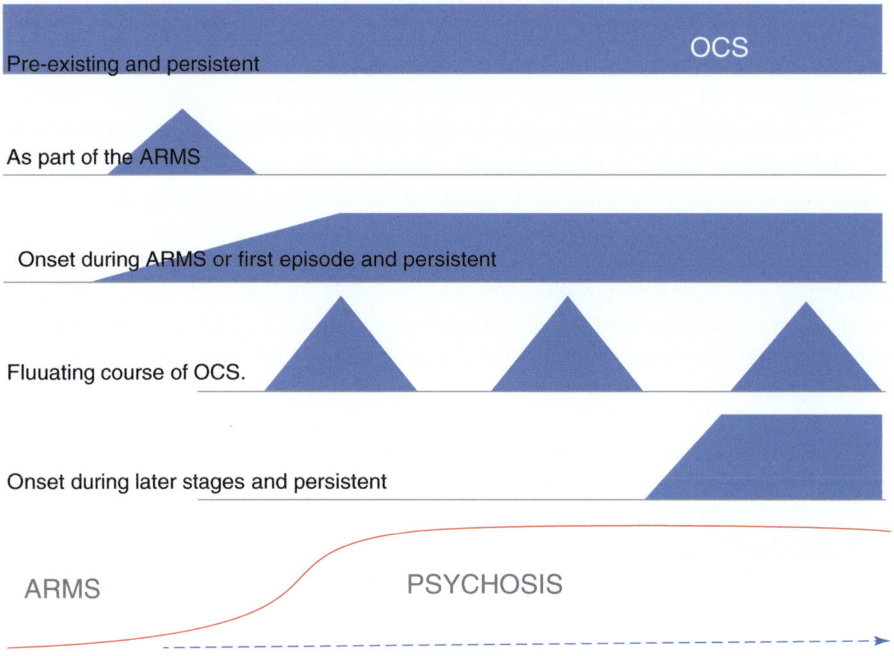

Fig. 4.5 Patterns of OCS onset and course during different stages of psychosis (Adapted from Schirmbeck and Zink (2013))

substantial remission of OCS and most importantly the exact time course of these events are still unknown. The diverse clinical course adds to the heterogeneous clinical presentation and suggests an involvement of different pathogenic pathways in the development of co-morbid OCS in schizophrenia.

4.3 Subgroups within the Co-morbid Sample

It seems very unlikely to assume that the high prevalence rates of OCS in psychotic disorders are simply due to a random association of two rather common psychiatric disorders (Pedersen et al. 2014). The heterogeneity of the clinical presentation suggests the involvement of several pathogenic mechanisms. Progress in understanding these mechanisms will most likely be achieved if studies focus on the identification of homogeneous subgroups within the co-morbid sample. This is especially important as different aetiologies may require different treatment approaches (see Chaps. 11 and 12).

Before introducing possible categorizations within the co-morbid sample, some notions on the assumption of OCS as an attempt to compensate psychotic symptoms seem appropriate. Furthermore, the often difficult differentiation between symptoms of schizophrenia and OCS (Chap. 3) should be addressed. Early concepts on the co-occurrence of OCS and psychotic disorders proposed that OCS might develop as an attempt to reduce psychotic symptoms, might have protective effects regarding psychotic disintegration and might indicate a favourable course of schizophrenia (Dowling et al. 1995; Stengel 1945). In contrast to these assumptions, subsequent research results mainly reported negative impacts of the co-occurrence of psychosis and OCS as shown in higher general illness severity, more social and functional impairment and an overall poor prognosis (Cunill et al. 2009; Ücok et al. 2011) (see Chap. 6). However, individual studies reported negative correlations between specific OCS and certain aspects of psychosis. Guillem et al. found negative associations between somatic obsessions as well as hoarding and the severity of psychotic disorganization in thinking and behaviour and proposed compensating mechanisms (Guillem et al. 2009).

As mentioned in Chap. 3, detailed diagnostic explorations and careful discrimination between symptoms of psychosis and OCS are of critical importance (see Chap. 3), not only for the sake of consensus concerning diagnostic categorizations but also for the development and adaptation of optimal treatment approaches (see Chaps. 11 and 12). One critical aspect concerns the distinction of catatonic symptoms of schizophrenia (Fink 2013), which phenotypically overlap with obsessions and compulsions (Fink and Taylor 2001). This fact limits the discriminative validity of psychometric scales such as the catatonia rating scale (CRS) (Bräunig et al. 2000) and the YBOCS (de Haan et al. 2006; Woody et al. 1995). Here, a more precise characterization and descriptions of the natural long-term course of symptoms should be considered, as, for instance, published by Leonhard (Beckmann et al. 2000). These descriptions allow clear discrimination between OCS and catatonic symptoms.

Detailed assessments may help to define homogeneous subgroups within the co-morbid sample. According to differences in time of first onset, clinical course and phenotypic presentation of OCS patients, we propose the following subgroups: (1) OCS as part of the at-risk mental state (ARMS) or as pre-existing independent OCD, (2) concurrent occurrence (OCS as a sub-syndrome of schizophrenia or as a co-occurring syndrome) and (3) subsequent development as antipsychotic-associated OCS.

4.3.1 Pre-existing: Part of the ARMS or Independent OCD

Devulpalli et al. evaluated the temporal sequence of clinical manifestation of OCS and psychotic symptoms ($n = 148$) excluding cases with antipsychotic-induced OCS. Results revealed that almost 50 % of schizophrenia patients retrospectively reported OCS onset prior to psychosis. Subsequent analyses showed that the majority of these patients reported OCS onset within 1 year prior to psychotic exacerbation. Authors therefore concluded that they could be a part of the prodromal phase, in particular the basic symptom cluster in the early course of schizophrenia (Ebel et al. 1989; Sullwold and Huber 1986). Similarly above-mentioned prevalence estimations in ARMS samples support the assumption that a relevant subgroup of patients experience co-occurring OCS during this time. Regarding the impact of OCS during the ARMS, findings have been heterogeneous. Whereas higher impairment of psychosocial functioning and more severe depressive symptoms have consistently been reported, findings regarding transition rates into psychosis and cognitive functioning remain contradicting (Zink et al. 2014). Because longitudinal studies are missing, little is known about the ongoing course of OCS in the ARMS and if they will resolve, attenuate or worsen after the onset of psychosis.

In comparison, the subgroup of patients primarily diagnosed with OCD and subsequent development of a psychotic disorder seems to be considerably small (de Haan et al. 2009; Murphy et al. 2010). However, recent large epidemiological studies reported an increased risk for OCD patients to develop psychotic disorders later on in life assuming a common etiological pathway (Cederlof et al. 2014; Meier et al. 2014). Some authors suggested that these pre-existing OCS most likely persist or worsen regardless of the development and progress in psychotic illness as an independent, co-existing disorder (Hwang et al. 2009).

4.3.2 Concurrent: OCS as a Sub-syndrome of Schizophrenia or Co-occurring Symptom Clusters

For those patients reporting concurrent psychotic and obsessive-compulsive symptoms, it has been suggested that the co-expression may mark a unique subgroup of patients, which has been referred to as the 'schizo-obsessive subtype' of schizophrenia (Bottas et al. 2005; Poyurovsky et al. 2012; Reznik et al. 2001). In addition to positive and/or negative symptoms, OCS are thought to represent a clinically meaningful dimension of this subtype of schizophrenia. Recently Poyurovsky et al. converged evidence suggesting that patients in this group can be characterized by distinct clinical and neurobiological features, treatment response and prognosis. The authors proposed diagnostic criteria for the identification of the subtype (Poyurovsky 2013; Poyurovsky et al. 2012). Attempts to validate this concept on a neurobiological level have not been conclusive (see Chaps. 7 and 9). Furthermore above-mentioned longitudinal studies showing large fluctuation of co-occurring OCS over time question the stability of this categorization as a true diagnostic entity. Therefore, other authors concluded that OCS may rather be similar to a range of other highly co-morbid diagnoses or symptom clusters that have been described in schizophrenia (e.g. depression, PTSS, panic disorder, substance abuse) (Meijer et al. 2012). Higher-than-chance co-morbidity may be caused by risk factors that are shared by both disorders (Buckley et al. 2009).

Based on inconclusive findings regarding the relationship between OCS and positive and negative symptoms, Lysaker et al. proposed yet another subdivision differentiating between a co-morbid group with high vs. low psychosocial functioning (see Chap. 6).

4.3.3 Subsequent: De Novo OCS After Initiation of Antipsychotic Treatment

As mentioned above and referred to in more detail in Chap. 10, it has been proposed that a significant subgroup of patients experience antipsychotic-induced OCS, in particular during treatment with clozapine. A remarkably simple clinical assessment of three important events allows for a screening of this group: (1) When did the first psychotic manifestation occur? (2) When was antipsychotic treatment initiated? (3) When did OCS develop or show marked aggravation? (Schirmbeck and Zink 2012, 2013).

The proposed subclassifications are certainly heuristic, and additional research and further large-scale follow-up studies are necessary to validate the existence of specific subgroups within the co-morbid sample and to elucidate possible neurobiological pathways.

4.4 Conclusion and Clinical Implications

Summarized findings show that obsessive-compulsive symptoms are a frequent co-morbid condition in patients with schizophrenia and other psychotic disorders causing additional impairment. Meta-analyses conclude that almost one out of six patients with schizophrenia fulfils the criteria for an additional OCD diagnosis, while almost 1/3 of patients experience any obsessions or compulsions. Because prevalence rates in the integrated individual studies largely differ, several approaches have been conducted to elucidate reasons for this high variability. Meta-regression analyses mainly revealed two moderating dimensions: (1) differences in sample characteristics, especially in illness duration (prevalence estimations increased in later disease stages of psychotic illness), and (2) methodological differences (studies which applied more comprehensive and OCS-specific diagnostic instruments reported higher prevalence rates).

These results indicate that OCS/OCD should be routinely explored during the intake of any patient suffering from psychosis. Assessments should be based on the general DSM criteria for OCD but should also include symptom-specific instruments such as the YBOCS to evaluate symptom content and severity in more detail. Furthermore, the time sequence of symptom onset and course over time should be explored. In the case of acute exacerbation, careful differentiation between presented psychotic and obsessive-compulsive symptoms should be based on proposed guidelines (Schirmbeck and Zink 2013) (Chap. 3). This detailed clinical characterization may result in more consensus diagnostic decisions and reduce heterogeneity between studies. Furthermore, collected information will help to identify subgroups of co-morbid patients.

The differentiation between subgroups, e.g. in accordance to symptom onset and course, seems necessary to elucidate specific underlying pathogenic mechanisms and define differential treatment needs and effective strategies. This approach has led to relevant insight into the de novo development and aggravation of OCD after the initiation of antipsychotic treatment. The exploration of the timeline of symptom onset and observed persistence of OCS helped to identify this subgroup. Subsequent research was able to identify genetic constellations indicating a possible risk factors for the development antipsychotic-associated OCS (see Chap. 10) and is now focusing on the exploration of effective pharmacological treatment approaches (see Chap. 11). Accordingly, the identification of factors which cause the observed fluctuation of OCS in a large proportion of co-morbid patients would help to understand symptom development in this particular group. Therefore, future prospective studies have to explore environmental and individual factors, which have an effect on the severity and course of co-morbid OCS. These might include daily hassles and important life events, as well as individual characteristics such as metacognitive beliefs and coping strategies. Furthermore, the interplay between psychotic, obsessive-compulsive and affective symptoms over time needs further investigation. It is plausible that treatment needs of individuals, who only experience occasional OCS significantly, differ from those reporting persistent OCS. While the first group might not need treatment at all or would profit from short psychoeducational or short cognitive-behavioural interventions, the development of effective pharmacological and psychotherapeutic approaches for the latter group seems highly necessary (Chaps. 11 and 12).

References

Achim A, Maziade M, Raymond E, Olivier D, Merette C, Roy M (2011) How prevalent are anxiety disorders in schizophrenia? A meta-analysis and critical review on a significant association. Schizophr Bull 37:811–821

Angst J, Gamma A, Endrass J, Goodwin R, Ajdacic V, Eich D, Rössler W (2004) Obsessive-compulsive severity spectrum in the community: prevalence, comorbidity, and course. Eur Arch Psychiatry Clin Neurosci 254:156–164

Bechdolf A, Mueller H, Stoetzer H, Wagner M, Maier W, Lautenschlager M, Heinz A, de Millas W, Janssen B, Gaebel W, Michel TM, Schneider F, Lambert M, Naber D, Bruene M, Krueger-Oezguerdal S, Wobrock T, Riedel M, Klosterk+Åtter J, PREVENT study group (2011) Rationale and Baseline Characteristics of PREVENT: a second-generation intervention trial in subjects at-risk (prodromal) of developing first-episode psychosis evaluating cognitive behavior therapy, aripiprazole, and placebo for the prevention of psychosis. Schizophr Bull 37:S111–S121

Beckmann H, Bartsch AJ, Neumärker K-J, Pfuhlmann B, Verdaguer MF, Franzek E (2000) Schizophrenia in the Wernicke-Kleist-Leonhard school. Am J Psychiatry 157:1024–1025

Bottas A, Cooke RG, Richter MA (2005) Comorbidity and pathophysiology of obsessive-compulsive disorder in schizophrenia: is there evidence for a schizo-obsessive subtype of schizophrenia? J Psychiatry Neurosci 30:187–193

Braga RJ, Reynolds GP, Siris SG (2013) Anxiety comorbidity in schizophrenia. Psychiatry Res 210:1–7

Bräunig P, Krüger S, Shugar G, Höffler J, Börner I (2000) The catatonia rating scale I–development, reliability, and use. Compr Psychiatry 41:147–158

Buckley P, Miller B, Lehrer D, Castle D (2009) Psychiatric comorbidities and schizophrenia. Schizophr Bull 35:383–402

Cederlof M, Lichtenstein P, Larsson H, Boman M, Ruck C, Landen M, Mataix-Cols D (2014) Obsessive-compulsive disorder, psychosis, and bipolarity: a longitudinal cohort and multigenerational family study. Schizophr Bull. doi:10.1093/schbul/sbu169

Craig T, Hwang MY, Bromet EJ (2002) Obsessive-compulsive and panic symptoms in patients with first-admission psychosis. Am J Psychiatry 159:592–598

Cunill R, Castells X, Simeon D (2009) Relationships between obsessive-compulsive symptomatology and severity of psychosis in schizophrenia: a systematic review and meta-analysis. J Clin Psychiatry 70:70–82

de Haan L, Linszen DH, Gorsira R (1999) Clozapine and obsessions in patients with recent-onset schizophrenia and other psychotic disorders. J Clin Psychiatry 60:364–365

de Haan L, Beuk N, Hoogenboom B, Dingemans P, Linszen D (2002) Obsessive-compulsive symptoms during treatment with olanzapine and risperidone: a prospective study of 113 patients with recent-onset schizophrenia or related disorders. J Clin Psychiatry 63:104–107

de Haan L, Oekeneva A, van Amelsvoort T, Linszen D (2004) Obsessive-compulsive disorder and treatment with clozapine in 200 patients with recent-onset schizophrenia or related disorders. Eur Psychiatry J Assoc Eur Psychiatrists 19:524

de Haan L, Hoogenboom B, Beuk N, van Amelsvoort T, Linszen D (2005) Obsessive-compulsive symptoms and positive, negative, and depressive symptoms in patients with recent-onset schizophrenic disorders. Can J Psychiatry Revue Canadienne de Psychiatrie 50:519–524

de Haan L, Hoogeboom B, Beuk N, Wouters L, Dingemans PM, Linszen DH (2006) Reliability and validity of the Yale-Brown Obsessive-Compulsive Scale in schizophrenia patients. Psychopharmacol Bull 39:25–30

de Haan L, Dudek-Hodge C, Verhoeven Y, Denys D (2009) Prevalence of psychotic disorders in patients with obsessive-compulsive disorder. CNS Spectr 14:415–417

de Haan L, Sterk B, Wouters L, Linszen DH (2012) The 5-year course of obsessive-compulsive symptoms and obsessive-compulsive disorder in first-episode schizophrenia and related disorders. Schizophr Bull 39:151–160

de Haan L, Sterk B, van der Valk R (2013) Presence of obsessive compulsive symptoms in first-episode schizophrenia or related disorders is associated with subjective well-being and quality of life. Early Interv Psychiatry 7:285–290

DeVylder JE, Oh AJ, Ben-David S, Azimov N, Harkavy-Friedman JM, Corcoran CM (2012) Obsessive compulsive symptoms in individuals at clinical risk for psychosis: association with depressive symptoms and suicidal ideation. Schizophr Res 140:110–113

Dowling FG, Pato MT, Pato CN (1995) Comorbidity of obsessive-compulsive and psychotic symptoms: a review. Harv Rev Psychiatry 3:75–83

Ebel H, Gross G, Klosterkotter J, Huber G, Ebel H, Gross G, Klosterkotter J, Huber G (1989) Basic symptoms in schizophrenic and affective psychoses. Psychopathology 22:224–232

Fineberg NA, Hengartner MP, Bergbaum CE, Gale TM, Gamma A, Ajdacic-Gross V, Rössler W, Angst J (2013) A prospective population-based cohort study of the prevalence, incidence and impact of obsessive-compulsive symptomatology. Int J Psychiatry Clin Pract 17:170–178

Fink M (2013) Rediscovering catatonia: the biography of a treatable syndrome. Acta Psychiatr Scand Suppl 127:1–47

Fink M, Taylor MA (2001) The many varieties of catatonia. Eur Arch Psychiatry Clin Neurosci 251(Suppl 1):I8–I13

Fontenelle LF, Lin A, Pantelis C, Wood SJ, Nelson B, Yung AR (2011) A longitudinal study of obsessive-compulsive disorder in individuals at ultra-high risk for psychosis. J Psychiatr Res 45:1140–1145

Fusar-Poli P, Nelson B, Valmaggia L, Yung AR, McGuire PK (2012) Comorbid depressive and anxiety disorders in 509 individuals with an at-risk mental state: impact on psychopathology and transition to psychosis. Schizophr Bull 40:120–131

Guillem F, Satterthwaite J, Pampoulova T, Stip E (2009) Relationship between psychotic and obsessive compulsive symptoms in schizophrenia. Schizophr Res 115:358–362

Hur JW, Shin NY, Jang JH, Shim G, Park HY, Hwang JY, Kim SN, Yoo JH, Hong KS, Kwon JS (2012) Clinical and neurocognitive profiles of subjects at high risk for psychosis with and without obsessive-compulsive symptoms. Aust N Z J Psychiatry 46:161–169

Hwang MY, Kim SW, Yum SY, Opler LA (2009) Management of schizophrenia with obsessive-compulsive features. Psychiatr Clin N Am 32:835–851

Lencz T, Smith CW, Auther A, Correll CU, Cornblatt B (2004) Nonspecific and attenuated negative symptoms in patients at clinical high-risk for schizophrenia. Schizophr Res 68:37–48

Lysaker PH, Whitney KA (2009) Obsessive-compulsive symptoms in schizophrenia: prevalence, correlates and treatment. Expert Rev Neurother 9:99–107

Meier SM, Petersen L, Pedersen MG, Arendt MC, Nielsen PR, Mattheisen M, Mors O, Mortensen PB (2014) Obsessive-compulsive disorder as a risk factor for schizophrenia: a nationwide study. JAMA Psychiatry 71:1215–1221

Meijer JH, Sweets M, Keeman S, Nieman DH, Meijer CJ, Consortium G (2012) Does a schizo-obsessive subtype exist from a cognitive perspective? Results from a large cross-sectional study in patients with psychosis and their unaffected relatives. J Nerv Ment Dis 201:30–35

Mukhopadhaya K, Krishnaiah R, Taye T, Nigam A, Bailey AJ, Sivakumaran T, Fineberg NA (2009) Obsessive-compulsive disorder in UK clozapine-treated schizophrenia and schizoaffective disorder: a cause for clinical concern. J Psychopharmacol 23:6–13

Murphy DL, Timpano KR, Wheaton MG, Greenberg BD, Miguel EC (2010) Obsessive-compulsive disorder and its related disorders: a reappraisal of obsessive-compulsive spectrum concepts. Dialogues Clin Neurosci 12:131–148

Niendam TA, Berzak J, Cannon TD, Bearden CE (2009) Obsessive compulsive symptoms in the psychosis prodrome: correlates of clinical and functional outcome. Schizophr Res 108:170–175

Pedersen C, Mors O, Bertelsen A et al (2014) A comprehensive nationwide study of the incidence rate and lifetime risk for treated mental disorders. JAMA Psychiatry 71:573–581

Poyurovsky M (2013) Schizo-obsessive disorder. Cambridge University Press, New York

Poyurovsky M, Fuchs C, Weizman A (1999) Obsessive-compulsive disorder in patients with first-episode schizophrenia. Am J Psychiatry 156:1998–2000

Poyurovsky M, Zohar J, Glick I, Koran LM, Weizman R, Tandon R, Weizman A (2012) Obsessive-compulsive symptoms in schizophrenia: implications for future psychiatric classifications. Compr Psychiatry 53:480–483

Reznik I, Mester R, Kotler M, Weizman A (2001) Obsessive-compulsive schizophrenia: a new diagnostic entity? J Neuropsychiatry Clin Neurosci 13:115–116

Rosen JL, Miller TJ, D'Andrea JT, McGlashan TH, Woods SW (2006) Comorbid diagnoses in patients meeting criteria for the schizophrenia prodrome. Schizophr Res 85:124–131

Rubino IA, Frank E, Croce NR, Pozzi D, di Lanza ST, Siracusano A (2009) A comparative study of axis I antecedents before age 18 of unipolar depression, bipolar disorder and schizophrenia. Psychopathology 42:325–332

Schirmbeck F, Zink M (2012) Obsessive-compulsive syndromes in schizophrenia: a case for polypharmacy? In: Ritsner M (ed) Polypharmacy in psychiatric practice. Springer, Dordrecht. ISBN 978-94-007-5798-1

Schirmbeck F, Zink M (2013) Comorbid obsessive-compulsive symptoms in schizophrenia: contributions of pharmacological and genetic factors. Front Pharmacol 4:99

Schirmbeck F, Esslinger C, Rausch F, Englisch S, Meyer-Lindenberg A, Zink M (2011) Antiserotonergic antipsychotics are associated with obsessive-compulsive symptoms in schizophrenia. Psychol Med 41:2361–2374

Schirmbeck F, Rausch F, Englisch S, Eifler S, Esslinger C, Meyer-Lindenberg A, Zink M (2013) Differential effects of antipsychotic agents on obsessive-compulsive symptoms in schizophrenia: a longitudinal study. J Psychopharmacol 27:349–357

Sevincok L, Akoglu A, Arslantas H (2006) Schizo-obsessive and obsessive-compulsive disorder: comparison of clinical characteristics and neurological soft signs. Psychiatry Res 145:241–248
Shioiri T, Shinada K, Kuwabara H, Someya T (2007) Early prodromal symptoms and diagnoses before first psychotic episode in 219 inpatients with schizophrenia. Psychiatry Clin Neurosc 61:348–354
Stengel E (1945) A study on some clinical aspects of the relationship between obsessional neurosis and psychotic reaction types. J Ment Sci 91:166–187
Sterk B, Lankreijer K, Linszen DH, de Haan L (2011) Obsessive-compulsive symptoms in first episode psychosis and in subjects at ultra high risk for developing psychosis; onset and relationship to psychotic symptoms. Aust N Z J Psychiatry 45:400–405
Strakowski SM, Tohen M, Stoll AL, Faedda GL, Mayer PV, Kolbrener ML, Goodwin DC (1993) Comorbidity in psychosis at first hospitalization. Am J Psychiatry 150:752–757
Strakowski SM, Keck PE Jr, McElroy SL, Lonczak HS, West SA (1995) Chronology of comorbid and principal syndromes in first-episode psychosis. Compr Psychiatry 36:106–112
Sullwold L, Huber G (1986) Basic schizophrenic disorders. Monographien aus dem Gesamtgebiete der Psychiatrie Psychiatry Series 42:1–177
Swets M, Dekker J, van Emmerik-van Oortmerssen K, Smid GE, Smit F, de Haan L, Schoevers RA (2014) The obsessive compulsive spectrum in schizophrenia, a meta-analysis and meta-regression exploring prevalence rates. Schizophr Res 152:458–468
Ücok A, Ceylan ME, Tihan AK, Lapcin S, Ger C, Tükel R (2011) Obsessive compulsive disorder and symptoms may have different effects on schizophrenia. Prog Neuropsychopharmacol Biol Psychiatry 35:429–433
Westphal K (1878) Ueber Zwangsvorstellungen. Arch Psychiatr Nervenkr 8:734–750
Woody SR, Steketee G, Chambless DL (1995) Reliability and validity of the Yale-Brown Obsessive-Compulsive Scale. Behav Res Ther 33:597–605
Zink M, Schirmbeck F, Rausch F, Eifler S, Elkin H, Solojenkina X, Englisch S, Wagner M, Maier W, Lautenschlager M, Heinz A, Gudlowski Y, Janssen B, Gaebel W, Michel TM, Schneider F, Lambert M, Naber D, Juckel G, Krueger-Oezguerdal S, Wobrock T, Hasan A, Riedel M, Müller H, Klosterkötter J, Bechdolf A (2014) Obsessive–compulsive symptoms in at-risk mental states for psychosis: associations with clinical impairment and cognitive function. Acta Psychiatr Scand 130:214–226

Obsessive-Compulsive Disorder with Schizotypal Personality Disorder (Schizotypal OCD)

5

Michael Poyurovsky

5.1 Schizotypal Personality Disorder

Schizotypal personality disorder (SPD) was initially introduced as a specific personality disorder in DSM-III (Spitzer et al. 1979) to encompass the attenuated schizophrenia-like symptoms consistently observed in the relatives of patients with schizophrenia. SPD retained its status as a distinct personality disorder in both DSM-IV (American Psychiatric Association 1994) and recently introduced DSM-5 (American Psychiatric Association 2013).

The term "schizotypal" means "like schizophrenia" and was chosen to represent the concept of "borderline schizophrenia" introduced by Kety and colleagues (1971) to describe subtle psychopathological characteristics that are stable over time and assumed to be genetically related to the schizophrenia-spectrum disorder. Earlier, seminal observations by Kraepelin and Bleuler revealed that biological relatives of schizophrenia patients often displayed subtle formal thought disorders and interpersonal oddities (Kraepelin 1919; Bleuler 1911/1950). Meehl (1990) proposed the term *schizotaxia* for the "genetically determined integrative defect, predisposing to schizophrenia", and the term *schizotypy* for a subtly deviant psychobehavioral organization, reflective of interactions of schizotaxic vulnerability with environmental factors. Schizotaxic individuals manifest schizotypy on a dynamic continuum ranging from various degrees of subclinical deviance to schizophrenia-spectrum personality disorders to full-blown schizophrenia (Meehl 1990).

Individuals with schizotypal personality disorder share common phenomenological characteristics with those who suffer from schizophrenia (Siever and Davis 2004; Raine 2006; Skodol et al. 2011). Three major psychopathological dimensions are common to schizotypal psychopathology and schizophrenia:

M. Poyurovsky
Research Unit, Tirat Carmel Mental Health Center, POB 90000, Tirat Carmel 30200, Israel
e-mail: poyurovs@tx.technion.ac.il

L. De Haan et al. (eds.), *Obsessive-Compulsive Symptoms in Schizophrenia*,
DOI 10.1007/978-3-319-12952-5_5

cognitive-perceptual/positive (magical thinking, unusual perceptual experiences, ideas of reference, paranoid ideations), *interpersonal/negative* (lack of close friends, constructed affect), and *disorganized* (odd/eccentric behavior, odd speech) (Reynolds et al. 2000; Raine 2006).

In addition to phenomenological similarities, patients with schizotypal personality disorder share a number of neurophysiological, neurocognitive, and brain imaging abnormalities found in schizophrenia patients. Shared information-processing abnormalities (e.g., a failure of prepulse inhibition) or the capacity to "gate" sensory input may result in sensory overload and cognitive disorganization (Siever and Davis 2004). Cognitive impairments in executive function, working memory, and verbal learning are also comparable to those found in schizophrenia patients. Nevertheless, overall IQ is preserved, and neurocognitive deficits are less severe and persistent than in schizophrenia (Raine 2006). These findings along with a lower striatal dopamine release mediated by amphetamine or by physiological stressors found in schizotypal personality disorder as compared to schizophrenia have been hypothesized to result in a significantly lower vulnerability for psychosis in patients with schizotypal personality disorder and may account for the relatively low rate of progression to schizophrenia exhibited by patients with schizotypal personality disorder (Abi-Dargham et al 2002; Siever et al. 2002; Mitropoulou et al. 2004; Skodol et al. 2011).

5.2 Schizotypal and Obsessive-Compulsive Symptoms on a Subclinical Level

Examination of the relationship between schizotypal and obsessive-compulsive phenomena in *nonclinical* samples provides unique insight into the strength and nature of the relationship while avoiding the intervening factors of symptom severity, medication use, and hospitalization that are typical to the clinical population.

The interrelationship between schizotypal and obsessive-compulsive symptoms (OCS) has been extensively investigated in *nonclinical* samples (Roth and Baribeau 2000; Dinn et al. 2002; Norman et al. 1996; Rossi and Daneluzzo 2002; Suhr et al. 2006; Chmielewski and Watson 2008; Fonseca-Pedrero et al. 2011). In general, factor and cluster analytic studies support an intercorrelation between the two psychopathological dimensions (Suhr et al. 2006; Chmielewski and Watson 2008; Fonseca-Pedrero et al. 2011). Notably, positive schizotypal symptoms but not negative symptoms were positively correlated with OCS. This in turn underscores a distinct pattern of association between positive/negative dimensions of schizotypy and OCS in a nonclinical population. In an attempt to explain this association, Lee and colleagues (2005) hypothesized that the magical thinking characteristic of schizotypy may increase the likelihood of *thought-action fusion* that would heighten the risk for OCS. According to the authors, thought-action fusion refers to a set of cognitive biases that involve faulty causal relationships between one's own thoughts and external reality, thereby increasing the sense of personal responsibility. For instance, the belief that having an unacceptable or disturbing thought will increase the likelihood that the content of the thought will occur in reality (e.g., "if I think of a friend losing his job, this increases the risk that he will indeed lose his job"). Furthermore, a cognitive model classified obsessions into two subtypes, "autogenous" and "reactive," based on the differences in their respective contents, emotional reactions, evaluative appraisals, control strategies, trigger stimuli, and relatedness to schizotypal traits (Lee and Telch 2005). Autogenous obsessions are characterized by aggressive, sexual, and blasphemous themes. They are activated without clear triggers, perceived as highly ego-dystonic, and are not associated with overt compulsive rituals. In contrast, "reactive obsessions" are relatively more realistic thoughts (e.g., contamination), and the perceived threat is not the obsession itself but the associated potential negative consequences. The significant association of autogenous, but not reactive obsessions, with schizotypal traits was shown in a nonclinical sample of college students, lending empirical support for the hypothesis (Lee and Telch 2005).

5.3 Schizotypal and Obsessive-Compulsive Symptoms on the Clinical Level

5.3.1 Prevalence

The rate of occurrence of schizotypal personality disorder in OCD is yet to be clarified. The observed rates vary substantially (0–50 %) (Rasmussen and Tsuang 1986; Jenike et al. 1986; Baer et al. 1990; Black et al. 1993; Eisen and Rasmussen 1993; Samuels et al. 2000; Sobin et al. 2000; Matsunaga et al. 2000; Torres et al. 2006; Brakoulias et al. 2014) (Table 5.1).

This may be accounted for by different definitions of schizotypal features (categorical vs. dimensional), methods of evaluation (structured interview vs. chart review), and the patient populations studied. The British National Survey of Psychiatric Morbidity 2000 (Torres et al. 2006), a large-scale epidemiological study, provided particularly compelling evidence for the strength of the association between OCD and schizotypal personality disorder. The prevalence of personality disorders was compared among participants with OCD ($N=108$), with other disorders within the ICD 10 F3 and F4 categories (generalized anxiety disorder, depressive disorder, phobias, panic disorder, and mixed anxiety and depressive disorder; $N=1,353$) and controls without these conditions ($N=6,938$). The prevalence of screen-positive personality disorders in the OCD group was substantial (74 %) and greater than in both comparison groups. Schizotypal personality disorder (24.9 %) was one of the most common personality disorders in OCD patients.

Overall, as many as *one-quarter* of all individuals with OCD may have comorbid symptoms of schizotypy with roughly 10 % who meet DSM-5 criteria for schizotypal personality disorder.

Table 5.1 Prevalence of schizotypal personality disorder in patients with OCD

Authors	Study sample	Study design and diagnostic criteria	Prevalence of SPD in OCD	Comments
Jenike et al. (1986)	43 OCD patients	Chart review, DSM-III for SPD	33 % (14/43)	OCD-SPD patients had poorer prognosis
Rasmussen and Tsuang (1986)	44 OCD patients	Semi-structured interview	0 %	
Baer et al. (1990)	96 OCD patients	SCID for DSM-III personality disorders	5 % (5/96)	SPD – a predictor of poor outcome in OCD
Steketee (1990)	26 OCD patients	PDQ-R, self-report questionnaire based on the DSM-III-R criteria for personality disorders	34.6 % (9/26)	SPD was among the most frequently occurred comorbidites, along with dependent and avoidant personality disorders
Black et al. (1993)	32 OCD patients; 33 controls	SCID for DSM-III personality disorders	18.8 % (6/32) in OCD. 3 % (1/33) in controls	OCD patients also had more cluster C personality disorders
Eisen and Rasmussen (1993)	475 OCD patients	Semi-structured interview, DSM-III-R criteria for OCD and SPD	3 % (14/475)	79 % of OCD-SPD patients were men and 69 % had a deteriorative course
Bejerot et al. (1998)	36 OCD patients	SCID-II for personality disorders	3 % (1/36)	One-third of the sample was diagnosed with Cluster A (schizoid, schizotypal, paranoid) personality disorders
Sobin et al. (2000)	119 OCD patients	SIS for schizotypy; self-rated	50 % had mild to severe positive schizotypy signs	OCD patients with schizotypy had earlier age of onset, more comorbid diagnoses and learning disability
Samuels et al. (2000)	72 OCD probands, 72 controls and their first-degree relatives	Direct interview, SADS-LA, SIDP-R	0 % (0/72) of OCD and 1.4 % (1/72) of control probands had SPD	OCD probands had a higher prevalence of OCPD

Table 5.1 (continued)

Authors	Study sample	Study design and diagnostic criteria	Prevalence of SPD in OCD	Comments
Matsunaga et al. (2000)	94 OCD patients	SCID-II for personality disorders	23 % (9/40) of men and 4 % (2/54) of women had SPD	
Torres et al. (2006)	108 OCD patients in the community	SCID-II for personality disorders	24.9 % (27/108)	SPD was among the most common personality disorders screened
Brakoulias et al. (2014)	177 OCD patients	MINI for OCD; SPQ for schizotypy	23.2 % had high levels of schizotypy; 12 % meet criteria for DSM-III-R SPD	Higher schizotypy level was associated with higher rates of symmetry/order obsessions, ordering/arranging compulsions, checking compulsions; MDD, PTSD, SUD, and general but not OCD-related psychopathology

Reproduced with modification from Poyurovsky (2013)
SCID Structured Clinical Interview for DSM-IV, *SADS-LA* the Schedule for Affective Disorders and Schizophrenia-Lifetime Anxiety, *SIDP-R* the Revised Structured Instrument for the Diagnosis of Personality Disorders, *SIS* the Structured Interview for Schizotypy, *SPD* schizotypal personality disorder, *PDQ-R* the Revised Personality Diagnostic Questionnaire, *OCD* obsessive-compulsive disorder, *MINI* Mini International Neuropsychiatric Interview, *SPQ* a scale for the assessment of schizotypal personality based on DSM-III-R criteria, *MDD* major depressive disorder, *PTSD* post-traumatic stress disorder, *SUD* substance use disorders

5.4 Clinical Characteristics

There is increasing evidence of differences in demographic and clinical characteristics of OCD patients with and without schizotypal features, supporting the clinical validity of a schizotypal subgroup of OCD (Eisen and Rasmussen 1993; Matsunaga et al. 2000; Sobin et al. 2000; Torres et al. 2006; Catapano et al. 2010; Brakoulias et al. 2014). Early age of onset, male gender, and a history of specific phobia have been shown to increase the risk of schizotypy in patients with OCD. In addition, schizotypal OCD patients are more likely to be single and unemployed. Similar to studies in nonclinical samples, most but not all clinical studies link positive symptoms of schizotypy with OCS (Einstein and Menzies 2004; Enright and Beech 1993; Lee and Telch 2005; Poyurovsky et al. 2008). Notably, marked intercorrelations have been found between positive schizotypal symptoms and indicators of OCD severity, including earlier age of onset, comorbid diagnoses, and treatment resistance (Moritz et al. 2004; Sobin et al. 2000). Compared to OCD patients, those with schizotypal OCD exhibit higher rates of symmetry/order obsessions, ordering/arranging, and checking and counting compulsions (Sobin et al. 2000; Brakoulias et al. 2014). Hoarding seems to be associated with somewhat higher levels of schizotypal features. Hoarders are significantly more likely to have more severe psychopathology, poorer insight, higher prevalence of comorbid schizotypal or obsessive-compulsive personality disorder, closer association with symmetry dimension, and poorer treatment outcome (Frost et al. 2000; Matsunaga et al. 2010).

Axis I comorbid psychiatric disorders are highly prevalent in patients with schizotypal OCD and are associated with additional morbidity. Similar to "pure" OCD patients, two-thirds of patients with schizotypal OCD have at least one additional comorbid disorder (Poyurovsky et al. 2008). Major depressive disorder appeared to be the most common (roughly 50 %), followed by anxiety disorders (panic disorder, social and simple phobias), and OCD-spectrum disorders (tic disorders, body dysmorphic disorder). Whether patients with schizotypal OCD are more susceptible for developing schizophrenia compared to their "pure" OCD counterparts are yet to be clarified and merit prospective investigations.

5.5 Neurobiological Underpinnings

5.5.1 Family Inheritance

Schizotypal OCD seems to have a distinct pattern of familial aggregation of schizophrenia-spectrum disorders compared to non-schizotypal OCD. Our research group obtained family information regarding OCD and schizophrenia-spectrum disorders for 100 and 31 first-degree relatives of OCD patients, with and without schizotypal personality disorder (Poyurovsky et al. 2008). As expected, there was a substantial aggregation of OCD cases in the relatives of both groups (13 % in each), supporting a well-established familial transmission of the disorder (Pauls 2008). In contrast, one-third of the schizotypal OCD patients had at least one first-degree relative with schizophrenia-spectrum disorders as compared to only 3 % in the "pure" OCD group ($\chi^2=5.48$, $P=0.019$). The fact that the schizotypal OCD group had a family load of schizophrenia-spectrum disorders indicates that in this subset of patients, OCD and schizophrenia-spectrum disorders co-transmit in families. From a clinical perspective, detection of schizophrenia-spectrum disorders in first-degree relatives may alert clinicians to better identification of schizotypal personality disorder in OCD patients.

5.5.2 Neurocognitive Dysfunction and Neuroimaging

Neurocognitive and neuroimaging findings lend some credence to the division of OCD into subgroups based on the presence of schizotypy. While patients with "pure" OCD display impaired performance on measures sensitive to the orbitofrontal cortex (alternation learning, response inhibition, delayed memory), patients with schizotypal OCD perform poorly on tests sensitive to both the orbitofrontal and dorsolateral prefrontal cortex (Harris and Dinn 2003; Shin et al. 2008). Similar to findings in schizophrenia patients, deficits in cognitive performance on tests sensitive to the dorsolateral prefrontal cortex are consistently found in patients with schizotypal personality disorder (Mitropoulou et al. 2002). OCD patients with schizotypal personality traits also showed a significant gray matter volume reduction compared to their "pure" OCD counterparts (Jin Lee et al. 2006). Consistent with neurocognitive findings, the schizotypal OCD group seems to occupy a "niche" between OCD without schizotypy and the schizophrenia groups. Replication of these findings in a larger sample with clinically defined schizotypal personality disorder is needed.

5.6 Treatment

Schizotypal personality disorder predicts poor response to standard pharmacological and behavioral intervention in OCD patients. Jenike et al. (1986) retrospectively examined characteristics of 43 treatment-resistant obsessive-compulsive patients and found that those with concomitant schizotypal personality disorder had a higher rate of treatment failure. Of the 29 treated OCD patients without schizotypal personality disorder, 26 (90 %) improved at least moderately, and only one of 14 (7 %) schizotypal OCD patients improved. The same authors conducted a controlled 12-week trial of clomipramine among 55 patients with OCD and confirmed that the presence of schizotypal personality disorder was a strong predictor of poor treatment outcome (Baer et al. 1992). These results were substantiated by Ravizza et al. (1995) who found that poorer response to either clomipramine or fluoxetine was predicted in a stepwise multiple regressions by (1) concomitant schizotypal personality disorder, (2) presence of compulsions, and (3) longer duration of illness. Similarly, in a 3-year prospective naturalistic study of OCD patients, significant predictors of poor outcome included longer duration of illness, a greater severity of obsessive-compulsive symptoms at intake, and the presence of comorbid schizotypal personality disorder (Catapano et al. 2006).

Not all studies found an association between schizotypal personality disorder and nonresponse to treatment in patients with OCD. It was hypothesized that a binary approach (presence vs. absence of schizotypal personality) may obscure the relation between schizotypal personality disorder and treatment outcome (Moritz et al. 2004). The authors investigated whether the predictive importance of schizotypal personality is confined to a subset of symptoms of schizotypy. In 53 patients with OCD who underwent multimodal cognitive behavioral therapy, stepwise regression analysis revealed that, indeed, elevated scores in the positive but not negative schizotypal factor, especially perceptual aberrations, strongly predicted treatment failure.

Overall, the presence of schizotypal personality disorder, particularly its positive psychopathological dimension, seems to increase the risk of treatment failure in OCD patients with as many as 25 % of schizotypal OCD patients failing to experience any improvement with treatment (Ravizza et al. 1995; Erzegovesi et al. 2001).

Two pharmacological augmentation strategies for nonresponders to serotonin reuptake inhibitors (SRIs) have been studied. The first strategy involved the use of serotonin-enhancing agents (e.g., lithium, clonazepam, or buspirone) to maximize treatment response and yielded unanimously discouraging results. The second involved the addition of low-dose dopamine antagonists to SRIs. The rationale for adding dopamine antagonists is based on the assumption of the involvement of the dopaminergic system in addition to the serotonergic system in the mediation of obsessive-compulsive symptoms and putative treatment resistance. This seems to be particularly relevant in schizotypal personality disorder comorbid to OCD (Coccaro 1998; Koenigsberg et al. 2003). Indeed, starting with small open-label studies, the presence of schizotypal personality disorder seemed to herald positive response to antipsychotic augmentation in SRI-resistant OCD.

McDougle et al. (1990) explicitly examined whether comorbid schizotypal personality disorder and tic spectrum disorders were associated with a positive response to the addition of a neuroleptic (pimozide, mean dose = 6.5 mg/day; thioridazine, mean dose = 87.5 mg/day; or thiothixene, 6 mg/day) in OCD patients who did not respond to fluvoxamine. On the basis of the Clinical Global Impression scale criterion of improvement, 9 (53 %) of 17 participants responded, 7 (88 %) of 8 patients with comorbid tic or schizotypal personality disorder responded; however, only 2 (22 %) of 9 patients without these disorders responded ($P = 0.02$, Fisher's exact test). The addition of antipsychotic agents however was not without cost. More than half of the patients experienced mild to moderate extrapyramidal side effects after the addition of the neuroleptic agent.

Promising results were also obtained when the efficacy of olanzapine addition to fluvoxamine-refractory OCD patients was investigated (Bogetto et al. 2000). Twenty-three OCD nonresponders to a 6-month, open-label trial with fluvoxamine (300 mg/day) entered a 3-month open-label trial of augmentation with olanzapine (5 mg/day). Ten patients (43.5 %) were rated as responders, and concomitant schizotypal personality disorder was the only factor significantly associated with response.

McDougle et al. (2000) conducted a double-blind placebo-controlled study of risperidone addition in OCD patients refractory to SRIs. Fifty percent of the risperidone-treated study completers (9 of 18) were responders (mean daily dose, 2.2 ± 0.7 mg/day) compared with none of 15 in the placebo addition group ($P < 0.005$). There was no difference, however, in response between OCD patients with and without comorbid diagnoses of schizotypal personality disorder.

Our comparative study of treatment-seeking OCD patients with and without schizotypal personality disorder revealed a significant difference between the two groups in the proportion of patients who required antipsychotic augmentation (Poyurovsky et al. 2008). Thus, 73 % (11 of 15 patients) in the schizotypal OCD group compared to 26 % (8 of 31 patients) were prescribed antipsychotic augmentation (haloperidol, 2.5 mg/day, risperidone, 0.5–1.5 mg/day, or olanzapine 5–10 mg/day). This study supported clinical experience that indicated that treatment-seeking schizotypal OCD patients most probably require an SRI and antipsychotic agent combination to address both components of their complex psychiatric condition.

Notably, the role of psychotherapy in the management of schizotypal OCD patients has not been addressed in this study.

In a comprehensive systematic review, Bloch et al. (2006) strongly supported the clinical utility of low-dose antipsychotic augmentation as an effective intervention for treatment-refractory OCD patients. However, the evaluation of the role of comorbid schizotypal personality disorder was notably absent in this and other more recent reviews (Bandelow et al. 2008; Muscatello et al. 2011) most probably because of the insufficient number of studies with randomized controlled trial methodology required to be included in the review.

Glutamatergic agents are the promising new candidates for the treatment of OCD. This seems to be particularly pertinent to schizotypal OCD in view of the revealed glutamatergic dysfunction in both OCD and schizophrenia-spectrum disorders. Agents that attenuate glutamatergic neurotransmission, memantine and riluzole, produced preliminary promising results, but none has achieved sufficient empirical evidence to become recommended in treatment guidelines (Bandelow et al. 2008). Further controlled investigations of these and other glutamatergic modulators (e.g., N-acetylcysteine, D-cycloserine) and agents with alternative mechanisms of actions for treatment-refractory OCD with and without schizotypal personality disorders are needed to clarify their clinical utility.

Finally, when there is no improvement with any of the available pharmacological strategies, and before considering invasive interventions (e.g., deep brain stimulation), clozapine therapy may be attempted in severe treatment-refractory OCD patients with schizotypal personality disorder. Clozapine monotherapy is beneficial in treatment-resistant schizophrenia but not OCD (McDougle et al. 1995) (see Chap. 10). An OCD-provoking effect of clozapine in schizophrenia patients is well established, but clozapine-related amelioration of schizophrenia-related obsessive-compulsive symptoms has also been revealed (Poyurovsky et al. 1998; Reznik et al. 2004). Indeed, relatively low doses of clozapine resulted in clinically significant improvement in some treatment-refractory OCD patients with comorbid schizotypal personality disorder (Poyurovsky et al. 2008).

The role of psychotherapeutic interventions in patients with schizotypal OCD is yet to be clarified. Minichiello et al. (1987) retrospectively reviewed the treatment outcome of OCD patients treated with behavior therapy either alone or in combination with pharmacotherapy and determined which patients met DSM-III criteria for schizotypal personality disorder. Eighty-four percent (16/19) of the OCD patients without schizotypal personality disorder and only 1/10 (10 %) of those with schizotypy achieved at least moderate improvement in their OCD symptoms with combined behavioral and pharmacological treatment. The number of schizotypal features strongly negatively correlated with treatment outcomes ($r=-0.68$; $p=0.001$). Schizotypal personality encompasses several factors that predict poor outcome. Most noticeably, a substantial proportion of these patients has poor insight and strongly believes that rituals are necessary to prevent the occurrence of terrible events. They frequently have difficulty complying with prescribed treatment and with record-keeping tasks assigned in CBT. The schizotypal OCD patients in this study did not benefit from cognitive behavioral treatment.

Some schizotypal OCD patients actually may become more dysfunctional following CBT (Walker et al. 1994).

In contrast, social skills training is a behavioral procedure based on shaping appropriate responses and extinguishing inappropriate or socially maladaptive behaviors and has proven to be an efficacious rehabilitative approach for schizophrenia-spectrum disorders. Conversation skills, appropriate facial expressions, eye contact, and reciprocity are some of the areas commonly targeted for social skills training. The utility of these techniques as well as metacognitive interventions recently developed by Moritz and colleagues (2013) in schizotypal OCD patients merits further evaluation.

5.7 Proposed Diagnostic and Treatment Recommendations

Overall, schizotypal OCD seems to have clinical and predictive validity and putative etiological specificity. Lacking evidence-based guidelines, the following may be considered when formulating diagnosis, treatment plan, and prognosis in patients with schizotypal OCD:

- Schizotypal personality disorder is commonly observed in patients with OCD. Clinicians should be aware that as many as *one-quarter* of all individuals with OCD may have comorbid symptoms of schizotypy. This high estimate, and the additional morbidity associated with the presence of schizotypal personality disorder in OCD patients, underscores the clinical relevance of schizotypal OCD.
- Diagnosis of schizotypal OCD is warranted for those patients who meet full DSM-5 criteria for both OCD and schizotypal personality disorder. Identification of schizophrenia-spectrum disorders in first-degree relatives of patients with OCD might contribute to the diagnosis.
- Differential diagnosis of schizotypal OCD from schizophrenia with obsessive-compulsive symptoms is challenging but critical for better delineation and effective treatment of these patients. Stringent adherence to DSM criteria for schizophrenia, schizotypal personality disorder, and OCD and repeated evaluations to establish diagnostic stability are crucial for correct diagnosis.
- Treatment of OCD patients with schizotypal personality disorder is challenging. Low-dose antipsychotic augmentation might be necessary for schizotypal OCD patients who have not responded to an adequate trial with an SRI. Administration of the lowest effective dose of antipsychotic medication is essential to minimize the risk for extrapyramidal side effects and akathisia to which patients with schizotypal OCD seem to be especially sensitive. Long-term gains and risks of adjunctive antipsychotic therapy for schizotypal OCD patients remain to be clarified.
- Social skills training might attenuate maladaptive behaviors associated with schizotypy and might potentially enable the initiation of exposure and ritual prevention to deal directly with obsessive-compulsive symptoms.

References

Abi-Dargham A, Mawlawi O, Lombardo I, Gil R, Martinez D, Huang Y, Hwang DR, Keilp J, Kochan L, Van Heertum R, Gorman JM, Laruelle M (2002) Prefrontal dopamine D1 receptors and working memory in schizophrenia. J Neurosci 22:3708–3719

American Psychiatric Association (1994) Diagnostic and statistical manual of mental disorders, 4th edn. American Psychiatric Association, Washington, DC

American Psychiatric Association (2013) Diagnostic and statistical manual of mental disorders, 5th edn. American Psychiatric Publishing, Arlington

Baer L, Jenike MA, Ricciardi JN 2nd, Holland AD, Seymour RJ, Minichiello WE, Buttolph ML (1990) Standardized assessment of personality disorders in obsessive-compulsive disorder. Arch Gen Psychiatry 47:826–830

Baer L, Jenike MA, Black DW, Treece C, Rosenfeld R, Greist J (1992) Effect of axis II diagnoses on treatment outcome with clomipramine in 55 patients with obsessive-compulsive disorder. Arch Gen Psychiatry 49:862–866

Bandelow B, Zohar J, Hollander E, Kasper S, Möller HJ, WFSBP Task Force on Treatment Guidelines for Anxiety, Obsessive-Compulsive and Post-Traumatic Stress Disorders, Zohar J, Hollander E, Kasper S, Möller HJ, Bandelow B, Allgulander C, Hindmarch I, Kaiya H, Klein DF, Lader M, Lecrubier Y, Lépine JP, Liebowitz MR, Lopez-Ibor JJ, Marazziti D, Miguel EC, Oh KS, Preter M, Rupprecht R, Sato M, Starcevic V, Stein DJ, van Ameringen M, Vega J (2008) World Federation of Societies of Biological Psychiatry (WFSBP) guidelines for the pharmacological treatment of anxiety, obsessive-compulsive and post-traumatic stress disorders – first revision. World J Biol Psychiatry 9:248–312

Bejerot S, Ekselius L, von Knorring L (1998) Comorbidity between obsessive-compulsive disorder (OCD) and personality disorders. Acta Psychiatr Scand 97:398–402

Black DW, Noyes R Jr, Pfohl B, Goldstein RB, Blum N (1993) Personality disorder in obsessive-compulsive volunteers, well comparison subjects, and their first-degree relatives. Am J Psychiatry 150:1226–1232

Bleuler E (1911/1950) Dementia praecox or the group of schizophrenias. J Zinkin (Trans International University Press), New York

Bloch MH, Landeros-Weisenberger A, Kelmendi B, Coric V, Bracken MB, Leckman JF (2006) A systematic review: antipsychotic augmentation with treatment refractory obsessive-compulsive disorder. Mol Psychiatry 11:622–632

Bogetto F, Bellini S, Vaschetto P, Ziero S (2000) Olanzapine augmentation of fluvoxamine-refractory obsessive-compulsive disorder (OCD): a 12-week open trial. Psychiatry Res 96: 91–98

Brakoulias V, Starcevic V, Berle D, Milicevic D, Hannan A, Viswasam K, Mann K (2014) The clinical characteristics of obsessive compulsive disorder associated with high levels of schizotypy. Aust N Z J Psychiatry 48(9):852–60

Catapano F, Perris F, Masella M, Rossano F, Cigliano M, Magliano L, Maj M (2006) Obsessive-compulsive disorder: a 3-year prospective follow-up study of patients treated with serotonin reuptake inhibitors: OCD follow-up study. J Psychiatr Res 40:502–510

Catapano F, Perris F, Fabrazzo M, Cioffi V, Giacco D, De Santis V, Maj M (2010) Obsessive-compulsive disorder with poor insight: a three-year prospective study. Prog Neuropsychopharmacol Biol Psychiatry 34:323–330

Chmielewski M, Watson D (2008) The heterogeneous structure of schizotypal personality disorder: item-level factors of the Schizotypal Personality Questionnaire and their associations with obsessive-compulsive disorder symptoms, dissociative tendencies, and normal personality. J Abnorm Psychol 117:364–376

Coccaro EF (1998) Clinical outcome of psychopharmacologic treatment of borderline and schizotypal personality disordered subjects. J Clin Psychiatry 59(Suppl 1):30–35

Dinn WM, Harris CL, Aycicegi A, Greene P, Andover MS (2002) Positive and negative schizotypy in a student sample: neurocognitive and clinical correlates. Schizophr Res 56:171–185

Einstein DA, Menzies RG (2004) Role of magical thinking in obsessive-compulsive symptoms in an undergraduate sample. Depress Anxiety 19:174–179
Eisen JL, Rasmussen SA (1993) Obsessive-compulsive disorder with psychotic features. J Clin Psychiatry 54:373–379
Enright SJ, Beech AR (1993) Reduced cognitive inhibition in obsessive-compulsive disorder. Br J Clin Psychol 32(Pt 1):67–74
Erzegovesi S, Cavallini MC, Cavedini P, Diaferia G, Locatelli M, Bellodi L (2001) Clinical predictors of drug response in obsessive-compulsive disorder. J Clin Psychopharmacol 21:488–492
Fonseca-Pedrero E, Paino M, Lemos-Giráldez S, Muñiz J (2011) Schizotypal traits and depressive symptoms in nonclinical adolescents. Compr Psychiatry 52(3):293–300
Frost RO, Steketee G, Williams LF, Warren R (2000) Mood, personality disorder symptoms and disability in obsessive compulsive hoarders: a comparison with clinical and nonclinical controls. Behav Res Ther 38:1071–1081
Harris CL, Dinn WM (2003) Subtyping obsessive-compulsive disorder: neuropsychological correlate. Behav Neurol 14:75–87
Jenike MA, Baer L, Minichiello WE, Schwartz CE, Carey RJ Jr (1986) Concomitant obsessive-compulsive disorder and schizotypal personality disorder. Am J Psychiatry 143:530–532
Jin Lee K, Wook Shin Y, Wee H, Youn Kim Y, Kwon JS (2006) Gray matter volume reduction in obsessive-compulsive disorder with schizotypal personality trait. Prog Neuropsychopharmacol Biol Psychiatry 30:1146–1149
Kety SS, Rosenthal D, Wender PH, Schulsinger F (1971) Mental illness in the biological and adoptive families of adopted schizophrenics. Am J Psychiatry 128:302–306
Koenigsberg HW, Reynolds D, Goodman M, New AS, Mitropoulou V, Trestman RL, Silverman J, Siever LJ (2003) Risperidone in the treatment of schizotypal personality disorder. J Clin Psychiatry 64:628–634
Kraepelin E (1919) Dementia praecox. Krieger, New York
Lee HJ, Telch MJ (2005) Autogenous/reactive obsessions and their relationship with OCD symptoms and schizotypal personality features. Anxiety Disord 19:793–805
Lee HJ, Cougle JR, Telch MJ (2005) Thought-action fusion and its relationship to schizotypy and OCD symptoms. Behav Res Ther 43:29–41
Matsunaga H, Kiriike N, Matsui T, Miyata A, Iwasaki Y, Fujimoto K, Kasai S, Kojima M (2000) Gender differences in social and interpersonal features and personality disorders among Japanese patients with obsessive-compulsive disorder. Compr Psychiatry 41:266–272
Matsunaga H, Hayashida K, Kiriike N, Maebayashi K, Stein DJ (2010) The clinical utility of symptom dimensions in obsessive-compulsive disorder. Psychiatry Res 30:25–29
McDougle CJ, Goodman WK, Price LH, Deldago PL, Kristal JH, Charney DS, Heninger GR (1990) Neuroleptic addition in fluvoxamine-refractory obsessive-compulsive disorder. Am J Psychiatry 147:652–654
McDougle CJ, Barr LC, Goodman WK, Pelton GH, Aronson SC, Anand A, Price LH (1995) Lack of efficacy of clozapine monotherapy in refractory obsessive-compulsive disorder. Am J Psychiatry 152:1812–1814
McDougle CJ, Epperson CN, Pelton GH, Wasylink S, Price LH (2000) A double-blind, placebo-controlled study of risperidone addition in serotonin reuptake inhibitor-refractory obsessive-compulsive disorder. Arch Gen Psychiatry 57:794–801
Meehl PE (1990) Toward an integrated theory of schizotaxia, schizotypy and schizophrenia. J Pers Disord 4:1–99
Minichiello WE, Baer L, Jenike MA (1987) Schizotypal personality disorder: a poor prognostic indicator for behavior therapy in the treatment of obsessive-compulsive disorder. J Anxiety Disord 1:273–276
Mitropoulou V, Harvey PD, Maldari LA, Moriarty PJ, New AS, Silverman JM, Siever LJ (2002) Neuropsychological performance in schizotypal personality disorder: evidence regarding diagnostic specificity. Biol Psychiatry 52:1175–1182
Mitropoulou V, Goodman M, Sevy S, Elman I, New AS, Iskander EG, Silverman JM, Breier A, Siever LJ (2004) Effects of acute metabolic stress on the dopaminergic and pituitary-adrenal axis activity in patients with schizotypal personality disorder. Schizophr Res 70:27–31

Moritz S, Fricke S, Jacobsen D, Kloss M, Wein C, Rufer M, Katenkamp B, Farhumand R, Hand I (2004) Positive schizotypal symptoms predict treatment outcome in obsessive-compulsive disorder. Behav Res Ther 42:217–227

Moritz S, Veckenstedt R, Bohn F, Hottenrott B, Scheu F, Randjbar S, Aghotor J, Köther U, Woodward TS, Treszl A, Andreou C, Pfueller U, Roesch-Ely D (2013) Complementary group Metacognitive Training (MCT) reduces delusional ideation in schizophrenia. Schizophr Res 151:61–69

Muscatello MR, Bruno A, Pandolfo G, Micò U, Scimeca G, Romeo VM, Santoro V, Settineri S, Spina E, Zoccali RA (2011) Effect of aripiprazole augmentation of serotonin reuptake inhibitors or clomipramine in treatment-resistant obsessive-compulsive disorder: a double-blind, placebo-controlled study. J Clin Psychopharmacol 31:174–179

Norman RM, Davies F, Malla AK, Cortese L, Nicholson IR (1996) Relationship of obsessive-compulsive symptomatology to anxiety, depression and schizotypy in a clinical population. Br J Clin Psychol 35:553–566

Pauls DL (2008) The genetics of obsessive compulsive disorder: a review of the evidence. Am J Med Genet C Semin Med Genet 148C(2):133–139

Poyurovsky M, Bergman Y, Shoshani D, Schneidman M, Weizman A (1998) Emergence of obsessive-compulsive symptoms and tics during clozapine withdrawal. Clin Neuropharmacol 21:97–100

Poyurovsky M (2013) Schizo-obsessive disorder. Cambridge University Press, Cambridge

Poyurovsky M, Faragian S, Pashinian A, Heidrach L, Fuchs C, Weizman R, Koran L (2008) Clinical characteristics of schizotypal-related obsessive-compulsive disorder. Psychiatry Res 159:254–258

Raine A (2006) Schizotypal personality: neurodevelopmental and psychosocial trajectories. Annu Rev Clin Psychol 2:291–326

Rasmussen SA, Tsuang MT (1986) Clinical characteristics and family history in DSM-III obsessive-compulsive disorder. Am J Psychiatry 143:317–322

Ravizza L, Barzega G, Bellino S, Bogetto F, Maina G (1995) Predictors of drug treatment response in obsessive-compulsive disorder. J Clin Psychiatry 56:368–373

Reynolds CA, Raine A, Mellingen K, Venables PH, Mednick SA (2000) Three-factor model of schizotypal personality: invariance across culture, gender, religious affiliation, family adversity, and psychopathology. Schizophr Bull 26:603–618

Reznik I, Yavin I, Stryjer R, Spivak B, Gonen N, Strous R, Mester R, Weizman A, Kotler M (2004) Clozapine in the treatment of obsessive-compulsive symptoms in schizophrenia patients: a case series study. Pharmacopsychiatry 37:52–66

Rossi A, Daneluzzo E (2002) Schizotypal dimension in normals and schizophrenic patients: a comparison with other clinical samples. Schizophr Res 1:67–75

Roth RM, Baribeau J (2000) The relationship between schizotypal and obsessive-compulsive features in university students. Pers Individ Differ 29:1083–1093

Samuels J, Nestadt G, Bienvenu OJ (2000) Personality disorders and normal personality dimensions in obsessive-compulsive disorder. Br J Psychiatry 177:457–462

Saxena S, Wang D, Bystritsky A, Baxter LR Jr (1996) Risperidone augmentation of SRI treatment for refractory obsessive-compulsive disorder. J Clin Psychiatry 57:303–306

Shin NY, Lee AR, Park HY, Yoo SY, Kang DH, Shin MS, Kwon JS (2008) Impact of coexistent schizotypal personality traits on frontal lobe function in obsessive-compulsive disorder. Prog Neuropsychopharmacol Biol Psychiatry 32:472–478

Siever LJ, Davis KL (2004) The pathophysiology of schizophrenia disorders: perspectives from the spectrum. Am J Psychiatry 161:398–413

Siever LJ, Koenigsberg HW, Harvey P, Mitropoulou V, Laruelle M, Abi-Dargham A, Goodman M, Buchsbaum M (2002) Cognitive and brain function in schizotypal personality disorder. Schizophr Res 54:157–167

Skodol AE, Bender DS, Morey LC, Clark LA, Oldham JM, Alarcon RD, Krueger RF, Verheul R, Bell CC, Siever LJ (2011) Personality disorder types proposed for DSM-5. J Pers Disord 25:136–169

Sobin C, Blundell ML, Weiller F, Gavigan C, Haiman C, Karayiorgou M (2000) Evidence of a schizotypy subtype in OCD. J Psychiatr Res 34:15–24

Spitzer RL, Endicott J, Gibbon M (1979) Crossing the border into borderline personality and borderline schizophrenia: the development of criteria. Arch Gen Psychiatry 36:17–24
Steketee G (1990). Personality traits and disorders in obsessive-compulsives. J Anxiety Disord 4:351–364
Suhr JA, Spitznagel MB, Gunstad J (2006) An obsessive-compulsive subtype of schizotypy: evidence from a nonclinical sample. J Nerv Ment Dis 194:884
Torres AR, Moran P, Bebbington P, Brugha T, Bhugra D, Coid JW, Farrell M, Jenkins R, Lewis G, Meltzer H, Prince M (2006) Obsessive-compulsive disorder and personality disorder: evidence from the British National Survey of Psychiatric Morbidity 2000. Soc Psychiatry Psychiatr Epidemiol 41:862–867
Walker WR, Freeman RF, Christensen DK (1994) Restricting environmental stimulation (REST) to enhance cognitive behavioral treatment for obsessive compulsive disorder with schizotypal personality disorder. Behav Ther 25:709–719

6 Associations of Comorbid Obsessive-Compulsive Symptoms with Psychotic and Affective Symptoms and General Functioning

Helen K. Hunter and Paul H. Lysaker

Descriptions of obsessive-compulsive symptoms (OCS) in patients with schizophrenia date back to the early the twentieth century. For example, Bleuler (1911/1950) stated, "compulsive thinking (obsession) is the most common of all the automatic phenomena." He characterized OCS in schizophrenia as "automatisms" that are similar to auditory or visual hallucinations – meaning that they are "hallucinations of thinking, striving, and wanting" (p. 450). Further, Bleuler went on to describe the clinical significant of OCS in schizophrenia, suggesting that OCS and positive symptoms may exacerbate each other. Hence, Bleuler noted the commonality and frequency of OCS in schizophrenia. Bleuler could be seen as the first to emphasize the clinical importance of OCS in schizophrenia rather than just noting the mere presence of OCS in schizophrenia.

Although early descriptions by Bleuler discussed OCS in schizophrenia, this association did not gain the wide attention that schizophrenia's positive and negative symptoms have received during Bleuler's time. The prevalence of OCS in schizophrenia mostly gained attention in the past 20 years. It has not been until the middle 1980s that large systematic studies have demonstrated that more than a third of individuals with schizophrenia also have OCS (Berman et al. 1995; Bland et al. 1987; Porto et al. 1997) and 10–25 % meet full criteria for obsessive-compulsive disorder (OCD; Achim et al. 2011; Cosoff and Hafner 1998; Eisen et al. 1997; Krüger et al. 2000; Nechmad et al. 2003; Ohta et al. 2003). Moreover, the prevalence rates of OCS in schizophrenia are much higher than the lifetime prevalence rate of 2.5 % in the general population (American Psychiatric Association 2000),

H.K. Hunter, MS
Department of Psychology, Indiana State University, Terre Haute, IN, USA

P.H. Lysaker, PhD (✉)
Department of Psychiatry, Roudebush VA Medical Center, Indiana University School of Medicine, 1481 West 10th Street, Indianapolis, IN 46202, USA
e-mail: plysaker@iupui.edu

L. De Haan et al. (eds.), *Obsessive-Compulsive Symptoms in Schizophrenia*,
DOI 10.1007/978-3-319-12952-5_6

which suggests OCS likely has an important influence on schizophrenia's clinical expression.

Further, this relationship between OCS and schizophrenia has just started to be empirically researched within the last 25 years. Whereas there have been many descriptions of the comorbidity between OCS and schizophrenia, the causes and consequences of this comorbidity remains unclear and leaves many questions unanswered. What is the relationship between OCS and positive and negative symptoms? What association does OCS in schizophrenia have on affective symptoms? If OCS does indeed cause more positive and/or negative symptoms as well as affective symptoms, what link does it have to general functioning? Is it possible that the presence of OCS in schizophrenia is a separate subtype of schizophrenia with its own pathophysiology and treatment implications? In order for one to begin to answer these questions, a review of the literature is required. Hence, this chapter will first present current findings on the relationship between OCS, psychotic and affective symptoms, and general functioning. Then the chapter will end with conceptualizations of OCS in schizophrenia.

6.1 OCS and Psychotic Symptoms

Investigation into the relationship between OCS and positive and negative is needed to understand whether, as noted by Lysaker and Whitney (2009), OCS may serve as an indicator for a separate subtype of schizophrenia (as will be further discussed in the conceptualization section) that has its own pathophysiology or as Bleuler (1911/1950) suggested, OCS may simply aggravate the symptoms of schizophrenia rather than be a separate form of schizophrenia. Additionally, it continues to be unclear whether or not OCS exacerbates schizophrenia symptoms or serves as a protective factor against further deterioration.

Early studies examining the relationship between OCS and positive and negative symptoms produced contradictory results. Some studies have found no significant correlations (Berman et al. 1997; Borkowska et al. 2003; Poyurovsky et al. 2001), whereas others have noted that schizophrenia with OCD in younger individuals is associated with lesser levels of negative symptoms (Poyurovsky et al. 1999; Tibbo et al. 2000). Furthermore, other early studies support an association between OCS and positive and negative symptoms (Hwang and Hollander 1993; Lysaker et al. 2000).

OCS and Positive Symptoms In a prospective study of 113 patients with recent-onset schizophrenia, de Haan et al. (2005) assessed OCS levels with the Yale-Brown Obsessive-Compulsive Scale (Y-BOCS; Goodman et al. 1989) and positive and negative symptoms with the Positive and Negative Syndrome Scale (PANSS; Kay et al. 1987). The results showed that patients with OCD did not have more severe positive symptoms compared to those patients without comorbid OCD. With 118 schizophrenia participants in an urban clinic, Ongür and Goff (2005) found that higher severity of OCS symptoms as measured by Y-BOCS scores were associated with more severe positive symptoms. Additionally, Kayahan et al. (2005) studied 100 patients with schizophrenia who were hospitalized or under treatment and found greater levels of OCS, as assessed with the Y-BOCS, to be significantly correlated with severity of positive symptoms, as assessed by the PANSS. Huppert and Smith (2005) found that higher levels of positive symptoms were correlated with higher self-reported obsessive and compulsive levels in an outpatient program for individuals with schizophrenia.

On the other hand, both Byerly et al. (2005) and Sevincok et al. (2007) did not find associations between positive symptoms and OCS and OCD in participants with schizophrenia. In examining the clinical profiles of 55 participants with comorbid schizophrenia and OCD, Rajkumar et al. (2008) found that they had more paranoia and first-rank symptoms than those without comorbid OCD. In a meta-analysis of 18 studies between 1998 and 2006, Cunill et al. (2009) found no significant differences in symptom severity between groups of individuals with schizophrenia with OCD and schizophrenia without OCD. However, when comparing schizophrenia with OCS and without OCS, Cunill et al. found schizophrenia with OCS to be associated with greater global and positive symptoms compared to schizophrenia without OCS. Tiryaki and Ozkorumak (2010) also found more severe psychotic symptoms in participants with schizophrenia and OCS compared to participants without OCS.

More recent studies have failed to find a significant relationships between OCS and positive symptoms. Nasrollahi et al. (2012) did not find a relationship between OCS and positive symptoms of schizophrenia as assessed by the Y-BOCS and PANSS, respectively, in participants in a psychiatric hospital. Further, in a prospective study of the 5-year course of comorbid OCS and OCD in 172 patients with first-episode schizophrenia and related disorders, de Haan et al. (2013b) did not find a relationship among positive symptoms of schizophrenia and OCD/OCS, as assessed by the Y-BOCS. In a 12-month longitudinal study, Schirmbeck et al. (2013) also used the Y-BOCS and PANSS and found that individuals with schizophrenia and comorbid OCS did not have significantly higher scores in positive symptoms than individuals without OCS.

OCS and Negative Symptoms In the previously mentioned study by de Haan et al. (2005), the authors did not find more severe negative symptoms in patients with comorbid OCD and schizophrenia. On the contrary, they found that patients with schizophrenia and mild OCS had less severe negative symptoms. Additionally, Ongür and Goff (2005) and Sevincok et al. (2007) found no correlation between negative symptoms and OCD in both inpatient and outpatient participants with schizophrenia. Ongür and Goff (2005) also did not find more negative symptoms in participants with schizophrenia and OCS who were being treated in an urban setting. Similarly to de Haan et al. (2005), Ongür and Goff (2005), Kayahan et al. (2005) and Byerly et al. (2005) did not find a correlation between OCS and negative symptoms as measured by the PANSS. The authors stated that the results support the notion that OCS and schizophrenia are two separate comorbid disorders which affect and influence one another. In the previously discussed meta-analysis by Cunill et al. (2009), it was found that OCS, but not OCD, was significantly correlated with negative symptoms.

Nasrollahi et al. (2012) found a significant negative correlation between negative symptoms of schizophrenia and obsessive symptoms as assessed by the PANSS and Y-BOCS, respectively. Further, the authors found that more obsessive symptoms predicted less negative symptoms. Nasrollahi and colleagues suggested that obsessions could serve as a protective factor against developing negative symptoms of schizophrenia, and obsessions do not necessarily mean poorer prognosis. De Haan et al. (2013b) did not find a correlation between positive symptoms of schizophrenia and comorbid OCD/OCS nor between negative and disorganized symptoms of schizophrenia and OCD/OCS in a study of first-episode schizophrenia patients followed for 5 years. On the contrary to the previously discussed studies, Schirmbeck et al. (2013) found individuals with schizophrenia and comorbid OCS had significantly higher scores in negative symptoms and general psychopathology, but not in their positive symptoms.

Overall, there no consistent relationship between OCS/OCD and psychotic symptoms has emerged from the literature. While some studies have found higher levels of OCS/OCD were linked with more severe positive symptoms others have failed to replicate this. The majority of studies, on the other hand, have found little evidence of a relationship between negative symptoms and OCS/OCD. Among the studies in support for a relationship between OCS/OCD and psychotic symptoms, the relationship between OCS and psychotic symptoms (i.e., both positive and negative symptoms) is more consistently found than between OCD and psychotic symptoms. Additionally, a few studies have supported a negative correlation between OCS and negative symptoms.

6.2 OCS and Affective Symptoms

The literature tends to be clearer in regard to the comorbidity of schizophrenia and OCS and affective symptoms, with the majority of studies supporting a positive correlation between OCS and depressive symptoms. Individuals with schizophrenia and OCS tend to demonstrate significant depressive symptoms, which is not surprising given that major depressive episodes are the most common comorbid disorder in OCD individuals (Murphy et al. 2010).

De Haan et al. (2005) found more severe depressive symptoms in patients with comorbid OCD as assessed with the Montgomery-Asberg Depression Rating Scale (MADRS; Montgomery and Asberg 1979). In the opposite direction, Sevincok et al.'s (2007) study that has been previously referred to found no relationship between OCD and depressive symptoms in individuals with schizophrenia in addition to finding no links with positive and negative symptoms. Ongür and Goff (2005) found schizophrenia participants with OCS had more depressive symptoms in addition to positive symptoms as previously mentioned. In regard to individuals with schizophrenia in an inpatient unit and/or under treatment, Kayahan et al. (2005) found that increased levels of OCS, as assessed with the Y-BOCS, had a significant relationship with depressive symptoms as assessed by the Calgary Depression Rating Scale for Schizophrenia (Addington 1990). In addition to Rajkumar et al. (2008) finding schizophrenia patients with comorbid OCD to have greater associations with more paranoia and first-rank symptoms compared to patients without OCD, they found that participants with both comorbid schizophrenia and OCD had greater depression scores on both the Hamilton Rating Scale for Depression (HAM-D; Hamilton 1960) and the depression subscale of the PANSS and more comorbid anxiety disorders.

In a prospective study of the 5-year course of comorbid OCS and OCD in 172 patients with first-episode schizophrenia and related disorders, de Haan et al. (2013b) found that comorbid OCD, but not OCS, as assessed by the Y-BOCS, was associated with more severe depressive symptoms at follow-ups. Additionally, Schirmbeck et al. (2013) found individuals with comorbid schizophrenia and OCS did not have increased levels of depressive symptoms compared to those without OCS.

Overall, the literature more clearly suggests a trend toward an association between the comorbidity of schizophrenia and OCS/OCD and depressive symptoms. Additionally, studies more frequently find correlations between depressive symptoms and persons with schizophrenia and OCD than with schizophrenia and OCS.

6.3 OCS and General Functioning

In regard to general functioning/psychosocial functioning, the research demonstrates that the relationship between OCS and functioning appears to be clearer than the relationship between OCS and symptoms; overall, OCS are associated with greater levels of impairment. This association between OCS and functional impairments may be explained by the fact that OCS can be debilitating in and of itself, which may hence exacerbate other symptoms. On the other hand, OCS in schizophrenia may be a separate subtype of schizophrenia with its own pathophysiology, which is linked with higher levels of maladaptive behaviors (Lysaker and Whitney 2009). In an early retrospective study, Fenton and McGlashan (1986) found OCS in schizophrenia to be associated with poorer social and global functioning as well as less employment. Additionally, the study demonstrated that persistent OCS in schizophrenia predicted poorer prognosis. These findings have been replicated in participants with chronic schizophrenia (Berman et al. 1995; Poyurovsky et al. 2001).

In order to further examine the effects of OCS in individuals with schizophrenia, Lysaker et al. (2006) examined participants' coping mechanism and hope. The study used the Y-BOCS to assess severity of OCS, the PANSS to assess severity of positive and negative symptoms, the Ways of Coping Questionnaire to assess coping preference (Folkman and Lazarus 1988), and the Beck Hopelessness Scale

(Beck et al. 1974) to assess hope. Lysaker and colleagues found that participants with greater levels of OCS were more likely to engage in an avoidance coping skills, have less hope for their future, and give up. Further, the participants with both negative symptoms and OCS had greater pessimistic views about their future and greater avoidance coping strategies than the participants with similar levels of negative symptoms but no OCS.

Regarding the issues of suicide, Sevincok et al. (2007) found inpatient and outpatient participants with comorbid OCD and schizophrenia ($N=24$) had more suicide attempts and ideations than those without comorbid OCD ($N=33$). Additionally, results showed that those with comorbid OCD and schizophrenia had a greater number of previous suicidal attempts and ideations. In participants with severe OCS as measured by the Y-BOCS, a positive correlation with suicide attempts was found. Hagen et al. (2013) found higher rates of suicidal ideations and attempts in participants with comorbid OCD and first-episode psychosis. Likewise, DeVylder et al. (2012) also found social impairments and more suicidal ideations in psychosis-risk participants with OCS than those without OCS. On the contrary, when comparing schizophrenia patients with and without OCS/OCD, Hosseini et al. (2012) found no association between OCS/OCD and suicidal ideations. Hosseini et al. (2012) also used the Y-BOCS and PANSS to assess severity of OCS and symptoms of schizophrenia. They used the Beck Scale for Suicide Ideation (Beck and Steer 1991).

Additional studies have continued to consistently find a relationship between lower levels of psychosocial functioning and OCS in schizophrenia. Considering life satisfaction, Huppert and Smith (2005) investigated the association between self-reported OCS using the Obsessive-Compulsive Inventory (Foa et al. 1998) and quality of life using the Lehman Quality of Life Interview (Lehman 1988). Results demonstrated that lower levels of OCS were related to greater quality of life. In addition, Tiryaki and Ozkorumak (2010) examined the quality of life of 62 schizophrenia patients with and without OCS. The study utilized the Scale for the Assessment of Negative Symptoms, Scale for the Assessment of Positive Symptoms, Y-BOCS, and the Quality of Life Scale (QOLS; Heinrichs et al. 1984). Tiryaki and Ozkorumak (2010) found that schizophrenia patients with OCS had lower quality of life scores compared to schizophrenia patients without OCS. Additionally, DeVylder et al. (2012) found lower levels of subjective quality of life in first-episode schizophrenia participants with OCS compared to those without OCS. Further, Zink et al. (2014) found patients with at-risk mental states for psychosis and OCS had higher levels of psychosocial impairments.

In the prospective first-episode study (previously discussed) by de Haan et al. (2013b), the authors also found that both individuals with schizophrenia and comorbid OCD and individuals with schizophrenia but without OCS were correlated with poor premorbid functioning and poor social functioning at 5-year follow-ups. In regard to social functioning, de Haan and colleagues suggested that mild OCS may serve as a protective factor against further social dysfunction, or it may be a marker of better social capacities, but that diagnosable OCD may lead to further decompensation in social functioning or that OCD develops in those with an already vulnerable social functioning. The authors noted that mild

OCS may be an adaptive response against stressful psychotic symptoms. Another interesting finding of the study is that approximately half of the patients reported experiencing OCS at least once during the 5-year course, suggesting that OCS are common but fluid, which may account for why the study did not find a correlation between negative and positive symptoms of schizophrenia and OCS/OCD. However, Schirmbeck et al. (2013) did find individuals with comorbid OCS to have lower psychosocial functioning scores.

In regard to first-episode schizophrenia, de Haan et al. (2013a) examined subjective well-being and quality of life in participants with first-episode schizophrenia and OCS. Participants with OCS were correlated with lower overall subjective well-being than participants without comorbid OCS. Additionally, those participants had lower scores on general and social quality of life, but it was not significant.

Zink et al. (2014) examined at-risk mental states for psychosis participants and found that those with subclinical OCS had more deficits in psychosocial functioning and greater levels of general psychopathology but less impairments in verbal working memory and verbal immediate memory. The authors noted that OCS could be viewed as a protective factor against some cognitive decline.

The comorbidity of OCS/OCD and schizophrenia has consistently demonstrated graver psychosocial and overall functioning. Greater levels of OCS among persons with schizophrenia have been linked to more pessimistic views and avoidance coping strategies. Additionally, comorbid OCS/OCD and schizophrenia have been associated with more suicide attempts and ideations. This comorbidity of OCS and schizophrenia is also related to lower perceived quality of life. In regard to premorbid functioning, at least one study supports an association between comorbid schizophrenia and OCD and poorer premorbid functioning, but not among those with schizophrenia and OCS.

6.4 Conceptualization of OCS in Schizophrenia and Related Issues

Overall, the literature shows an association between lower perceived quality of life and social dysfunctioning with comorbid OCS and OCD. Further, individuals with both OCS and schizophrenia appear to have pessimistic views about their life, less effective coping skills, and more suicidal ideations compared to those with schizophrenia without OCS. However, the relationship between schizophrenia symptoms and OCS is more equivocal. The association between OCS and positive symptoms of schizophrenia appears to be very mixed. On the other hand, the link between OCS and negative symptoms demonstrates a trend toward no association with some studies even finding less severe negative symptoms in patients with comorbid OCS (de Haan et al. 2005, 2013b; Nasrollahi et al. 2012). One could argue that having OCS and more severe positive symptoms may be better than having significant negative symptoms because positive symptoms may allow persons to have social contact whereas persons with substantial negative symptoms tend to present as very barren and difficult to engage socially. In regard to relationship between affective symptoms and OCS in schizophrenia, a relatively consistent association is found in that OCS in schizophrenia is linked to more depressive symptoms.

So why are the results concerning the association between OCS and other psychopathological symptoms variable and inconsistent? There are several possible answers. The mixed results in the literature may be due to methodological issues among studies. The fact that most studies separate the participants into one group with OCS and one group without OCS may be a cause for the inconsistent findings. In the meta-analysis previously discussed by Cunill et al. (2009), the results found OCS but not OCD to be associated with more severe psychotic symptoms (e.g., positive and negative symptoms). However, the authors noted that the results depended on the use of dimensional or categorical definitions for OCS/OCD – OCD definitions are stricter and thus more participants would fall into the OCS group if dimensional definitions were used and the non-OCD group if a categorical definition was used. Overall, Cunill and colleagues' meta-analysis supports that OCS exacerbates psychosis. Their results support the perspective of a subtype of schizophrenia with OCS that may have its own etiology, course, and prognosis.

The phase of illness is another issue that could affect the presentation of OCS in schizophrenia. Studies have used participants with chronic schizophrenia, first-episode schizophrenia, and at-risk individuals as well as participants in stable and acute phases, which may be a reason for the equivocal results regarding the relationships between OCS and symptoms. Furthermore, it may be that the presentation of OCS in schizophrenia changes depending on the stage and/or phase of illness. Treatment side effects such as OCS due to medications (Poyurovsky et al. 2004) could also be among the confounding effects of studies that used participants with chronic schizophrenia. Many individuals with schizophrenia also experience symptom remission, and the relationships OCS and schizophrenia during periods of positive and negative symptom remission. In addition, most studies utilize the rational scoring system for the PANSS although research demonstrates that the rational scoring scheme is problematic due to disorganization symptoms being combined with both positive and negative symptoms of schizophrenia (Bell et al. 1994).

Furthermore, there are different approaches to conceptualizing OCS in schizophrenia (see Chap. 4). In a case series analysis, Reznik et al. (2004) described three possible groups of individuals with OCS in schizophrenia: the "OCD-schizophrenia" group that represents OCD patients who later develop schizophrenia, the "schizo-obsessive" group that represents patients with treatment-resistant schizophrenia in which delusions and behaviors may possess compulsive characteristics, and the group of individuals who develop OCS as a result of certain circumstances such as treatment with clozapine.

On the other hand, Lysaker et al. (2004) proposed that there are two distinct groups of individuals with schizophrenia and OCS; one group whose symptoms are associated with graver deficits and one group whose symptoms are associated with better functioning. The study utilized the Y-BOCS to assess OCS, the QOLS to measure social functioning, the PANSS to examine negative symptoms, and the

Wisconsin Card Sorting Test to measure executive functioning (Heaton et al. 1993). According to a cluster analysis, the authors found four different groups of participants with schizophrenia spectrum disorders: "high OCS/good function," "high OCS/poor function," "non-OCS/poor function," and "non-OCS/moderate function." Additionally, they found that both the OCS/good function group and the non-OCS/moderate function group had fewer negative symptoms than the poor function groups. The OCS poor function group also had poorer neurocognitive function performance than either non-OCS groups. Thus, the authors' results add support to the proposal that there may be two subgroups of individuals with schizophrenia and OCS, one with less negative symptoms and one with worse neurocognitive deficits but more negative symptoms. This perspective could help explain the trend toward finding less of an association of OCS and negative symptoms. It could be that the previously mentioned studies incorporated participants who would fall into the subgroup of schizophrenia and OCS with less negative symptoms. This interpretation is also concordant with the finding of an association between mild OCS and less severe negative symptoms (de Haan et al. 2005).

Conclusion

The majority of studies examining OCS in schizophrenia have produced inconsistent findings especially in regard to the relationship with positive and negative symptoms. Although, the exact relationship between OCS and symptoms is still unclear, research suggests that OCS in schizophrenia causes greater difficulties in everyday functioning more often than not. Furthermore, it is important to mention yet again that the prevalence rates of OCS in schizophrenia are greater than that in the general population, which points to the need to further examine this phenomenon. Concerning whether OCS and schizophrenia are a distinct subgroup of schizophrenia. Reznik et al. (2004) proposed three distinct groups of individuals with OCS and schizophrenia, whereas Lysaker et al. (2004) proposed two distinct groups of individuals with OCS. There has also been the suggestion that mild OCS serves as a protective factor. Could it be that there is yet another subtype of individuals with schizophrenia and OCS – one where OCS serves as a protective factor against further deterioration? Or does the protective aspect of OCS only last for a certain amount of time during the course of the illness?

Additionally, what is the diagnostic priority of OCS and schizophrenia? Should treatment focus on the OCS or schizophrenia symptoms first? Should one just treat the symptoms that are causing the most distress or impairment? What happens if OCS is treated before other symptoms? Does it make the positive and/or negative symptoms easier or more difficult to treat? These are all questions that future research could investigate in order to gain a better understanding of OCS in schizophrenia. Importantly, there is evidence showing that comorbid OCS may fluctuate during the early course of schizophrenia; however, a significant proportion of schizophrenia patients (around 13 %) have enduring and relatively severe OCS. It also remains a question whether interventions should differ depending on the subtype of OCS in schizophrenia. If indeed there are distinct groups of individuals with

OCS and schizophrenia, it is possible that treatments need to be tailored specifically for each type. For example, it may be beneficial to intervene with cognitive remediation for the subtype of OCS with poor neurocognitive function but not for the subtype of OCS with less negative symptoms.

References

Achim AM, Maziade M, Raymond E, Olivier D, Mérette C, Roy M-A (2011) How prevalent are anxiety disorders in schizophrenia? A meta-analysis and critical review on a significant association. Schizophr Bull 37:811–821. doi:10.1093/schbul/sbp148

Addington DA (1990) A depression rating scale for schizophrenia. Schizophr Res 3:247–251

American Psychiatric Association (2000) Diagnostic and statistical manual of mental disorders, Revised 4th edn. American Psychiatric Association, Washington, DC

Beck AT, Steer RA (1991) Manual for the beck scale for suicide ideation. Psychological Corporation, San Antonio

Beck AT, Weisman A, Lester D, Trexler L (1974) The measurement of pessimism: the hopelessness scale. J Consult Clin Psychol 42:861–865

Bell MD, Lysaker PH, Beam-Goulet JL, Milstein RM, Lindenmayer J-P (1994) Five-component model of schizophrenia: assessing the factorial invariance of the positive and negative syndrome scale. Psychiatry Res 52:295–303. doi:10.1016/0165-1781(94)90075-2

Berman I, Kalinowski A, Berman SM, Lengua J, Green AI (1995) Obsessive and compulsive symptoms in chronic schizophrenia. Compr Psychiatry 36:6–10. doi:10.1016/0010-440x(95)90092-a

Berman I, Pappas D, Bermam S (1997) Obsessive-compulsive symptoms in schizophrenia: are they manifestations of a distinct subclass of schizophrenia disorders. CNS Spectr 2:45–48

Bland RC, Newman SC, Orn H (1987) Schizophrenia: lifetime co-morbidity in a community sample. Acta Psychiatrica Scandinavica 75:383–391

Bleuler E (1911/1950) Dementia Praecox of the group of schizophrenias (trans: Zinkin J). International Universities Press, New York

Borkowska A, Pilaczyñska E, Rybakowski JK (2003) The frontal lobe neuropsychological tests in patients with schizophrenia and/or obsessive-compulsive disorder. J Neuropsychiatry Clin Neurosci 15:359–362

Byerly M, Goodman W, Acholonu W, Bugno R, Rush AJ (2005) Obsessive compulsive symptoms in schizophrenia: frequency and clinical features. Schizophr Res 76:309–316

Cosoff SJ, Hafner RJ (1998) The prevalence of comorbid anxiety in schizophrenia, schizoaffective disorder and bipolar disorder. Aust N Z J Psychiatry 32:67–72

Cunill R, Castells X, Simeon D (2009) Relationships between obsessive-compulsive symptomatology and severity of psychosis in schizophrenia: a systematic review and meta-analysis. J Clin Psychiatry 70:70–82

de Haan L, Hoogenboom B, Beuk N, van Amelsvoort T, Linszen D (2005) Obsessive-compulsive symptoms and positive, negative, and depressive symptoms in patients with recent-onset schizophrenic disorders. Can J Psychiatry (Revue Canadienne De Psychiatrie) 50:519–524

de Haan L, Sterk B, van der Valk R (2013a) Presence of obsessive compulsive symptoms in first-episode schizophrenia or related disorders is associated with subjective well-being and quality of life. Early Interv Psychiatry 7:285–290. doi:10.1111/j.1751-7893.2012.00377.x

de Haan L, Sterk B, Wouters L, Linszen DH (2013b) The 5-year course of obsessive-compulsive symptoms and obsessive-compulsive disorder in first-episode schizophrenia and related disorders. Schizophr Bull 39:151–160. doi:10.1093/schbul/sbr077

DeVylder JE, Oh AJ, Ben-David S, Azimov N, Harkavy-Friedman JM, Corcoran CM (2012) Obsessive compulsive symptoms in individuals at clinical risk for psychosis: association with depressive symptoms and suicidal ideation. Schizophr Res 140:110–113. doi:10.1016/j.schres.2012.07.009

Eisen JL, Beer DA, Pato MT, Venditto TA, Rasmussen SA (1997) Obsessive-compulsive disorder in patients with schizophrenia or schizoaffective disorder. Am J Psychiatry 154:271–273
Fenton WS, McGlashan TH (1986) The prognostic significance of obsessive-compulsive symptoms in schizophrenia. Am J Psychiatry 143:437–441
Foa EB, Kozak MJ, Salkovskis PM, Coles ME, Amir N (1998) The validation of a new obsessive-compulsive disorder scale: the obsessive-compulsive inventory. Psychol Assess 10:206–214
Folkman S, Lazarus RS (1988) Ways of coping questionnaire (manual). Consulting Psychologists Press, Palo Alto
Goodman WK, Price LH, Rasmussen SA et al (1989) The Yale Brown Obsessive Compulsive Scale I: development, use, and reliability. Arch Gen Psychiatry 46:1006–1101
Hagen K, Hansen B, Joa I, Larsen TK (2013) Prevalence and clinical characteristics of patients with obsessive-compulsive disorder in first-episode psychosis. BMC Psychiatry 13:156. doi:10.1186/1471-244x-13-156
Hamilton M (1960) A rating scale for depression. J Neurol Neurosurg Psychiatry 23:56–62
Heaton RK, Chelune GJ, Talley JL, Kay GG, Curtiss G (1993) Wisconsin card sorting test manual. Psychological Assessment Resources, Lutz
Heinrichs DW, Hanlon TE, Carpenter WT (1984) The quality of life scale: an instrument for rating the schizophrenic deficit syndrome. Schizophr Bull 10:388–398
Hosseini SH, Zarghami M, Moudi S, Mohammadpour AR (2012) Frequency and severity of obsessive-compulsive symptoms/disorders, violence and suicidal in schizophrenic patients. Iran Red Crescent Med J 14:345–351
Huppert JD, Smith TE (2005) Anxiety and schizophrenia: the interaction of subtypes of anxiety and psychotic symptoms. CNS Spectr 10:721–731
Hwang MY, Hollander E (1993) Schizo-obsessive disorders. Psychiatric Annuls 23:396–401
Kay SR, Fiszbein A, Opler L (1987) The Positive and Negative Syndrome Scale for schizophrenia. Schizophrenia Bulletin 13:261–276
Kayahan B, Ozturk O, Veznedaroglu B, Eraslan D (2005) Obsessive-compulsive symptoms in schizophrenia: prevalence and clinical correlates. Psychiatry Clin Neurosci 59:291–295
Krüger S, Bräunig P, Höffler J, Shugar G, Börner I, Langkrär J (2000) Prevalence of obsessive-compulsive disorder in schizophrenia and significance of motor symptoms. J Neuropsychiatry Clin Neurosci 12:16–24
Lehman AF (1988) A quality of life interview for the chronically mentally ill. Eval Program Plann 11:51–62
Lysaker PH, Whitney KA (2009) Obsessive-compulsive symptoms in schizophrenia: prevalence, correlates and treatment. Expert Rev Neurother 9:99–107. doi:10.1586/14737175.9.1.99
Lysaker PH, Marks KA, Picone JB, Rollins AL, Fastenau PS, Bond GR (2000) Obsessive and compulsive symptoms in schizophrenia: clinical and neurocognitive correlates. J Nerv Ment Dis 188:78–83
Lysaker PH, Lancaster RS, Nees MA, Davis LW (2004) Patterns of obsessive-compulsive symptoms and social function in schizophrenia. Psychiatry Res 125:139–146
Lysaker PH, Whitney KA, Davis LW (2006) Obsessive compulsive and negative symptoms in schizophrenia: Associations with coping preference and hope. Psychiatry Research 141:253–259
Montgomery SA, Aspber M (1979) A new depression scale designed to be sensitive to change. Br J Psychiatry 134:382–389
Murphy DL, Timpano KR, Wheaton MG, Greenberg BD, Miguel EC (2010) Obsessive-compulsive disorder and its related disorders: a reappraisal of obsessive-compulsive spectrum concepts. Dialogues Clin Neurosci 12:131–148
Nasrollahi N, Bigdelli I, Mocbrhammadi MR, Hosseini SM (2012) The relationship between obsessions and compulsions and negative and positive symptoms in schizophrenia. Iran J Psychiatry 7:140–145
Nechmad A, Ratzoni G, Poyurovsky M, Meged S, Avidan G, Fuchs C, Weizman R (2003) Obsessive-compulsive disorder in adolescent schizophrenia patients. Am J Psychiatry 160:1002–1004

Ohta M, Kokai M, Morita Y (2003) Features of obsessive-compulsive disorder in patients primarily diagnosed with schizophrenia. Psychiatry Clin Neurosci 57:67–74

Ongür D, Goff DC (2005) Obsessive-compulsive symptoms in schizophrenia: associated clinical features, cognitive function and medication status. Schizophr Res 75:349–362

Porto L, Bermanzohn P, Siris S, Pollack S, Morrissey R (1997) A profile of obsessive compulsive symptoms in schizophrenia. Schizophrenia Research 24:20–20. doi: 10.1016/s0920-9964(97)82054-3

Poyurovsky M, Fuchs C, Weizman A (1999) Obsessive-compulsive disorder in patients with first-episode schizophrenia. Am J Psychiatry 156:1998–2000

Poyurovsky M, Hramenkov S, Isakov V, Rauchverger B, Modai I, Schneidman M, Weizman A (2001) Obsessive-compulsive disorder in hospitalized patients with chronic schizophrenia. [Research Support, Non-U.S. Gov't]. Psychiatry Res 102:49–57. doi:10.1016/s0165-1781(01)00238-4

Poyurovsky M, Weizman A, Wiezman R (2004) Obsessive-compulsive disorder in schizophrenia: clinical characteristics and treatment. CNS Drugs 18:989–1010

Rajkumar RP, Reddy YCJ, Kandavel T (2008) Clinical profile of "schizo-obsessive" disorder: a comparative study. Compr Psychiatry 49:262–268. doi:10.1016/j.comppsych.2007.09.006

Reznik I, Yavin I, Stryjer R, Spivak B, Gonen N, Strous R, Kotler M (2004) Clozapine in the treatment of obsessive-compulsive symptoms in schizophrenia patients: a case series study. Pharmacopsychiatry 37:52–56

Schirmbeck F, Rausch F, Englisch S, Eifler S, Esslinger C, Meyer-Lindenberg A, Zink M (2013) Stable cognitive deficits in schizophrenia patients with comorbid obsessive-compulsive symptoms: a 12-month longitudinal study. Schizophr Bull 39(6):1261–1271

Sevincok L, Akoglu A, Kokcu F (2007) Suicidality in schizophrenic patients with and without obsessive-compulsive disorder. Schizophr Res 90:198–202

Tibbo P, Kroetsch M, Chue P, Warneke L (2000) Obsessive-compulsive disorder in schizophrenia. J Psychiatric Res 34:139–146

Tiryaki A, Ozkorumak E (2010) Do the obsessive-compulsive symptoms have an effect in schizophrenia? Compr Psychiatry 51:357–362. doi:10.1016/j.comppsych.2009.10.007

Zink M, Schirmbeck F, Rausch F, Eifler S, Elkin H, Solojenkina X, Englisch S, Wagner M, Maier W, Lautenschlager M, Heinz A, Gudlowski Y, Janssen B, Gaebel W, Michel TM, Schneider F, Lambert M, Naber D, Juckel G, Krueger-Oezguerdal S, Wobrock T, Hasan A, Riedel M, Müller H, Klosterkötter J, Bechdolf A (2014) Obsessive-compulsive symptoms in at-risk mental states for psychosis: associations with clinical impairment and cognitive function. Acta Psychiatr Scand 130(3):214–226

Part III

Neurobiology

The Neurocognitive and Behavioural Impact of Comorbid Obsessive–Compulsive Syndrome in Schizophrenia

7

Yana Varlakova, Devina D. Patel, Kaushik Mukhopadhaya, Keith R. Laws, Eilam David, Kaur Sukwinder, and Naomi A. Fineberg

Y. Varlakova
School of Life and Medical Sciences, University of Hertfordshire, Hertfordshire, England, UK

Highly Specialized Obsessive Compulsive and Related Disorders Service, Hertfordshire Partnership University NHS Foundation Trust, Rosanne House, 2nd floor, Parkway, Welwyn Garden City, Hertfordshire AL8 7JE, UK

D.D. Patel
School of Life and Medical Sciences, University of Hertfordshire, Hertfordshire, England, UK

Highly Specialized Obsessive Compulsive and Related Disorders Service, Hertfordshire Partnership University NHS Foundation Trust, Rosanne House, 2nd floor, Parkway, Welwyn Garden City, Hertfordshire AL8 7JE, UK

School of Health and Human Studies, University of Essex, Wivenhoe Park, Colchester CO4 3SQ, England, UK

K. Mukhopadhaya • K. Sukwinder
Highly Specialized Obsessive Compulsive and Related Disorders Service, Hertfordshire Partnership University NHS Foundation Trust, Rosanne House, 2nd floor, Parkway, Welwyn Garden City, Hertfordshire AL8 7JE, UK

K.R. Laws
School of Life and Medical Sciences, University of Hertfordshire, Hertfordshire, England, UK

E. David
Department of Zoology, Tel-Aviv University, Tel-Aviv, Ramat-Aviv 69978, Israel

N.A. Fineberg (✉)
Highly Specialized Obsessive Compulsive and Related Disorders Service, Hertfordshire Partnership University NHS Foundation Trust, Rosanne House, 2nd floor, Parkway, Welwyn Garden City, Hertfordshire AL8 7JE, UK

School of Life and Medical Sciences, Postgraduate Medical School, University of Hertfordshire, College Lane, Hatfield, Hertfordshire AL10 9AB, UK
e-mail: naomi.fineberg@hpft.nhs.uk

L. De Haan et al. (eds.), *Obsessive-Compulsive Symptoms in Schizophrenia*,
DOI 10.1007/978-3-319-12952-5_7

Vignette

Miss N. is a 41-year-old single university graduate who works part time in a supermarket. She first presented to mental health services in her late 20s and was diagnosed with schizophrenia. As she experienced unremitting auditory hallucinations, she was eventually prescribed clozapine. The paranoia and hallucinations improved, and she was even able to start working full time. Approximately 5 years later, she started to experience distressing repeated intrusive thoughts and urges to make racist or homophobic comments. She worried she would act on her compulsive urges. As a result, she spent most of her leisure time at home and became fearful of leaving the house. She became increasingly withdrawn and isolated. She broke a long-term relationship with her partner and reduced her working hours significantly. More recently, she started compulsively checking taps and doors whenever leaving the house. Miss N does not experience paranoia, apathy, blunting of affective response or poverty of thought. The decline in her social and occupational functioning appears to be secondary to obsessive–compulsive symptoms. To what extent might neurocognitive changes contribute to her problems, and could a better understanding help direct future pharmacological and/or psychological treatment and prognostication?

7.1 Introduction

Obsessive–compulsive disorder (OCD) and schizophrenia are each associated with considerable executive and functional impairment (Bokat and Goldberg 2003; Chamberlain et al. 2005; Heinrichs and Zakzanis 1998; Henry and Crawford 2005; Johnson-Selfridge and Zalewski 2001; Kashyap et al. 2013; Laws 1999; Menzies et al. 2008; Mesholam-Gately et al. 2009). Compared to bipolar and depressive disorder, the cognitive deficit in schizophrenia is more severe and widespread, affecting domains including memory, abstract thinking and planning (Buchanan et al. 2005). The finding that the severity of the cognitive deficit is the best predictor for social functioning (Krivoy et al. 2012) has been frequently replicated and appears to be robust, highlighting the clinical importance of neurocognitive function in this disorder. Moreover, current pharmacotherapy for schizophrenia does not ameliorate the cognitive deficit, which has become the focus of ongoing research evaluating novel compounds (Barnett et al. 2010).

Compared to non-comorbid schizophrenia, many (though not all, e.g. Rajkumar et al. 2008) studies in patients with schizophrenia comorbid with OCD or obsessive–compulsive syndrome (OCS), defined as the presence of obsessions and compulsions not severe enough to meet the diagnostic criteria of OCD, have found higher levels of positive and emotional discomfort symptoms on the Positive and Negative Syndrome Scale (PANSS) (Hwang et al. 2000; Lysaker et al. 2000; Tibbo et al. 2000). These patients were also found to have a poorer prognosis in terms of global functioning and illness severity (Fenton and McGlashan 1986), greater psychosocial dysfunction, poorer quality of life, poorer treatment response, poorer long-term outcome, greater functional impairment, a greater number of suicide attempts (Lysaker et al. 2004; Poyurovsky et al. 2001) as well as a smaller social network (de Haan et al. 2011; Lysaker and Whitney 2009) (for details, see Chap. 6). Importantly, patients with schizophrenia and comorbid OCD made greater use of health service resources compared to those with schizophrenia alone and required a longer duration of hospitalisation (Berman et al. 1995; Fenton and McGlashan 1986; Hwang et al. 2000). Symptoms of OCD in the presence of schizophrenia may be relatively unresponsive to pharmacotherapy or cognitive behaviour therapy (CBT) (Mukhopadhaya et al. 2009). Thus, the impact and burden of OCD/OCS occurring with schizophrenia, in terms of personal distress, disability and health service cost, is high.

The reported prevalence rates of OCD, OCS and obsessive–compulsive symptoms in schizophrenia are also strikingly high. OCS may occur in as many as 64 % patients with schizophrenia (Kayahan et al. 2005), whereas reported OCD comorbidity varies between 0 and 59 % across studies (Achim et al. 2011; Bland et al. 1987; Buckley et al. 2009; Fabisch et al. 2001). Buckley et al. (2009) calculated a weighted average from 36 studies and estimated the prevalence of OCS to be 25 % and OCD to be 23 %. In a more recent meta-analysis (Swets et al. 2014), OCD showed a 13.6 % prevalence after meta-regression and a higher prevalence in chronically symptomatic cases. In contrast, the prevalence of obsessive–compulsive symptoms, defined as any obsession or compulsion, was as high as 30 % after meta-regression. Overall, these rates of OCD/OCS substantially exceed those in the general population where the lifetime prevalence for OCD is estimated at 1.6 % (Kessler et al. 2005) (see Chap. 4). Yet, OCD is poorly recognised in the presence of schizophrenia. For example, in the study by Mukhopadhaya et al. (2009), whereas roughly one quarter of a cohort of clozapine-treated patients with schizophrenia/schizoaffective disorder in active care were found to suffer with clinically relevant OCD, in approx. 50 % of these cases, the OCD was previously undiagnosed (Mukhopadhaya et al. 2009).

The term 'schizo-obsessive' was coined by Hwang and Opler in 1994 and refers to a dual diagnosis of schizophrenia and obsessive–compulsive disorder (OCD) or obsessive–compulsive symptoms (OCSs). Alternative explanations for the exaggerated overlap have included (a) OCD naturally occurring as a sub-syndrome within the schizophrenia spectrum (Poyurovsky et al. 2001), (b) treatment for schizophrenia unmasking OCD previously hidden by schizophrenic symptoms (Ertugrul and Demir 2005), (c) treatment for schizophrenia causing OCD de novo (Mukhopadhaya et al. 2009; Schirmbeck and Zink 2012) or (d) a factor, as yet unidentified, predisposing individuals to both OCD and schizophrenia as a 'true' comorbidity (Patel et al. 2010). It has been proposed, for example, that the neurobiology underpinning some forms of OCD may overlap with that of schizophrenia in the form of monoaminergic dysfunction in cortico-striatal tracts (Tibbo and Warneke 1999). In line with this hypothesis, schizophrenia with OCD has been found to be associated with a higher-than-expected frequency of neurological soft signs and motor abnormalities thought to be associated with cortico-striatal dysfunction, such as tic (Poyurovsky et al. 2006; Sevincok et al. 2004), extrapyramidal motor signs (Kruger et al. 2000; Mukhopadhaya et al. 2009; Ohta et al. 2003), motor symptoms including catatonia and loss of motor ability or hyperactive motor activity (Tibbo et al. 2000). A recent study, however, failed to identify a greater predominance of neurological or motor symptoms in schizophrenia with OCD compared to OCD (Poyurovsky et al. 2007). Ma et al. (2007) found low blood serotonin levels in OCD and in schizophrenia with comorbid OCD, implicating an alteration in serotonin metabolism as a common biological characteristic in these groups. Structural magnetic resonance imaging (MRI) studies have identified significantly reduced volume in the left hippocampus, frontal lobes (Aoyama et al. 2000) and anterior horn of the lateral and third ventricle (Goldstein et al. 1999) in patients with schizophrenia and OCS compared with schizophrenia counterparts without OCS (for details, see Chap. 9).

7.1.1 Aims

The existence of specific cognitive and behavioural deficits in psychiatric disorder may have important implications for classification, diagnosis and treatment (Melcher et al. 2008). Studies investigating neurocognitive function have reported overlapping domains of impairment in OCD and schizophrenia that are thought to involve frontal cortex or fronto-striatal brain mechanisms (Berman et al. 1998; Hwang et al. 2000; Lysaker et al. 2000, 2002; Whitney et al. 2004). In this chapter, we review the results of neurocognitive and behavioural studies in patients with OCD and schizophrenia, alone and combined. We use these data to attempt to identify the key neuropsychological mechanisms. A better understanding of the neurocognitive changes associated with this comorbidity may shed light on the neural mechanisms underpinning illness-related functional impairment and inform the modification of existing treatment strategies or even the development of new-targeted treatments for this prominently disabled, relatively treatment-resistant group. We additionally explore the extent to which the associated neuro-behavioural changes may characterise schizo–OCD as a distinct and clinically relevant schizophrenia subgroup (subtype), a more severe form of schizophrenia or a true comorbidity that integrates the psychopathology of both its parent disorders. We suggest directions for future research.

7.2 Determining the Cognitive Deficit in Schizo–OCD

Patients with schizophrenia show deficits relative to controls across a wide range of neuropsychological domains including memory, language, attention and executive function (Fioravanti et al. 2005). Neuropsychological assessment using standardised neurocognitive tasks with well-understood neural underpinnings allows evaluation of the different neural contributions in schizophrenia with OCD. Some tasks are relatively non-specific for neural circuitry or cognitive domains (e.g. Wisconsin Card Sorting Test (WCST); see next section), and poor scores on these tasks reflect abnormalities that may exist across a variety of neuropsychological processes; others are more domain-specific (Barnett et al. 2010). The former tasks may provide information on the magnitude of global functional impairment, from which we may infer impact on psychosocial disability; the latter tasks may be more useful for pinpointing specific areas of cognitive dysfunction.

7.2.1 Non-Specific Cognitive Tasks

The cognitive test domain that has most frequently shown impairment in schizo–OCS patients is cognitive flexibility, associated with the WCST. The WCST is a neuropsychological measure of multiple domains of executive function and is sensitive to frontal lobe dysfunction. The WCST allows assessment of the following key functions: strategic planning, organised searching, using environmental feedback to shift cognitive sets, directing behaviour toward achieving a goal and modulating impulsive responding (Monchi et al. 2001). Set-shifting, i.e. the ability to display flexibility in the face of changing schedules of reinforcement, is essential to cognitive flexibility and relies on frontal lobe function. Several studies of schizophrenia, OCD and schizo–OCD have used the WCST as a test of attentional set-shifting and have found impairment in this domain in all three clinical groups (reviewed in Patel et al. 2010). A meta-analysis of five such studies suggested that patients with schizophrenia and OCD/OCS sort fewer WCST categories than those with schizophrenia alone (Patel et al. 2010). However, the mean effect size was small ($d=0.20$, 95 % confidence interval from −0.02 to 0.50) and marginally nonsignificant, almost certainly because of the limited number of studies in the meta-analysis and because only one study produced a large effect size (Öngür and Goff 2005). Another, more recent meta-analysis (Cunill et al. 2013) that reviewed seven studies (Berman et al. 1998; Hermesh et al. 2003; Hwang et al. 2000; Lysaker et al. 2000, 2004; Öngür and Goff 2005; Schirmbeck and Zink 2012) also showed that schizophrenia patients with OCS/OCD were more impaired in the 'categories completed' component of the set-shift task of the WCST (overall effect: $Z=2.59$; $p=0.010$). The effect size was small (0.37), but considering that the control group comprised patients with schizophrenia, who would be expected to be impaired in this domain, the result could be considered clinically relevant. The finding of poorer set-shifting in this group implies an area of neurocognitive overlap with OCD.

In the most recent study, 40 patients with schizophrenia (20 with and 20 without OCS) were compared with 20 healthy controls on several tests of cognitive functioning tapping the domains of processing speed, executive function and visuospatial memory (Michalopoulou et al. 2014). Whereas both the schizo–OCD and schizophrenia-only groups of patients performed significantly worse than healthy controls on several tasks, the results did not indicate a significant between-group (schizo–OCD versus schizophrenia group) difference on the WCST, although positive correlations were found between perseverative errors in WCST and the Yale–Brown Obsessive Compulsive Scale (Y-BOCS; an OCD severity measure) total and compulsion scores, suggesting a relationship between performance in this domain and OCS severity in schizo–OCD. It is noteworthy that in this study, the schizophrenia (but not schizo–OCD) group showed significantly poorer scores than healthy controls in measures of premorbid IQ, which may have biased the analysis toward better performance in schizo–OCD. Another potential source of confound in studies such as these relates to the difficulty matching the severity of illness and the concurrent medication across both schizophrenia groups.

In a 12-month longitudinal study by Schirmbeck et al. (2013) that investigated the course of the cognitive deficit, patients with schizophrenia and comorbid OCS ($n=37$) showed significantly (compared to schizophrenia without comorbid OCD, $n=43$) more frequent perseverative errors on the WCST, more pronounced deficits in visuospatial perception and visual memory (block design, Rey–Osterrieth Figure Test), lower inhibitory control (Stroop task, Go/No-Go tasks), poorer cognitive flexibility (Trail Making Test, B, set-shift task) and poorer immediate recall of verbal stimuli (measured by Auditory Verbal Learning Test) at baseline. Impairment in these cognitive domains correlated with OCS severity. One year later, the repeated cross-sectional neuropsychological assessment showed similar results within the smaller sample of completers (OCS+: $n=20$, OCS–: $n=30$), suggesting persistence, though not all group comparisons (including set-shifting) remained significant, possibly owing to a lack of statistical power. Nevertheless, the authors concluded that OCS in schizophrenia is associated with specific and longitudinally stable cognitive deficits, emphasising the magnitude and breadth of executive impairment in this patient population and arguing for at least partially overlapping neurobiological mechanisms with OCD (Schirmbeck et al. 2013).

These findings contrast with those of a large study by Meijer et al. (2013) that evaluated cognitive performance in 984 patients with non-affective psychosis (222 with OCS), 973 unaffected siblings (75 with OCS), 851 parents (35 with OCS) and 573 controls (26 with OCS). The study was unable to demonstrate a clear association between the presence OCS and cognitive performance using either cross-trait, cross-relative or within-subject analysis using tests including the Response Shifting Task (a modified version of the Competing Programs Task) to assess set-shifting ability; this task previously showed impairment in schizophrenia patients compared to healthy controls in a number of studies (Meijer et al. 2012; Nolan et al. 2004). However, poorer set-shifting ability (on the Response Shifting Task) was associated with an increased severity of subclinical OCS in the parents of the schizophrenia patients (but not the patients themselves), though the effect sizes were small ($d=0.10$). This may be explained by the greater psychopathology associated with schizophrenia mitigating the effect of OCS on set-shifting performance through a ceiling effect in the patient group (Meijer et al. 2013).

Taken together, the results suggest a greater impairment in attentional set-shift performance in schizo–OCD compared with schizophrenia and provide some support for the 'pathophysiological double jeopardy' hypothesis, which proposes that patients with schizo–OCD show greater cognitive deficits in domains impaired both in OCD and schizophrenia because of the overlap in the structural and functional abnormalities associated with each disorder (Bottas et al. 2005; Lysaker et al. 2000; Tibbo and Warneke 1999). Thus, when OC features are present in schizophrenia, the cognitive impairments associated with OCD (e.g. set-shift deficit) may aggravate those existing in schizophrenia (Whitney et al. 2004). Attempts have been made to identify the neuroanatomical basis of these changes. A functional neuroimaging (fMRI) study (Bleich-Cohen et al. 2014) did not find significant differences between schizophrenia patients with and without OCD in behavioural or imaging responses while performing a working memory (N-back) task. Regardless of the presence of OCS, schizophrenia patients had reduced activation of the right dorsolateral prefrontal cortex (DLPFC) and right caudate in response to increasing working memory load compared to healthy controls (for details, see Chap. 9).

7.2.2 Domain-Specific Tasks

Tasks such as the WCST can be criticised for their non-specific nature, tapping a wide range of neurocognitive processes including attentional set-shifting, error-based learning, feedback processing and working memory (Laws 1999). The National Institute of Mental Health-sponsored Measurement and Treatment Research to Improve Cognition in Schizophrenia (MATRICS) programme (http://www.matrics.ucla.edu/) was established to promote regulatory acceptance of cognition as a pharmaceutical target and to focus research onto remediating cognitive function in schizophrenia (Barnett et al. 2010). Key candidate cognitive domains and tests for schizophrenia were identified, based on expert opinion, analysis of the existing literature and a multisite pilot study in schizophrenia (Nuechterlein et al. 2008). The results formed the basis for the final selection of tests covering seven domains of cognitive function (speed of processing, attention/vigilance, working memory, verbal learning, visual learning, reasoning and problem solving, social cognition) that are contained in the MATRICS Consensus Cognitive Battery (MCCB) (Kern et al. 2008; Nuechterlein et al. 2008).

The Cambridge Neuropsychological Test Automated Battery (CANTAB; www.cambridgecognition.com/) is another well-established computerised neuropsychological touch-screen test battery that examines a range of discrete, domain-specific neurocognitive functions, including the domains pinpointed in the MATRICS consortium. In contrast to the MCCB tests, which were selected initially through expert consensus, and subsequently on their psychometric performance in patients with schizophrenia, the CANTAB was developed based on the neural validation and translational utility of each test and its known sensitivity to pharmacological manipulation (Barnett et al. 2010). The CANTAB tasks tap functional integrity in specific areas of the frontal cortex and the subcortical connections, for which the underpinning neuroanatomy is relatively well defined (see below). The largely nonverbal nature of the tests makes CANTAB practical for use across multisite and multilingual clinical trials and allows for direct translation of the results into animal models and neuroimaging forms of the tests. To date, little published literature exists on the use of CANTAB in patients with schizo–OCD; however, patients with schizophrenia (for a review of the use of CANTAB in schizophrenia, see Levaux et al. 2007; Barnett et al. 2010) and OCD (reviewed in Fineberg et al. 2010) have been subject to considerable study using tests derived from the CANTAB and found to be impaired in several domains, implying this battery has utility in evaluating these patient groups (Patel et al. 2010; Table 7.1).

Table 7.1 Neuropsychological performance in schizophrenia and OCD on CANTAB tasks

	Schizophrenia vs control		OCD vs control	
Task	Author	Deficits	Author	Deficits
ID–ED	Elliott et al. (1998)	More perseverative errors	Veale et al. (1996)	More failures at each stage
	Pantelis et al. (1999)	More errors at ID and ED shift	Purcell et al. (1998a)	IDS lower score
	Shamay-Tsoory et al. (2007)	More trials to reach criterion at ID reversal, ED shift and ED reversal	Chamberlain et al. (2006)	More trials to reach criterion on ED shift trials
	Joyce et al. (2002)	75 % of patients were unable to perform an extra-dimensional shift	Purcell et al. (1998b)	No difference on IDS and EDS trial scores
	Hutton et al. (1998)	First-episode schizophrenia patients had intact ability to switch attention	Nielen et al. (2003)	Require the same number of trials to complete the task, no difference in ID or ED errors
	Tyson et al. (2004)	Fewer stages reached, more errors up to ED shift and at ED shift	Watkins et al. (2005)	More errors at ED stage, more patients failed to complete all stages
	Jazbec et al. (2007)	Selective difficulties on C_D and EDS stages	Fenger et al. (2005)	Deficit in shifting attention, reversing response, performed more poorly on IDS and EDS trials
	Braw et al. (2008)	More errors, fewer stages completed	Chamberlain et al. (2007b)	More trials to reach criterion on ED shift trials
	Elliott et al. (1998)	More errors, more perseverative errors on ED and ID shift	Patel et al. (2010)	Marginally significant difference showing more errors in OCD patients for EDS stage
	Ceaser et al. (2008)	More errors across all stages ID–ED; not shared with unaffected first-degree relatives		
	Yun et al. (2011)	More errors in acute schizophrenia, compared to remitted patients		

SOC	Pantelis et al. (1997)	More moves, fewer perfect solutions, longer to execute, longer subsequent thinking time	Veale et al. (1996)	Longer generating solutions, more errors at each stage
	Hutton et al. (1998)			
	Elliott et al. (1998)	Fewer correct on higher move problems	Purcell et al. (1998a, b)	Longer initial movement time, longer subsequent movement time
	Joyce et al. (2002)	More failures at ED stage, reached lower stages	Watkins et al. (2005)	One-touch TOL found intact planning ability
	Tyson et al. (2004)	Solved fewer minimum move problems	Purcell et al. (1998b)	Longer, initial and subsequent movement times
	Braw et al. (2008)	Longer initial thinking times, longer subsequent thinking times, solved fewer problems in minimum moves	Chamberlain et al. (2006b)	Lower strategy scores, generated fewer novel sequences after training
			Pantelis et al. (1997)	Fewer perfect solutions, required more moves for completion, slower movement times and slower subsequent thinking latencies
			Nielen and Den Boer (2003)	Fewer minimum move solutions, longer subsequent thinking time and longer time spent initiating and completing one sequence
			Van del Heuvel et al. (2005)	More time generating alternative strategies following an incorrect move on the same task
			Patel et al. (2010)	No significant difference
CGT	Hutton et al. (1998)	Fewer perfect solutions, total solutions and more moves per solution	Watkins et al. (2005)	Unimpaired on choosing the most likely outcome and OCD did not influence bet size or latency
	Hutton et al. (2002)	Longer decision-making latencies, poorer quality of decision-making in chronic schizophrenia	Chamberlain et al. (2007a)	No difference on percentage of rational decisions made or percentage of points gambled
			Patel et al. (2010)	No difference was found
AGN	No studies to date		Chamberlain et al. (2007a)	More omission errors for sad words
			Watkins et al. (2005)	More false-positive errors following switch
			Patel et al. (2010)	No difference was found

Adapted from Patel et al. (2010). Cambridge University Press. Reproduced with kind permission of Cambridge University Press

ID–ED intra-dimensional–extra-dimensional set-shift task, *SOC* Stockings of Cambridge task, *CGT* Cambridge Gamble Task, *AGN* Affective Go/No-Go task

Patel et al. (2010) used tasks derived from the CANTAB to compare the performance of a group of clozapine-treated patients with schizophrenia alone to a group of IQ, symptom-severity and treatment-matched patients with schizo–OCD derived from the same clinical service. Patients were administered four domain-specific tests (see below), two of which were fronto-striatal tasks, derived from the CANTAB schizophrenia battery and chosen to evaluate executive functioning known to be affected in schizophrenia and OCD (*Intra-dimensional–Extra-dimensional Set-Shift*, *Stockings of Cambridge*). The additional tasks (*Cambridge Gamble Task*, *Affective Go/No-Go task*) measure aspects of motivational function and emotional processing, respectively, and tap ventral and medial–prefrontal (including orbitofrontal) areas of the cortex and the limbic and subcortical connections with this region. A detailed description of the tasks, rationale and results are provided below.

7.2.2.1 Intra- and Extra-Dimensional Set-Shift Task

The intra- and extra-dimensional (ID–ED) phases of the ID–ED set-shift test assess reversal learning and set-shifting, respectively. In humans, the former task is thought to depend upon the integrity of orbitofrontal neurocircuitry and the latter on ventrolateral prefrontal cortex circuits (Hampshire and Owen 2006). During the conceptually crucial extra-dimensional shift (EDS) stage, divergent thinking is required in order to shift attention away from a previously correct stimulus dimension to a novel (previously irrelevant) one. The total number of errors on the ID–ED and the number of errors at the EDS stage are used as the principal measures of attentional set-shifting (see Fig. 7.1).

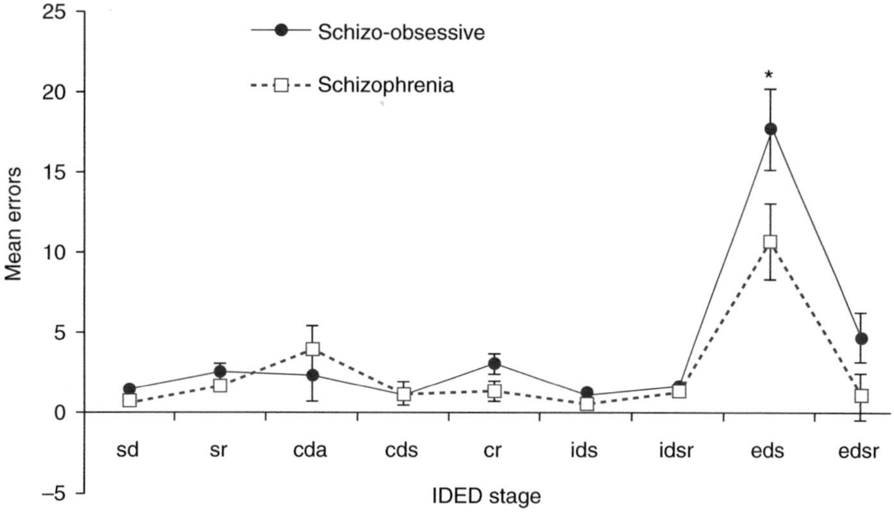

Fig. 7.1 Mean error at each stage of the intra-dimensional–extra-dimensional set-shift task, comparing schizophrenia with OCD ($n=12$) and schizophrenia ($n=16$) (Adapted from Patel et al. (2010). Cambridge University Press. Reproduced with kind permission of Cambridge University Press). *SD* simple discrimination, *SR* simple reversal, *CDA* compound discrimination adjacent, *CDS* compound discrimination superimposed, *CR* compound reversal, *IDS* intra-dimensional shift, *IDSR* intra-dimensional shift reversal, *EDS* extra-dimensional shift, *EDSR* extra-dimensional shift reversal, *SE* error bars

Compared with healthy controls, patients with schizophrenia exhibit significant deficits that include high levels of perseverative error on both elements of the task (Ceaser et al. 2008; Elliott et al. 1998; Tyson et al. 2004). Yun et al. (2011) showed that patients with non-remitted schizophrenia produced a significantly greater number of errors that occurred before the EDS (i.e. pre-ED errors) on this task, compared to remitted patients with schizophrenia and healthy controls (F=5.6, p=0.005). Interestingly, differences in the pre-ED errors and total adjusted errors on the ID–ED task became insignificant when scores on the Beck Anxiety Inventory were entered as the covariate, whereas other significant differences (e.g. stop signal reaction time and lower intelligence by WAIS) remained constant when these scores were entered, suggesting they reflect 'state' symptom severity and strengthening the importance of matching illness severity across schizophrenia groups when testing for set-shifting deficits. Importantly, in the study by Ceaser et al. (2008), the set-shift deficit seen in schizophrenia patients was not shared by unaffected relatives, again suggesting that this impairment represents the effect of illness state on performance and not an intermediate phenotype (endophenotype) of schizophrenia. In contrast, patients with OCD and their first-degree relatives show robust performance deficits, restricted to the EDS stage of the task (see Table 7.1) (Chamberlain et al. 2006a, 2007a; Veale et al. 1996; Watkins et al. 2005). Taken together, these results suggest that unlike in schizophrenia, in OCD, the cognitive inflexibility associated with EDS impairment represents a neurocognitive endophenotype.

Figure 7.1 shows the mean number of errors (and the standard error) at each stage of the ID–ED task in the study by Patel et al. (2010). Inspection of ID–ED errors at different task stages showed patients with schizophrenia and comorbid OCD separated from matched controls with schizophrenia at the two most difficult stages of attentional set-shift, i.e. EDS (extra-dimensional shift), in which the relevant stimulus dimension alters, and EDS reversal, in which a rule learnt needs to be inhibited and reversed. Although the error bars separated, when the correction for multiple comparisons was applied, the result for the EDS was marginally significant ($F_{(1,26)}=4.03, p=.05$). However, there was no significant difference between the number of errors on the extra-dimensional shift reversal (EDSR) stage between the two groups ($F_{(1,26)}=2.96, p=0.09$). The EDS stage is the critical stage of the ID/ED and is thought to represent the category shift in the Wisconsin Card Sorting Test (Downes et al. 1989). The number of errors made at this stage represents attentional set-shifting ability. There was no evident relationship between ED impairment and schizophrenia or OCD symptom severity, and the deficits in those with schizo–OCD were present despite treatment with SSRI in 74 % of cases, implying trait rather than state-marker status and hinting that the EDS abnormality holds endophenotype status (see below).

7.2.2.2 Stockings of Cambridge (SOC)

The SOC assesses spatial planning and motor control. The task involves placing balls in sockets to match a given pattern within a specified number of moves. A low score on the measure 'number of problems solved in minimum moves' reflects inability to plan ahead. This task is thought to involve the dorsolateral prefrontal cortex and its subcortical connections in the dorsal striatum.

Patients with schizophrenia typically make fewer correct solutions and require more moves on the SOC task (see Table 7.1) (Braw et al. 2008; Elliott et al. 1998; Hutton et al. 1998; Pantelis et al. 1997; Tyson et al. 2004). In contrast, Purcell et al. (1998a, b) found that compared with controls, OCD patients spent more time engaged in movements on the SOC test, suggesting motor initiation and execution problems, but they showed no increase in thinking latencies nor increased error rates. Veale and colleagues (1996) reported that patients with OCD spend more time generating alternative strategies following an incorrect move on the same task. Similarly, Chamberlain et al. (2007a) found OCD patients made more attempts to correct a solution on the SOC task. A functional MRI study in patients with OCD using a version of the SOC found poorer planning, which was associated with decreased dorsolateral prefrontal cortex and caudate nucleus activity when compared with controls (van den Heuvel et al. 2005). However, no significant difference was found in performance of the SOC task when patients with schizophrenia and schizophrenia plus OCD were compared (Patel et al. 2010; $p=0.14$), though the latter group showed poorer performance on this task.

7.2.2.3 Cambridge Gamble Task (CGT)

This task assesses impulse control, risk-taking and decision-making and is sensitive to the integrity of orbitofrontal neurocircuitry (Murphy et al. 2001; Rahman et al. 1999; Rogers et al. 1999). The participant is presented with a row of boxes, some of which are coloured red and others blue. Participants start by guessing whether a token is hidden in a red or blue box. In the gambling stages, subjects are given 100 points and can place a bet on the location of the token (either rising or falling offers) based on their confidence. The ratio of red to blue boxes is manipulated to present different levels of uncertainty of winning, and the aim is to accumulate as many points as possible. A higher score on the CGT risk-taking measure is indicative of more risk-taking. The task also measures the average latency to make a decision when placing bets.

Patients with schizophrenia showed longer decision-making latencies and poorer decision-making compared with healthy controls (Table 7.1; Hutton et al. 2002). Unlike patients with schizophrenia, however, studies in individuals with OCD do not usually demonstrate abnormal performance on the CGT (Chamberlain et al. 2007a; Watkins et al. 2005). In the study by Patel et al. (2010), no difference in CGT task performance was found between patients with schizophrenia with or without OCD (Table 7.1). Interestingly, however, in the schizo–OCD group, correlational analysis revealed that an increased severity of motor tic positively correlated with CGT decision latency ($r=0.65$, $n=11$, $p=0.03$) (for further discussion, see later).

7.2.2.4 Affective Go/No-Go Task (AGN)

The AGN assesses information-processing biases for positive and negative stimuli and response inhibition (Murphy et al. 1999) and is sensitive to mood and orbitofrontal cortex function (Barnett et al. 2010). A series of words, either positive, negative or neutral, are rapidly presented. The participant is given a target category, e.g. negative, and is asked to respond whenever they see a word that matches the category. The AGN total omissions (e.g. failure to respond to sad words in sad word blocks) measure affective bias, whereas the total commissions measure response inhibition, where more errors would be indicative of motor impulsivity, i.e. an inability to inhibit motoric responses. Before the study by Patel and colleagues (2010), we are not aware of studies that used the AGN task in patients with schizophrenia. In contrast, patients with OCD are known to make more omission errors for sad words than matched controls, suggesting a selective attentional bias toward negative stimuli (Chamberlain et al. 2007a; Watkins et al. 2005). In the study by Patel et al. (2010), no significant difference was found between schizophrenia with and without OCD. Therefore, taking these results together with the CGT data, no between-group difference in performance appears to exist on tasks thought to probe ventral cortico-striatal circuitry function (GGT and AGN).

7.2.2.5 Other Potential Sources of Confound

Depressive symptoms are known to impair cognition and may confound interpretation of neurocognitive data. In the study by Patel and colleagues (2010), no correlation was found between level of impairment and OCD or depressive symptoms, consistent with neurocognitive impairment holding trait rather than state-marker status. Tic may represent another potential source of confound. In the same study, patients with schizo–OCD exhibited a trend toward increased motor tic, emphasising a neurological contribution to schizo–OCD ($M=9.92$, $SD=15.08$, $p=0.04$). Furthermore, motor tic was related to longer decision latency on the CGT. This single significant correlation might simply reflect a chance finding. However, considering the results from the study by Watkins et al. (2005), in which patients with Tourette's syndrome showed greater impairment on decision-making tasks, compared with OCD and normal controls, such a result may implicate longer decision latency on the CGT as a neurocognitive marker related to the presence of motor tic.

7.3 Neurocognitive Endophenotypes in Schizo–OCD

Patients with schizo–OCD appear to exhibit significantly greater impairment in executive function compared to patients with schizophrenia, and this dysfunction is particularly apparent in tests of cognitive flexibility such as the category shift of the WCST and the EDS of the ID–ED task. The specific EDS deficit found in the small study by Patel et al. (2010) merits further validation, as all patients were antipsychotic resistant and were taking clozapine. Therefore, the result cannot necessarily be generalised to all cases of schizophrenia.

Evidence from studies in unaffected first-degree relatives of tic-free OCD patients with predominantly washing and checking rituals suggests that EDS impairment may represent a neurocognitive endophenotype (Chamberlain et al. 2006a, 2007b). In the study by Chamberlain et al. (2007b), non-affected relatives of OCD probands exhibited the abnormality in EDS impairment, which was unrelated to symptom severity and endured despite treatment, suggesting EDS represents a trait marker (familial vulnerability marker, unrelated to state illness or medication confounds) reflecting genetic vulnerability to OCD. Chamberlain et al. (2007b) proposed that the inability to shift attentional focus may result in functional cognitive inflexibility and contribute to the generation of compulsive symptoms.

Furthermore, EDS deficits are found to occur across a range of compulsive disorders and may underpin the generation of compulsive symptoms across traditional diagnostic groupings. For example, impaired EDS has been identified in patients with obsessive–compulsive personality disorder (Fineberg et al. 2007) and body dysmorphic disorder (Jefferies et al. 2012; Labuschagne et al. 2013). We may therefore extend this hypothesis to propose EDS cognitive inflexibility as a candidate endophenotype for schizo–OCD; replication of this result in the unaffected relatives of patients with schizo–OCD would indicate (a) that this association is not merely state related and (b) that there may be a shared genetic vulnerability for both schizophrenia and OCD in this grouping (Poyurovsky and Koran 2005). Further support could therefore be derived from further investigation of the non-affected first-degree relatives of patients with schizo–OCD. So far, the only study to investigate cognitive inflexibility in the unaffected relatives of patients with psychosis used a set-shift task (Response Shifting Task) that was unable to discriminate the psychotic patients with OCD from those without (Meijer et al. 2013). However, regression analysis indicated that in the unaffected parents, the severity of subclinical OCSs (Y-BOCS score) was significantly correlated with poorer set-shifting ability (based on Response Shifting Task accuracy), although the effect size was small ($d'=-0.10$). Thus, in individuals with increased vulnerability to psychosis, there is some weak evidence that impaired set-shift performance may be associated with the presence of OCS.

The evidence of trans-diagnostic impairment in cognitive flexibility that characterises a range of compulsive disorders and that may extend to schizo–OCD suggests that in schizo–OCD, a form of 'true' overlap exists (rather than schizo–OCD representing a subset of schizophrenia or an artefact of treatment). This raises further important questions, such as: What is the mediating neurobiology? Are there treatment implications? Could a wider range of tests identify additional behavioural features unique to schizo–OCD?

7.4 Probing the Mediating Neuropsychology and Treatment Implications

According to studies using fMRI in healthy subjects, 'cognitive flexibility' or 'cognitive inhibition' as measured by EDS performance is selectively associated with activation in the circuits connecting the bilateral ventrolateral prefrontal cortex with subcortical structures (Hampshire and Owen 2006). Using another task-switching fMRI activation paradigm, Gu and colleagues (2008) investigated a group of 21 patients with OCD compared with 21 healthy subjects of matching age, IQ and sex. In the healthy subjects, the task-switch produced activation in widespread networks both in cortical and subcortical brain regions including the fronto-striatal circuit, which was reduced significantly in OCD patients during the same task. Significant between-group differences were also observed in the ventromedial prefrontal and right orbitofrontal cortices. According to the authors, these findings provide neural correlates related to a task-switching deficit in OCD and suggest that impaired task-switching ability in OCD might be associated with an imbalance in brain activation between dorsal and ventral fronto-striatal circuits (Gu et al. 2008). However, compared with the healthy subjects, patients with OCD exhibited a significantly higher error rate in task-switch trials ($p<0.05$), which may have introduced a source of confound in the imaging results. Indeed, correlational analysis indicated that the activation of orbitofrontal cortex was related to task performance in both groups and also with the activation of anterior cingulate cortex in the OCD group.

While fMRI has localised certain brain regions involved in set-shifting, it does not capture the millisecond timing of neurocognitive processes. Magneto-encephalography (MEG) is a modality that provides improved temporal resolution for examining the timing of activations across brain regions during cognitive tasks. A recent study (Oh et al. 2014) that explored the location and timing of frontal and parietal activations during an ID–ED task found that activations related to EDS were detected in left inferior frontal gyrus, left middle frontal gyrus and right middle frontal gyrus between 100 and 350 ms, followed by superior frontal gyrus between 250 and 500 ms. EDS also activated right parietal areas – areas previously implicated in OCD (Chamberlain et al. 2008; Oh et al. 2014).

Pharmacological probe work in healthy volunteers suggests that the EDS can be modulated by compounds with dopamine receptor antagonist effects (Mehta et al. 1999). Patients with schizo–OCD are usually receiving treatment with dopamine antagonist agents, which therefore may contribute toward this problem. Multiple lines of evidence also implicate glutamate signalling in the dorsal striatum as a mechanism for regulating behavioural flexibility. Animal research implicates interaction between the striatal metabotropic glutamate receptor (mGlu5R) and the ionotropic N-methyl-D-aspartate receptor (NMDAR) in modulating aspects of cognitive flexibility in instrumental learning, based on the contingency-dependent attribution of goal-directed versus habitual activity (Lovinger 2010). Modulation of the mGlu5R in rats using a selective positive allosteric modulator has been shown to produce beneficial effects in the treatment of perseverative and set-shifting deficits (Gastambide et al. 2012). In another study, modafinil, a central nervous system wakefulness-promoting agent, was found to remediate the EDS decrement in patients with schizophrenia (Turner et al. 2004). The mode of action of modafinil remains somewhat unclear, but its cognitive-enhancing properties might result from glutamatergic and/or dopaminergic increased neuronal activation in the hippocampus and in the prefrontal cortex, respectively (Scoriels et al. 2012). Investigation of new treatment targets, such as the pharmacological manipulation of dopamine, NMDAR or mGluR function in disease states, might be of particular relevance in remediating cognitive inflexibility in schizo–OCD and the associated severe executive dysfunction associated with the disorder.

Cognitive inflexibility negatively impacts upon evidence-based treatment for compulsive disorder such as CBT and may partly explain the relatively treatment-resistant nature of schizo–OCD (reviewed in Mukhopadhaya et al. 2009; Schirmbeck and Zink 2012). Often, it is the compulsive symptoms themselves that become the most intransigent and impairing problem for patients with schizo–OCD (see our vignette). New treatments targeting cognitive inflexibility are under investigation in compulsive disorders such as OCD and eating disorder and have yielded promise of efficacy in small trials, with potential to improve treatment outcomes. These include psychological (cognitive remediation therapy (CRT)) and brain stimulation strategies (repetitive transcranial magnetic stimulation (rTMS)).

CRT has been developed for and tested in eating disorder, targets set-shifting, helps patients adopt flexible behaviour strategies, increases motivation and perceived ability to change and enhances success when combined with usual forms of treatment. Two small-scale trials in OCD employing CRT were effective in improving compulsive symptoms as well as executive skills and cognitive flexibility, respectively (Buhlmann et al. 2006; Park et al. 2006). A recent randomised controlled trial (RCT) in eating disorder showed individual CRT given with CBT improved quality of life and dropout rates compared with CBT alone. Poor baseline EDS predicted a better response to CRT (Dingemans et al. 2014). These results strongly suggest that individual CRT may be a beneficial adjunct to usual treatment in other compulsive disorders characterised by cognitive inflexibility, such as schizo–OCD.

Repetitive (r)TMS has produced variable results in compulsivity. In OCD, rTMS of the dorsolateral PFC was not found to be effective, though two small RCTs have reported promising results for low-frequency rTMS applied to the pre-supplementary motor area and the orbitofrontal cortex, respectively (Jaafari et al. 2012). Better targeting of fronto-striatal neurocircuitry, using coils that can induce stimulation in deeper brain areas, higher stimulus intensities and longer treatment course (3–6 weeks), has been suggested as a means to improve therapeutic outcome. Consequently, TMS studies using deep H-coils are ongoing in several disorders of compulsivity and are starting to produce positive results for OCD and addiction (Carmi et al. 2013; Dinur-Klein et al. 2014). There would be grounds to consider the future investigation of rTMS or deep TMS as an adjunct to usual treatment in patients with schizo–OCD.

7.5 Dissecting Motor and Spatial Activity in Schizophrenia and OCD

Aside from traditional laboratory-based neurocognitive tests, a recent innovative study used motor tracking computer software to investigate the motor behaviour of patients with schizophrenia comorbid with OCD and patients with OCD in their natural environment, e.g. at home (Gershoni et al. 2014). The study compared the performance of the patient with the performance of the same motor task by a matching control individual. The motor behaviour in patients with schizo–OCD and OCD differed from that of controls in terms of excessive repetition and addition of superfluous acts, thus validating a similar obsessive–compulsive behavioural facet. There was, however, an additional significant between-patient group difference in the spatial organisation of the behaviour. Patients with schizo–OCD travelled around with less focused activity, as is typical for schizophrenia and in contrast to the OCD

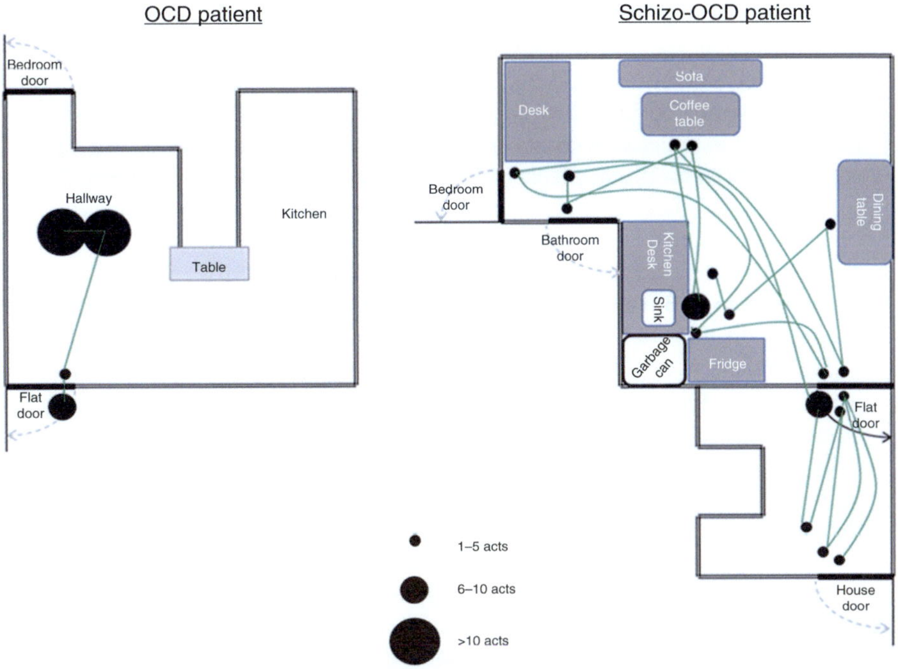

Fig. 7.2 Trajectories and acts; comparing exemplar patients with OCD and schizo–OCD, each performing the motor task of 'going out of the home' (Adapted from Gershoni et al. (2014). Cambridge University Press. Reproduced with kind permission of Cambridge University Press) The location of each *circle* represents a location/object. The *size of the circle* represents the number of acts that took place at that location/object. The *green line* represents the trajectories of each individual between the locations

group, who were more focused and travelled less distance within a confined area (Fig. 7.2). Thus, whilst patient with schizo–OCD and OCD may share many ritualistic attributes, they also differ, inasmuch as there is a greater spread of activity in schizo–OCD. Considering that behaviour is a direct manifestation of brain activity, the authors suggested that the focused and confined activity in OCD compared with the divergent activity over a large area in schizo–OCD is a reflection of the focused attention in the former and the continuously shifting attention in the latter. In other words, the attentional deficit in schizo–OCD is an overt schizophrenia feature that overrides the narrow focussed repetition of acts in OCD.

Conclusion

A recent meta-analysis of 43 studies (Swets et al. 2014) estimates around 13 % of patients with schizophrenia meet the diagnostic threshold for OCD, while a higher proportion (around 31 %) display obsessive or compulsive symptoms (OCSs). Whereas schizophrenia is associated with global impairment in a wide range of neurocognitive domains, schizo–OCD may be associated with additional executive deficits (neurocognitive double jeopardy) featuring impaired performance on specific executive tasks, notably tasks measuring attentional set-shifting and cognitive flexibility and likely to involve fronto-striatal neurocircuitry known to be linked to OCD (Patel et al. 2010). Furthermore, the EDS impairment associated with schizo–OCD resembles that reported for 'archetypal' OCD (washers and checkers without tic) (Chamberlain et al. 2006a, 2007a, b), as well as other compulsive disorders, e.g. body dysmorphic disorder and obsessive–compulsive personality disorder. In other words, the EDS deficit appears to reflect a trans-diagnostic aspect of 'compulsivity'. Such an overlap has important implications for understanding the neurobiology of this complex, disabling disorder and generating new candidate pharmacological and psychological treatment targets.

Whereas neurocognitive profiling suggests a simple overlap between OCD compulsions and schizophrenia, other behavioural tests (e.g. Gershoni et al. 2014) imply a separate pathology for schizo–OCD. Therefore, whilst patients with schizo–OCD and OCD share most OC ritualistic attributes, they differ in the greater spread of activity in schizo–OCD. The behavioural differences imply a separate phenotype for the compulsions of schizo–OCD. This finding questions the simple 'overlap' model and suggests an added and previously unrecognised degree of complexity. The behavioural difference represents an easily evaluable clinical sign that could contribute toward an improved nosological classification of a range of OC spectrum disorders.

Looking ahead, prospective, longitudinal studies investigating cognitive and behavioural changes in patients with at-risk and prodromal mental states could be expected to help decipher the interaction between neurocognitive impairment and the clinical manifestation of schizophrenia and OC syndromes as they develop. This, in turn, could facilitate the definition of patients at high risk for developing schizo–OCD, an early detection of subclinical disorder, therapeutic intervention and clinical monitoring.

Chapter Summary

1. Schizo–OCD (schizophrenia co-occurring with OCD) represents a relatively common and severely impairing illness that remains undiagnosed in around 50 % of cases.
2. The key neuropsychological mechanisms underpinning schizo–OCD are not completely understood.
3. Research shows impaired cognitive flexibility in patients with schizo–OCD, manifested as poor performance on set-shift tasks, and implies an area of neurocognitive overlap between schizophrenia and OCD.
4. Poor set-shifting characterises OCD and a range of other compulsive disorders and may represent a neurocognitive endophenotype of compulsivity.
5. The rituals of schizo–OCD differ from those of 'pure' OCD on behavioural analysis and may represent a pathognomonic sign of this disorder.

References

Achim AM, Maziade M, Raymond E, Olivier D, Mérette C, Roy MA (2011) How prevalent are anxiety disorders in schizophrenia? A meta-analysis and critical review on a significant association. Schizophr Bull 37(4):811–821

Aoyama F, Iida J, Inoue M, Iwasaka H, Sakiyama S, Hata K, Kishimoto T (2000) Brain imaging in childhood- and adolescence-onset schizophrenia associated with obsessive-compulsive symptoms. Acta Psychiatr Scand 102(1):32–37

Barnett JH, Robbins TW, Leeson VC, Sahakian BJ, Joyce EM, Blackwell AD (2010) Assessing cognitive function in clinical trials of schizophrenia. Neurosci Biobehav Rev 34(8):1161–1177. doi:10.1016/j.neubiorev.2010.01.012

Berman I, Kalinowski A, Berman SM, Lengua J, Green AI (1995) Obsessive and compulsive symptoms in chronic schizophrenia. Compr Psychiatry 36(1):6–10

Berman I, Merson A, Viegner B, Losonczy MF, Pappas D, Green AI (1998) Obsessions and compulsions as a distinct cluster of symptoms in schizophrenia: a neuropsychological study. J Nerv Ment Dis 186(3):150–156

Bland RC, Newman SC, Orn H (1987) Schizophrenia: lifetime co-morbidity in a community sample. Acta Psychiatr Scand 75(4):383–391

Bleich-Cohen M, Hendler T, Weizman R, Faragian S, Weizman A, Poyurovsky M (2014) Working memory dysfunction in schizophrenia patients with obsessive-compulsive symptoms: an fMRI study. Eur Psychiatry 29(3):160–166. http://dx.doi.org/10.1016/j.eurpsy.2013.02.004

Bokat CE, Goldberg TE (2003) Letter and category fluency in schizophrenic patients: a meta-analysis. Schizophr Res 64(1):73–78

Bottas A, Cooke RG, Richter MA (2005) Comorbidity and pathophysiology of obsessive-compulsive disorder in schizophrenia: is there evidence for a schizo-obsessive subtype of schizophrenia? J Psychiatry Neurosci 30(3):187–193

Braw Y, Bloch Y, Mendelovich S, Ratzoni G, Gal G, Harari H, Levkovitz Y (2008) Cognition in young schizophrenia outpatients: comparison of first-episode with multiepisode patients. Schizophr Bull 34(3):544–554. doi:10.1093/schbul/sbm115

Buchanan RW, Ball MP, Weiner E, Kirkpatrick B, Gold JM, McMahon RP, Carpenter WT Jr (2005) Olanzapine treatment of residual positive and negative symptoms. Am J Psychiatry 162(1):124–129. doi:10.1176/appi.ajp.162.1.124

Buckley PF, Miller BJ, Lehrer DS, Castle DJ (2009) Psychiatric comorbidities and schizophrenia. Schizophr Bull 35(2):383–402. doi:10.1093/schbul/sbn135

Buhlmann U, Deckersbach T, Engelhard I, Cook LM, Rauch SL, Kathmann N, Savage CR (2006) Cognitive retraining for organizational impairment in obsessive-compulsive disorder. Psychiatry Res 144(2–3):109–116. doi:10.1016/j.psychres.2005.10.012

Carmi L, Alyagon U, Zangen A, Dar R, Zohar J (2013) General error monitoring system dysfunction in obsessive compulsive disorder patients: an event-related potential study. Poster abstract. European College of Neuropsychopharmacology, Spain

Ceaser AE, Goldberg TE, Egan MF, McMahon RP, Weinberger DR, Gold JM (2008) Set-shifting ability and schizophrenia: a marker of clinical illness or an intermediate phenotype? Biol Psychiatry 64(9):782–788. doi:10.1016/j.biopsych.2008.05.009

Chamberlain SR, Blackwell AD, Fineberg NA, Robbins TW, Sahakian BJ (2005) The neuropsychology of obsessive compulsive disorder: the importance of failures in cognitive and behavioural inhibition as candidate endophenotypic markers. Neurosci Biobehav Rev 29(3):399–419

Chamberlain SR, Fineberg NA, Blackwell AD, Robbins TW, Sahakian BJ (2006a) Motor inhibition and cognitive flexibility in obsessive-compulsive disorder and trichotillomania. Am J Psychiatry 163(7):1282–1284

Chamberlain SR, Blackwell AD, Fineberg NA, Robbins TR, Sahakian BJ (2006b) Strategy implementation in obsessive-compulsive disorder and trichotilomania. Psychological Medicine 36: 91–97

Chamberlain SR, Fineberg NA, Blackwell AD, Clark L, Robbins TW, Sahakian BJ (2007a) A neuropsychological comparison of obsessive-compulsive disorder and trichotillomania. Neuropsychologia 45(4):654–662. doi:10.1016/j.neuropsychologia.2006.07.016

Chamberlain SR, Fineberg NA, Menzies LA, Blackwell AD, Bullmore ET, Robbins TW, Sahakian BJ (2007b) Impaired cognitive flexibility and motor inhibition in unaffected first-degree relatives of patients with obsessive-compulsive disorder. Am J Psychiatry 164(2):335–338

Chamberlain SR, Menzies L, Hampshire A, Suckling J, Fineberg NA, del Campo N, Sahakian BJ (2008) Orbitofrontal dysfunction in patients with obsessive-compulsive disorder and their unaffected relatives. Science 321(5887):421–422. doi:10.1126/science.1154433

Cunill R, Huerta-Ramos E, Castells X (2013) The effect of obsessive-compulsive symptomatology on executive functions in schizophrenia: a systematic review and meta-analysis. Psychiatry Res 210(1):21–28. doi:10.1016/j.psychres.2013.05.029

de Haan L, Sterk B, Wouters L, Linszen DH (2011) The 5-year course of obsessive-compulsive symptoms and obsessive-compulsive disorder in first-episode schizophrenia and related disorders. Schizophr Bull. doi:10.1093/schbul/sbr077

Dingemans AE, Danner UN, Donker JM, Aardoom JJ, van Meer F, Tobias K, van Furth EF (2014) The effectiveness of cognitive remediation therapy in patients with a severe or enduring eating disorder: a randomized controlled trial. Psychother Psychosom 83(1):29–36

Dinur-Klein L, Dannon P, Hadar A, Rosenberg O, Roth Y, Kotler M, Zangen A (2014) Smoking cessation induced by deep repetitive transcranial magnetic stimulation of the prefrontal and insular cortices. Biol Psychiatry 76(9):742–749

Downes JJ, Roberts AC, Sahakian BJ, Evenden JL, Morris RG, Robbins TW (1989) Impaired extra-dimensional shift performance in medicated and unmedicated Parkinson's disease: evidence for a specific attentional dysfunction. Neuropsychologia 27(11–12):1329–1343

Elliott R, McKenna PJ, Robbins TW, Sahakian BI (1998) Specific neuropsychological deficits in schizophrenic patients with preserved intellectual function. Cogn Neuropsychiatry 3(1):45–69. doi:10.1080/135468098396242

Ertugrul A, Demir B (2005) Clozapine-induced tardive dyskinesia: a case report. Prog Neuropsychopharmacol Biol Psychiatry 29(4):633–635. doi:10.1016/j.pnpbp.2005.01.014

Fabisch K, Fabisch H, Langs G, Huber HP, Zapotoczky HG (2001) Incidence of obsessive-compulsive phenomena in the course of acute schizophrenia and schizoaffective disorder. Eur Psychiatry 16(6):336–341

Fenger MM, Gade A, Adams KH, Hansen ES, Bolwig TG, Knudsen GM (2005) Cognitive deficits in obsessive-compulsive disorder on tests of frontal lobe functions. Nord J Psychiatry 59(1):39–44. doi:10.1080/08039480510018814

Fenton WS, McGlashan TH (1986) The prognostic significance of obsessive-compulsive symptoms in schizophrenia. Am J Psychiatry 143(4):437–441

Fineberg NA, Sharma P, Sivakumaran T, Sahakian B, Chamberlain SR (2007) Does obsessive-compulsive personality disorder belong within the obsessive-compulsive spectrum? CNS Spectr 12(6):467–482

Fineberg NA, Potenza MN, Chamberlain SR, Berlin HA, Menzies L, Bechara A, Hollander E (2010) Probing compulsive and impulsive behaviors, from animal models to endophenotypes: a narrative review. Neuropsychopharmacology 35(3):591–604. doi:10.1038/npp.2009.185

Fioravanti M, Carlone O, Vitale B, Cinti M, Clare L (2005) A meta-analysis of cognitive deficits in adults with a diagnosis of schizophrenia. Neuropsychol Rev 15(2):73–95. doi:10.1007/s11065-005-6254-9

Gastambide F, Cotel MC, Gilmour G, O'Neill MJ, Robbins TW, Tricklebank MD (2012) Selective remediation of reversal learning deficits in the neurodevelopmental MAM model of schizophrenia by a novel mGlu5 positive allosteric modulator. Neuropsychopharmacology 37(4):1057–1066

Gershoni A, Hermesh H, Fineberg NA, Eilam D (2014) Spatial behavior reflects the mental disorder in OCD patients with and without comorbid schizophrenia. CNS Spectr 19(1):90–103. doi:10.1017/S1092852913000424

Goldstein JM, Goodman JM, Seidman LJ, Kennedy DN, Makris N, Lee H, Tsuang MT (1999) Cortical abnormalities in schizophrenia identified by structural magnetic resonance imaging. Arch Gen Psychiatry 56(6):537–547

Gu BM, Park JY, Kang DH, Lee SJ, Yoo SY, Jo HJ, Kwon JS (2008) Neural correlates of cognitive inflexibility during task-switching in obsessive-compulsive disorder. Brain 131(Pt 1):155–164. doi:10.1093/brain/awm277

Hampshire A, Owen AM (2006) Fractionating attentional control using event-related fMRI. Cereb Cortex 16(12):1679–1689. doi:10.1093/cercor/bhj116

Heinrichs RW, Zakzanis KK (1998) Neurocognitive deficit in schizophrenia: a quantitative review of the evidence. Neuropsychology 12(3):426–445

Henry JD, Crawford JR (2005) A meta-analytic review of verbal fluency deficits in schizophrenia relative to other neurocognitive deficits. Cogn Neuropsychiatry 10(1):1–33

Hermesh H, Weizman A, Gur S, Zalsman G, Shiloh R, Zohar J, Gross-Isseroff R (2003) Alternation learning in OCD/schizophrenia patients. Eur Neuropsychopharmacol 13(2):87–91

Hutton SB, Puri BK, Duncan LJ, Robbins TW, Barnes TR, Joyce EM (1998) Executive function in first-episode schizophrenia. Psychol Med 28(2):463–473

Hutton SB, Murphy FC, Joyce EM, Rogers RD, Cuthbert I, Barnes TR, Robbins TW (2002) Decision making deficits in patients with first-episode and chronic schizophrenia. Schizophr Res 55(3):249–257

Hwang MY, Morgan JE, Losconzcy MF (2000) Clinical and neuropsychological profiles of obsessive-compulsive schizophrenia: a pilot study. J Neuropsychiatry Clin Neurosci 12(1):91–94

Jaafari N, Rachid F, Rotge JY, Polosan M, El-Hage W, Belin D, Pelissolo A (2012) Safety and efficacy of repetitive transcranial magnetic stimulation in the treatment of obsessive-compulsive disorder: a review. World J Biol Psychiatry 13(3):164–177. doi:10.3109/15622975.2011.575177

Jazbec S, Pantelis C, Robbins T, Weickert T, Weinberger DR, Goldberg TE (2007) Intra-dimensional/extra-dimensional set-shifting performance in schizophrenia: impact of distractors. Schizophr Res 89(1–3):339–349. doi:10.1016/j.schres.2006.08.014

Jefferies K, Laws KR, Fineberg NA (2012) Superior face recognition in body dysmorphic disorder. J Obsess Compuls Rel Disord 1(3):175–179

Johnson-Selfridge M, Zalewski C (2001) Moderator variables of executive functioning in schizophrenia: meta-analytic findings. Schizophr Bull 27(2):305–316

Joyce E, Hutton S, Mutsatsa S, Gibbins H, Webb E, Paul S, Barnes T (2002) Executive dysfunction in first-episode schizophrenia and relationship to duration of untreated psychosis: the West London Study. Br J Psychiatry 181(43):s38–s44. doi:10.1192/bjp.181.43.s38

Kashyap H, Kumar JK, Kandavel T, Reddy YCJ (2013) Neuropsychological functioning in obsessive-compulsive disorder: are executive functions the key deficit? Compr Psychiatry 54(5):533–540

Kayahan B, Ozturk O, Veznedaroglu B, Eraslan D (2005) Obsessive-compulsive symptoms in schizophrenia: prevalence and clinical correlates. Psychiatry Clin Neurosci 59(3):291–295. doi:10.1111/j.1440-1819.2005.01373.x

Kern RS, Nuechterlein KH, Green MF, Baade LE, Fenton WS, Gold JM, Marder SR (2008) The MATRICS consensus cognitive battery, part 2: co-norming and standardization. Am J Psychiatry 165(2):214–220. doi:10.1176/appi.ajp.2007.07010043

Kessler RC, Berglund P, Demler O, Jin R, Merikangas KR, Walters EE (2005) Lifetime prevalence and age-of-onset distributions of dsm-iv disorders in the national comorbidity survey replication. Arch Gen Psychiatry 62(6):593–602. doi:10.1001/archpsyc.62.6.593

Krivoy A, Fischel T, Weizman A (2012) [The cognitive deficit in schizophrenia]. Harefuah 151(5):277–280, 319

Kruger S, Braunig P, Hoffler J, Shugar G, Borner I, Langkrar J (2000) Prevalence of obsessive-compulsive disorder in schizophrenia and significance of motor symptoms. J Neuropsychiatry Clin Neurosci 21:38–42

Labuschagne I, Rossell SL, Dunai J, Castle DJ, Kyrios M (2013) A comparison of executive function in body dysmorphic disorder (BDD) and obsessive-compulsive disorder (OCD). J Obsess Compuls Rel Disord 2(3):257–262. http://dx.doi.org/10.1016/j.jocrd.2013.05.003

Laws KR (1999) A meta-analytic review of Wisconsin Card Sort studies in schizophrenia: general intellectual deficit in disguise? Cogn Neuropsychiatry 4(1):1–30; discussion 31–35. doi:10.1080/135468099396025

Levaux MN, Potvin S, Sepehry AA, Sablier J, Mendrek A, Stip E (2007) Computerized assessment of cognition in schizophrenia: promises and pitfalls of CANTAB. Eur Psychiatry 22(2):104–115. doi:10.1016/j.eurpsy.2006.11.004

Lovinger DM (2010) Neurotransmitter roles in synaptic modulation, plasticity and learning in the dorsal striatum. Neuropharmacology 58(7):951–961. http://dx.doi.org/10.1016/j.neuropharm.2010.01.008

Lysaker PH, Whitney KA (2009) Obsessive–compulsive symptoms in schizophrenia: prevalence, correlates and treatment. Expert Rev Neurother 9(1):99–107. doi:10.1586/14737175.9.1.99

Lysaker PH, Marks KA, Picone JB, Rollins AL, Fastenau PS, Bond GR (2000) Obsessive and compulsive symptoms in schizophrenia: clinical and neurocognitive correlates. J Nerv Ment Dis 188(2):78–83

Lysaker PH, Bryson GJ, Marks KA, Greig TC, Bell MD (2002) Association of obsessions and compulsions in schizophrenia with neurocognition and negative symptoms. J Neuropsychiatry Clin Neurosci 14(4):449–453

Lysaker PH, Lancaster RS, Nees MA, Davis LW (2004) Patterns of obsessive-compulsive symptoms and social function in schizophrenia. Psychiatry Res 125(2):139–146. doi:10.1016/j.psychres.2003.12.007

Ma N, Tan LW, Wang Q, Li ZX, Li LJ (2007) Lower levels of whole blood serotonin in obsessive-compulsive disorder and in schizophrenia with obsessive-compulsive symptoms. Psychiatry Res 150(1):61–69. doi:10.1016/j.psychres.2005.10.005

Mehta MA, Sahakian BJ, McKenna PJ, Robbins TW (1999) Systemic sulpiride in young adult volunteers simulates the profile of cognitive deficits in Parkinson's disease. Psychopharmacology (Berl) 146(2):162–174

Meijer J, Simons CJ Fau, Quee PJ, Quee PJ Fau, Verweij K, Verweij K (2012) Cognitive alterations in patients with non-affective psychotic disorder and their unaffected siblings and parents. Acta Psychiatrica Scandinavica 215(1):66–76

Meijer JH, Swets M, Keeman S, Nieman DH, Meijer CJ (2013) Is a schizo-obsessive subtype associated with cognitive impairment? Results from a large cross-sectional study in patients with psychosis and their unaffected relatives. J Nerv Ment Dis 201:30–35 (1539-736X (Electronic))

Melcher T, Falkai P, Gruber O (2008) Functional brain abnormalities in psychiatric disorders: Neural mechanisms to detect and resolve cognitive conflict and interference. Brain Research Reviews 59(1):96–124

Menzies L, Chamberlain SR, Laird AR, Thelen SM, Sahakian BJ, Bullmore ET (2008) Integrating evidence from neuroimaging and neuropsychological studies of obsessive-compulsive disorder: the orbitofronto-striatal model revisited. Neurosci Biobehav Rev 32(3):525–549. http://dx.doi.org/10.1016/j.neubiorev.2007.09.005

Mesholam-Gately RI, Giuliano AJ, Goff KP, Faraone SV, Seidman LJ (2009) Neurocognition in first-episode schizophrenia: a meta-analytic review. Neuropsychology 23(3):315–336

Michalopoulou PG, Konstantakopoulos G, Typaldou M, Papageorgiou C, Christodoulou GN, Lykouras L, Oulis P (2014) Can cognitive deficits differentiate between schizophrenia with and without obsessive–compulsive symptoms? Compr Psychiatry 55(4):1015–1021. http://dx.doi.org/10.1016/j.comppsych.2013.12.004

Monchi O, Petrides M, Petre V, Worsley K, Dagher A (2001) Wisconsin Card Sorting revisited: distinct neural circuits participating in different stages of the task identified by event-related functional magnetic resonance imaging. J Neurosci 21(19):7733–7741

Mukhopadhaya K, Krishnaiah R, Taye T, Nigam A, Bailey A, Sivakumaran T, Fineberg N (2009) Obsessive-compulsive disorder in UK clozapine-treated schizophrenia and schizoaffective disorder: a cause for clinical concern. J Psychopharmacol 23(1):6–13. doi:10.1177/0269881108089582

Murphy FC, Sahakian BJ, Rubinsztein JS, Michael A, Rogers RD, Robbins TW, Paykel ES (1999) Emotional bias and inhibitory control processes in mania and depression. Psychol Med 29(6):1307–1321

Murphy FC, Rubinsztein JS, Michael A, Rogers RD, Robbins TW, Paykel ES, Sahakian BJ (2001) Decision-making cognition in mania and depression. Psychol Med 31(4):679–693

Nielen MM, Den Boer JA (2003) Neuropsychological performance of OCD patients before and after treatment with fluoxetine: evidence for persistent cognitive deficits. Psychol Med 33(5):917–925

Nolan KA, Bilder Rm Fau, Lachman HM, Lachman Hm Fau, Volavka J, Volavka J (2004) Catechol O-methyltransferase Val158Met polymorphism in schizophrenia: differential effects of Val and Met alleles on cognitive stability and flexibility. Am J Psychiatry 161(2):359–361

Nuechterlein KH, Green MF, Kern RS, Baade LE, Barch DM, Cohen JD et al (2008) The MATRICS consensus cognitive battery, part 1: test selection, reliability, and validity. Am J Psychiatry 165(2):203–213. doi:10.1176/appi.ajp.2007.07010042

Oh A, Vidal J, Taylor MJ, Pang EW (2014) Neuromagnetic correlates of intra- and extra-dimensional set-shifting. Brain Cogn 86:90–97. doi:10.1016/j.bandc.2014.02.006

Ohta M, Kokai M, Morita Y (2003) Features of obsessive–compulsive disorder in patients primarily diagnosed with schizophrenia. Psychiatry Clin Neurosci 57(1):67–74. doi:10.1046/j.1440-1819.2003.01081.x

Öngür D, Goff DC (2005) Obsessive-compulsive symptoms in schizophrenia: associated clinical features, cognitive function and medication status. Schizophr Res 75(2–3):349–362

Pantelis C, Barber FZ, Barnes TR, Nelson HE, Owen AM, Robbins TR (1999) Comparison of set-shifting ability in patients with chronic schizophrenia and frontal lobe damage. Schizophrenia Research 37:251–270

Pantelis C, Barnes TR, Nelson HE, Tanner S, Weatherley L, Owen AM, Robbins TW (1997) Frontal-striatal cognitive deficits in patients with chronic schizophrenia. Brain 120(Pt 10):1823–1843

Park HS, Shin YW, Ha TH, Shin MS, Kim YY, Lee YH, Kwon JS (2006) Effect of cognitive training focusing on organizational strategies in patients with obsessive-compulsive disorder. Psychiatry Clin Neurosci 60(6):718–726. doi:10.1111/j.1440-1819.2006.01587.x

Patel DD, Laws KR, Padhi A, Farrow JM, Mukhopadhaya K, Krishnaiah R, Fineberg NA (2010) The neuropsychology of the schizo-obsessive subtype of schizophrenia: a new analysis. Psychol Med 40(6):921–933. doi:10.1017/s0033291709991255

Poyurovsky M, Koran LM (2005) Obsessive–compulsive disorder (OCD) with schizotypy vs. schizophrenia with OCD: diagnostic dilemmas and therapeutic implications. J Psychiatr Res 39(4):399–408. http://dx.doi.org/10.1016/j.jpsychires.2004.09.004

Poyurovsky M, Hramenkov S, Isakov V, Rauchverger B, Modai I, Schneidman M et al (2001) Obsessive-compulsive disorder in hospitalized patients with chronic schizophrenia. Psychiatry Res 102(1):49–57

Poyurovsky M, Bergman J, Weizman R (2006) Obsessive-compulsive disorder in elderly schizophrenia patients. J Psychiatr Res 40(3):189–191

Poyurovsky M, Faragian S, Pashinian A, Levi A, Viosburd A, Stryjer R, Weizman A (2007) Neurological soft signs in schizophrenia patients with obsessive-compulsive disorder. J Neuropsychiatry Clin Neurosci 19(2):145–150. doi:10.1176/appi.neuropsych.19.2.145

Purcell R, Maruff P, Kyrios M, Pantelis C (1998a) Cognitive deficits in obsessive-compulsive disorder on tests of frontal-striatal function. Biol Psychiatry 43(5):348–357

Purcell R, Maruff P, Kyrios M, Pantelis C (1998b) Neuropsychological deficits in obsessive-compulsive disorder: a comparison with unipolar depression, panic disorder, and normal controls. Arch Gen Psychiatry 55(5):415–423

Rahman S, Sahakian BJ, Hodges JR, Rogers RD, Robbins TW (1999) Specific cognitive deficits in mild frontal variant frontotemporal dementia. Brain 122(Pt 8):1469–1493

Rajkumar RP, Reddy YCJ, Kandavel T (2008) Clinical profile of "schizo-obsessive" disorder: a comparative study. Compr Psychiatry 49(3):262–268

Rogers RD, Everitt BJ, Baldacchino A, Blackshaw AJ, Swainson R, Wynne K, Robbins TW (1999) Dissociable deficits in the decision-making cognition of chronic amphetamine abusers, opiate abusers, patients with focal damage to prefrontal cortex, and tryptophan-depleted normal volunteers: evidence for monoaminergic mechanisms. Neuropsychopharmacology 20(4):322–339. doi:10.1016/s0893-133x(98)00091-8

Schirmbeck F, Zink M (2012) Clozapine-induced obsessive-compulsive symptoms in schizophrenia: a critical review. Curr Neuropharmacol 10(1):88–95. doi:10.2174/157015912799362724

Schirmbeck F, Rausch F, Englisch S, Eifler S, Esslinger C, Meyer-Lindenberg A, Zink M (2013) Stable cognitive deficits in schizophrenia patients with comorbid obsessive-compulsive symptoms: a 12-month longitudinal study. Schizophr Bull 39(6):1261–1271. doi:10.1093/schbul/sbs123

Scoriels L, Barnett J, Soma P, Sahakian B, Jones P (2012) Effects of modafinil on cognitive functions in first episode psychosis. Psychopharmacology (Berl) 220(2):249–258. doi:10.1007/s00213-011-2472-4

Sevincok L, Akoglu A, Topaloglu B, Aslantas H (2004) Neurological soft signs in schizophrenic patients with obsessive–compulsive disorder. Psychiatry Clin Neurosci 58(3):274–279. doi:10.1111/j.1440-1819.2004.01231.x

Shamay-Tsoory SG, Shur S, Harari H, Lekovitz Y (2007) Neurocognitive basis of impaired empathy in schizophrenia. Neuropsychology 21:431–438

Swets M, Dekker J, van Emmerik-van Oortmerssen K, Smid GE, Smit F, de Haan L, Schoevers RA (2014) The obsessive compulsive spectrum in schizophrenia, a meta-analysis and meta-regression exploring prevalence rates. Schizophrenia Res 152(2–3):458–468. http://dx.doi.org/10.1016/j.schres.2013.10.033

Tibbo P, Warneke L (1999) Obsessive-compulsive disorder in schizophrenia: epidemiologic and biologic overlap. J Psychiatry Neurosci 24(1):15–24

Tibbo P, Kroetsch M, Chue P, Warneke L (2000) Obsessive-compulsive disorder in schizophrenia. J Psychiatr Res 34(2):139–146

Turner DC, Clark L Fau, Pomarol-Clotet E, Pomarol-Clotet E Fau, McKenna P, McKenna P Fau, Robbins TW, Robbins Tw Fau, Sahakian BJ, Sahakian BJ (2004) Modafinil improves cognition and attentional set shifting in patients with chronic schizophrenia. Neuropsychopharmacology 21(7):1363–1373

Tyson PJ, Laws KR, Roberts KH, Mortimer AM (2004) Stability of set-shifting and planning abilities in patients with schizophrenia. Psychiatry Res 129(3):229–239

van den Heuvel OA, Veltman DJ, Groenewegen HJ, Cath DC, van Balkom AJ, van Hartskamp J, van Dyck R (2005) Frontal-striatal dysfunction during planning in obsessive-compulsive disorder. Arch Gen Psychiatry 62(3):301–309. doi:10.1001/archpsyc.62.3.301

Veale DM, Sahakian BJ, Owen AM, Marks IM (1996) Specific cognitive deficits in tests sensitive to frontal lobe dysfunction in obsessive-compulsive disorder. Psychol Med 26(6):1261–1269

Watkins LH, Sahakian BJ, Robertson MM, Veale DM, Rogers RD, Pickard KM, Robbins TW (2005) Executive function in Tourette's syndrome and obsessive-compulsive disorder. Psychol Med 35(4):571–582

Whitney KA, Fastenau PS, Evans JD, Lysaker PH (2004) Comparative neuropsychological function in obsessive-compulsive disorder and schizophrenia with and without obsessive-compulsive symptoms. Schizophr Res 69(1):75–83. doi:10.1016/j.schres.2003.08.013

Yun DY, Hwang SSH, Kim Y, Lee YH, Kim YS, Jung HY (2011) Impairments in executive functioning in patients with remitted and non-remitted schizophrenia. Prog Neuropsychopharmacol Biol Psychiatry 35(4):1148–1154. http://dx.doi.org/10.1016/j.pnpbp.2011.03.018

Gene–Environment Interactions in the Pathogenesis of Obsessive–Compulsive Symptoms in Schizophrenia

8

Kyung Sue Hong

8.1 Introduction

Obsessive–compulsive disorder (OCD) is a common neuropsychiatric disorder with an estimated lifetime prevalence of ~2–3 % (Sadock and Sadock 2007). It is well known that a much higher rate of OCD was demonstrated in schizophrenia patients compared to the general population. In a recent review by Schirmbeck and Zink (2013), the lifetime risk of obsessive–compulsive symptoms (OCSs) and OCD in patients suffering from chronic schizophrenia was estimated as 25 and 12.1 %, respectively. OCSs can be observed in schizophrenia patients in different stages of the disease (Bottas et al. 2005; Byerly et al. 2005; Schirmbeck and Zink 2013), i.e., from before the onset of illness as a frank comorbid OCD, only in the prodromal phase, only in the active psychotic phase overlapping with psychotic symptoms, and after stabilization by pharmacotherapy. Sometimes, neuroleptics, especially second-generation antipsychotics (SGAs), aggravate or even induce OCSs or OCD (Lykouras et al. 2003; Lim et al. 2007).

Despite the large amount of knowledge about the neurobiological underpinnings of OCD and schizophrenia that might overlap partially, the mechanism underlying the link and combination of the two conditions remains unclear (Bottas et al. 2005; Hwang et al. 2009). It is well known that schizophrenia is a highly heritable disease with an estimated heritability of up to 80 % (Sullivan et al. 2003). Genetic epidemiologic studies demonstrate that OCD is also a multifactorial genetic condition with an approximate heritability of 40 % (Nestadt et al. 2000; Hettema et al. 2001; Mataix-Cols et al. 2013; Pauls et al. 2014). Therefore, one important approach to the pathogenesis of OCSs in schizophrenia would be

K.S. Hong
Department of Psychiatry, Sungkyunkwan University School of Medicine, Samsung Medical Center, Seoul, Korea
e-mail: hongks@skku.edu

L. De Haan et al. (eds.), *Obsessive-Compulsive Symptoms in Schizophrenia*,
DOI 10.1007/978-3-319-12952-5_8

genetic studies. Considering the abovementioned heterogeneity in the clinical presentation of OCSs in schizophrenia, heterogeneity and complexity of its genetic basis is expected.

Genetic epidemiologic studies and recent genome-wide association studies (GWASs) showed no clear relationship or shared genetic etiology between OCD and schizophrenia (Kendler and Diehl 1993; Sullivan et al. 2003; Poyurovsky et al. 2005a; The Schizophrenia Psychiatric Genome-Wide Association Study Consortium 2011; Cross-Disorder Group of the Psychiatric Genomics Consortium 2013; Stewart et al. 2013; Mattheisen et al. in press). Considering the independent genetic susceptibility to schizophrenia and OCD, we can assume the following scenarios regarding the genetic mechanism of OCSs in schizophrenia (Fig. 8.1). Schizophrenia patients with OCSs might have genetic vulnerabilities to both schizophrenia (G_{SCZ}) and OCD (G_{OC}). Risk variants for OCD (G_{OC}) can be expressed in any stage of the schizophrenic process. From a schizophrenia-centered perspective, OCD-related genes (G_{OC}) would be the modifier genes that diversify the clinical manifestations. From an OCD-centered perspective, higher expression of its susceptibility genes in schizophrenia patients compared to the general population implies that schizophrenia-related environmental factors might trigger the expression of OCD genes (G_{OC}). Some of the environmental factors might overlap with those triggering the expression of schizophrenia genes (E_{Common}). Either progressive biological changes in the brains of schizophrenia patients ($E_{OC\text{-}B}$) or psychological processes defending against psychotic

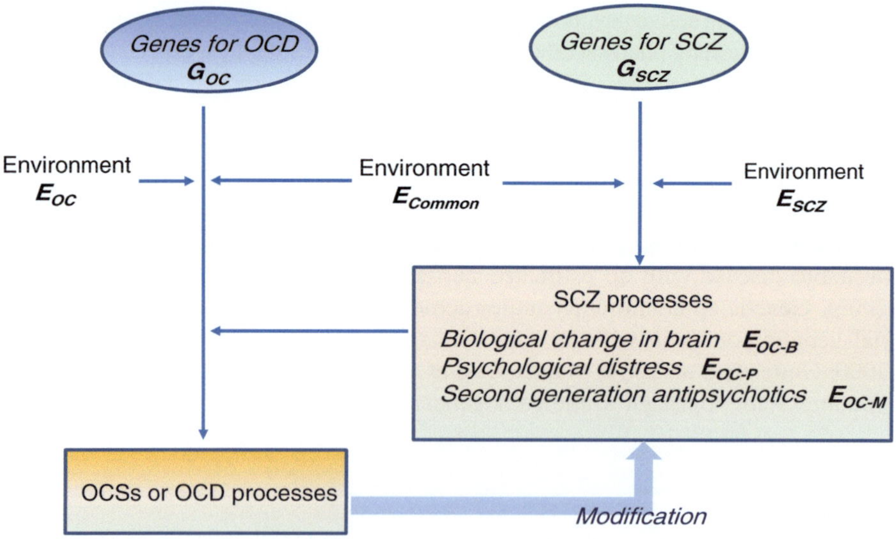

Fig. 8.1 Hypothetical mechanism of gene and environment interactions in the development of obsessive–compulsive symptoms in schizophrenia. *OCSs* obsessive–compulsive symptoms, *OCD* obsessive–compulsive disorder, *SCZ* schizophrenia, *E* environment, *G* gene

decompensation (Hwang et al. 2009) (E_{OC-P}) might also be the environmental factors that induce the expression of OCSs or OCD. SGAs seem to be a strong environmental factor (E_{OC-M}) that triggers the OCD genes (G_{OC}).

On the other hand, as both schizophrenia and OCD are expected to have a heterogeneous genetic basis with a large number of susceptibility genes, some degree of their co-occurrence might be explained by the presence of common genes with a pleiotropic effect that have not been identified so far. Also, considering the phenomenological similarity between obsession and delusion (Bottas et al. 2005) (for details on the similarities and differences between delusion and obsession, see Chap. 3), OCSs occurring only in the context of psychosis might be a special manifestation of the psychotic processes that are not related to the vulnerability to OCD.

Considering that most of the specific genetic and environmental factors in schizophrenia and OCD have not been identified as yet and that the biological mechanism of gene–environment interactions in psychiatric illness is not well established, testing the abovementioned hypotheses in the field of neurobehavioral genetics requires many prerequisite steps. According to a recent meta-analysis of twin studies (Taylor 2011) on OCD, additive genetic factors explained ~37–41 % of phenotypic variance, and non-shared (individual-specific) environment accounted for ~50–52 % of the variance. Several environmental factors including perinatal events, infections, traumatic life events, and stressors have been suggested to trigger OCSs (Geller et al. 2008; Grisham et al. 2011; Lafleur et al. 2011; Landau et al. 2011; Murphy et al. 2010). Compared to these factors, SGAs would be an environmental factor that is less complicated and can be reliably measured. Therefore, genetic studies on the SGA-induced OCSs could provide an important insight into the gene–environment interaction mechanism. For genetic studies of OCSs in schizophrenia, detailed characterization and subgrouping of OCSs in schizophrenia is also required. Until now, only a small number of studies have generated genetic data regarding OCSs in schizophrenia. These were mostly candidate gene association studies, and the phenotype was OCSs in general or SGA-induced OCSs manifested in schizophrenia. Although these are mostly unreplicated studies with a small sample size, these studies would be an important initial step for exploring the complete genetic architecture of OCSs in schizophrenia.

8.2 Genetic Studies on Obsessive–Compulsive Symptoms in Schizophrenia

Studies in twin pairs with schizophrenia found greater resemblance for symptomatic profile in monozygotic twins than in dizygotic twins, which suggests the influence of genetic factors on clinical features of schizophrenia (Cardno et al. 2001, 2002). Some family studies reported that various factorial dimensions of schizophrenia showed significant within-family correlations (Wickham et al. 2001; Choi et al. 2007; Vassos et al. 2008). However, in contrast to vigorous exploration of disease susceptibility genes, genetic approaches for exploring the genes related to specific symptoms or sub-phenotypes of schizophrenia are very limited. Until now, the most commonly investigated symptom dimensions in genetic linkage or association studies are reality distortion (positive), psychomotor poverty (negative), disorganization, and manic or depressive dimensions (Fanous et al. 2007, 2012; Hamshere et al. 2011). OCS or comorbid OCD has seldom been measured in large-scale genetic studies exploring modifier genes for comprehensive clinical symptom dimensions of schizophrenia.

In a recent genome-wide quantitative trait locus (QTL) linkage analysis, our group (Ryu et al. 2013) assessed clinical symptoms of a total of 315 schizophrenia patients on a lifetime basis. From 42 indicators measured using the Korean version of the Diagnostic Interview for Genetic Studies (DIGS) (Joo et al. 2004), eight quantitative phenotypes representing symptom dimensions were identified through the principal component factor analysis, i.e., "auditory hallucination factor," "Schneiderian first-rank symptom factor," "paranoid factor," "non-paranoid delusion factor," "somatic preoccupation factor," "prodromal impairment factor," "negative symptom factor," and "disorganization factor." In this study, lifetime OCSs were loaded on the "somatic preoccupation factor" together with tactile, gustatory, and olfactory hallucinations and somatic delusions. The loading value of OCSs on this dimension was 0.47, which was lower than that of tactile hallucination (0.69) and somatic delusion (0.60) and comparable to that of gustatory hallucination (0.49) and olfactory hallucination (0.45). This phenotype dimension could not be genetically validated in our QTL linkage analyses, which showed no significant linkage signal for this dimension (Ryu et al. 2013). In a recent clinical analysis of schizophrenia patients, our group observed that this symptom dimension was associated with earlier age of onset (unpublished data). Further validation of this dimension as a unique sub-phenotype of schizophrenia is warranted. In future studies, heterogeneity of the OCSs manifested in the lifetime course of schizophrenia needs to be considered.

In selecting candidate genes for association studies on schizophrenia with OCD or OCSs, previous findings of genetic studies for OCD could be considered. The results of GWASs and meta-analyses of candidate gene studies suggest that the genes involved in the glutamatergic, serotonergic, and dopaminergic systems and neurotrophic factors may contribute to the risk of OCD (Pauls et al. 2014). There were genetic association studies specifically focusing on schizophrenia with OCD. The catechol-O-methyltransferase (COMT) gene was the first candidate gene tested due to its crucial role in dopaminergic neurotransmission and prefrontal cognitive functions (Denys et al. 2004). Poyurovsky and colleagues (Poyurovsky et al. 2005b) investigated the association of Val158Met polymorphism of the COMT gene with comorbid OCD in schizophrenia in the Israeli population and reported negative results. In a subsequent study, Zinkstok and colleagues (Zinkstok et al. 2008) observed a significant effect of the COMT genotype on the Yale–Brown Obsessive–Compulsive Scale (Y-BOCS) (Goodman et al. 1989) scores in male patients with recent-onset schizophrenia in the Netherlands. The Val/Val genotype of COMT Val158Met polymorphism, the genotype of high activity, was associated with high Y-BOCS scores. The authors suggested that the COMT gene may be a modifier gene for the symptomatology of schizophrenia.

The brain-derived neurotrophic factor (BDNF) gene was another candidate gene for OCSs in schizophrenia. It is involved in the brain development and neurotransmitter systems known to be implicated in schizophrenia and OCD (Wang et al. 2011; Favalli et al. 2012). In a recent study by Hashim et al. (2012), the BDNF Val66Met polymorphism was significantly associated with OCSs in the Egyptian patients with schizophrenia. The Val allele was significantly higher in the with-OCS group compared to the without-OCS group. The mean Y-BOCS scores were significantly different among the three genotype groups: Val/Val > Val/Met > Met/Met.

Until now, genetic studies on OCSs in schizophrenia provided limited information due to a small sample size and few replication trials. However, these studies have shown the possibility of OCSs being a meaningful phenotype in the exploration of the genetic basis of course and symptom modifications in schizophrenia. Many more candidate genes related to the biological mechanism of schizophrenia and/or OCD need to be tested. Larger-scale linkage analysis and GWAS for this phenotype are also warranted. To construct a reliable basis of replication and meta-analyses, a more standardized definition for the phenotype should be applied in future studies.

8.3 Antipsychotic-Induced Obsessive–Compulsive Symptoms as a Phenotype

Since the introduction of clozapine and other SGAs, case reports (Lykouras et al. 2003) and clinical studies (Baker et al. 1992; de Haan et al. 1999; Ertugrul et al. 2005; Mahendran et al. 2007; Scheltema Beduin et al. 2012) have described the de novo onset of OCSs during treatment with these drugs (for details see Chap. 10). Our group previously screened 209 clinically stable schizophrenia outpatients receiving SGAs and detected OCSs in 44 patients (21.1 %) (Lim et al. 2007). OCSs associated with SGAs were identified in 26 patients (12.4 % of total patients and 59.1 % of patients with OCSs) (Lim et al. 2007). In this study, patient diagnosis was performed through a direct interview using the Korean versions of the Structured Clinical Interview Schedule for DSM-IV Axis I Disorders (K-SCID-I) (Hahn et al. 2000) and the Y-BOCS (Kim et al. 2004). We proposed the following criteria for SGA-induced OCSs: (1) meet all of the criteria of DSM-IV OCD except for criteria C (descriptions of severity) and E (exclusion of drug-induced cases); (2) OCSs are not the direct result of delusions, and their contents are clearly different from their residual psychotic symptoms; and (3) OCSs were developed de novo while receiving SGAs. Patients with a history of transient OCSs in childhood or adolescence were considered to have de novo OCSs if they experienced substantial OCS-free periods before the onset of psychotic illness. Although only 35.9 % of the study cohort was taking clozapine at the time of the evaluation, 76.9 % of SGA-induced OCSs were associated with clozapine treatment.

Among the various subgroups of comorbid OCSs in schizophrenia, SGA-induced OCSs might be more homogeneous in terms of biological mechanisms. It could also be a valid phenotype for pharmacogenetic studies aiming at individualized medicine. Since the SGA-induced OCSs are delayed adverse effects that cause great distress to the patients (Lim et al. 2007), and there are differences in the OCS-inducing propensity among SGAs, i.e., high in clozapine and olanzapine and low in amisulpride and aripiprazole (Schirmbeck et al. 2013), evaluation of an individual's susceptibility to SGA-induced OCSs in the early stage of medication would be highly helpful in the pharmacotherapy of schizophrenia.

It is widely accepted that genetic factors play an important role in an individual's response to specific drugs (Malhotra 2002; Arranz and de Leon 2007). However, heritability data for drug responses are extremely limited. Our group previously described clozapine-induced OCSs that emerged concordantly in a pair of monozygotic twins (Hong et al. 2008). More case reports and data from clinical surveys need to be accumulated to clarify the role of genetic factors. Another indirect evidence of genetic control of SGA-induced OCSs is the strong heritability of OCD reported in family and twin studies (Hanna et al. 2005; van Grootheest et al. 2005; Mataix-Cols et al. 2013; Pauls et al. 2014).

If there is a genetic vulnerability to SGA-induced OCSs, would it be related to the vulnerability to OCD? An indirect approach to find an answer to this question would be analyses of the phenomenological similarity between SGA-induced OCSs and OCD. For determining whether SGA-induced OCSs have the same symptom characteristics as those displayed in OCD, our group evaluated the frequencies and dimensions of SGA-induced OCSs measured using the Y-BOCS (Kim et al. 2004) in schizophrenia patients (Kim et al. 2012). Frequencies of 13 symptom categories were very similar to those in Korean OCD patients (Ha et al. 2004), showing statistically significant intraclass correlation ($ICC = 0.77$, $P < 0.01$) (Fig. 8.2, adopted from the study by Kim et al. 2012). The factor structure yielded from the principal component analysis was to a large extent comparable not only to that demonstrated in the previous study among Korean OCD patients (Ha et al. 2004) (Table 8.1, adopted from Kim et al. 2012) but also to that reported in other studies of OCD patients (Leckman et al. 1997; Hasler et al. 2005, 2007; Bloch et al. 2008), suggesting that a common biological mechanism underlies the two clinical conditions. In contrast, in a previous study of schizophrenia patients with comorbid OCD (Faragian et al. 2009) that excluded patients with drug-induced OCSs from their study, a somewhat different symptom structure was generated. In that study, only the cleaning factor was comparable to that in previous studies of pure OCD. Other factors were constructed by a combination of symptoms from different dimensions in previous OCD studies (Leckman et al. 1997; Hasler et al. 2005, 2007; Bloch et al. 2008).

Pharmacogenetic studies would not only be important for the individualized treatment but also for uncovering the biological mechanism of SGA-induced OCSs. To promote the progress of these studies, more clinical concerns regarding this phenotype and more heritability data including assessment of concordance between twin pairs or relative pairs are required. Analyses of phenomenological similarities between SGA-induced OCSs and OCD or other subgroups of OCSs in schizophrenia are also helpful to clearly determine the boundary of the phenotype.

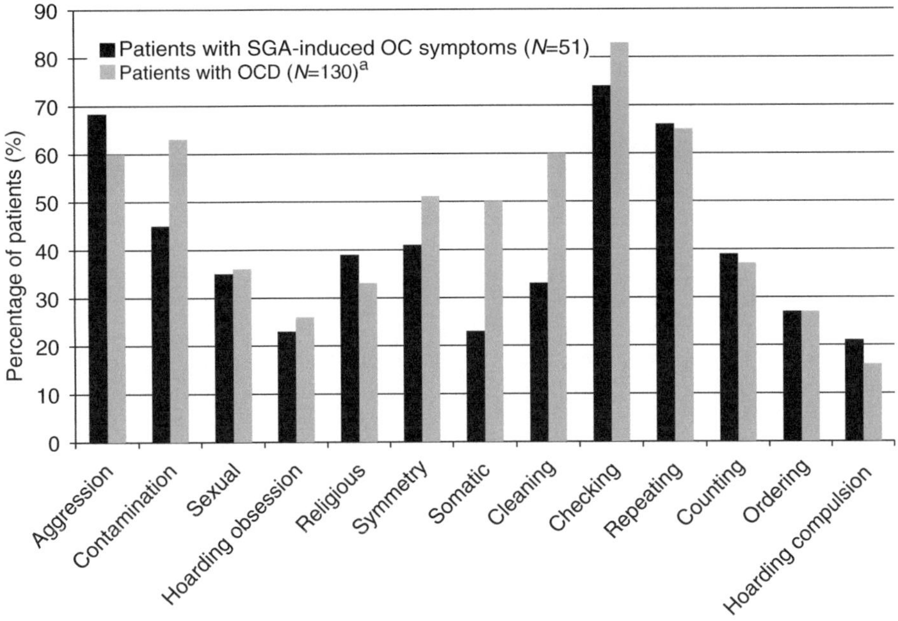

Fig. 8.2 Symptom frequencies for 13 categories of the Y-BOCS symptom checklist in patients with SGA-induced obsessive–compulsive symptoms and patients with OCD. Each category of the Y-BOCS symptom checklist was scored as 0 = absent or 1 = present. The symptom frequency (*y*-axis) was defined as the percentage of patients scored as "1" in the category. Symptom frequencies showed a significant correlation between two groups (ICC = 0.77, $P < 0.001$) (Reproduced from Kim et al. 2012). *Y-BOCS* yale–brown obsessive–compulsive scale, *SGA* second-generation antipsychotics, *OCD* obsessive–compulsive disorder, *ICC* intraclass correlation coefficient. [a]Ha et al. (2004)

8.4 Pharmacogenetic Studies on Antipsychotic-Induced Obsessive–Compulsive Symptoms

To date, several pharmacogenetic studies on SGA-induced OCSs have been performed. Owing to the short history of genetic researches on this topic and difficulties in large-scale patient recruitment, these are all candidate gene association studies with a small sample size. Genes coding for proteins involved in both the pharmacodynamic actions of SGAs and neurobiological processes of OCD, i.e., genes related to serotonergic, dopaminergic, and glutamatergic neurotransmission (Lopez-Gil et al. 2010), could be reasonable candidate genes. A few genes involved in the glutamatergic system have shown positive association with SGA-induced OCSs.

Our group investigated the glutamate transporter gene, *SLC1A1*, that was regarded as one of the most promising candidate genes for OCD (Arnold et al. 2006; Dickel et al. 2006; Stewart et al. 2007). Subjects included 94 clinically stable Korean patients with schizophrenia under SGA treatment. The obsessive–compulsive (OC)

Table 8.1 Comparison of factor structures and loadings for the Yale–Brown Obsessive–Compulsive Scale symptom categories between schizophrenia patients with second-generation antipsychotic-induced obsessive–compulsive symptoms and patients with obsessive–compulsive disorder

	SGA-induced OC symptoms ($N=51$)					Obsessive–compulsive disorder (Ha et al. 2004[a])				
Symptom category	Forbidden thoughts	Hoarding	Cleaning	Symmetry	Counting	Contamination/ cleaning	Symmetry/ ordering	Pure obsessions	Hoarding	Repeating/ counting
Aggressive	**0.80**	0.33	0.01	−0.06	0.19	−0.19	−0.19	**0.71**	0.10	−0.10
Contamination	0.37	−0.12	**0.80**	−0.13	−0.03	**0.92**	−0.05	0.05	0.05	−0.04
Sexual	**0.62**	0.05	0.12	0.16	−0.54	0.15	−0.07	**0.78**	−0.01	0.00
Hoarding[b]	0.18	**0.85**	−0.08	−0.07	−0.01	0.08	0.12	0.04	**0.86**	0.10
Religious	**0.55**	0.37	0.15	0.24	−0.23	0.32	0.11	**0.51**	−0.04	0.15
Symmetry	0.24	−0.16	0.14	**0.76**	0.02	0.01	**0.80**	0.03	0.10	0.23
Somatic	**0.60**	−0.33	−0.02	0.26	−0.07	0.01	0.38	0.34	0.19	−0.13
Cleaning	0.02	0.22	**0.84**	0.18	0.15	**0.89**	0.11	−0.01	0.09	−0.03
Checking	**0.74**	0.28	0.08	−0.00	0.16	−0.20	0.39	0.49	0.03	0.00
Repeating	0.23	0.20	−0.29	**0.59**	0.04	−0.06	0.24	0.04	0.10	**0.79**
Counting	0.19	0.04	0.16	0.10	**0.83**	0.02	−0.02	−0.06	0.15	**0.83**
Ordering	−0.27	0.22	0.48	**0.66**	−0.01	0.12	**0.84**	−0.17	0.02	0.07
Hoarding[c]	0.21	**0.80**	0.27	0.20	0.04	0.05	0.05	0.04	**0.86**	0.16
Percent variance (%)	19.35	15.81	14.21	12.59	8.80	14.41	13.71	13.66	12.20	11.27

Reproduced from Kim et al. (2012)
SGA second-generation antipsychotics, *OC* obsessive–compulsive
The highest loading for each symptom category in each study is bolded
[a]130 Korean patients with obsessive–compulsive disorder
[b]Hoarding obsession
[c]Hoarding compulsion

group was defined based on the criteria proposed in our previous study (Lim et al. 2007) (described in the previous section), and the non-OC group consisted of patients who had received SGA for more than 24 months and did not develop OCSs. Ten SNPs of *SLC1A1* were selected based on the previous reports on OCD, and the genotype- and haplotype-based association was tested using a logistic regression model considering age, sex, and medication type as covariates. We observed trends of association in rs2228622 and rs3780412 (nominal $P<0.05$, adjusted permutation $P<0.1$) for the dominant model that was the best inheritance model fitting our data. In the haplotype-based analysis, the A/C/G haplotype at rs2228622-rs3780413-rs3780412 showed a significant association with SGA-induced OCSs, and this association withstood multiple test correction (nominal $P=0.011$, adjusted permutation $P=0.038$, OR=3.955, 95 % CI 1.366–11.452, for dominant model) (Fig. 8.3). The same nature of association was observed in the separate analysis of the subgroup of patients receiving clozapine treatment. This was the first study that provided preliminary evidence of the involvement of glutamatergic neurotransmission in the pathogenesis of SGA-induced OCSs.

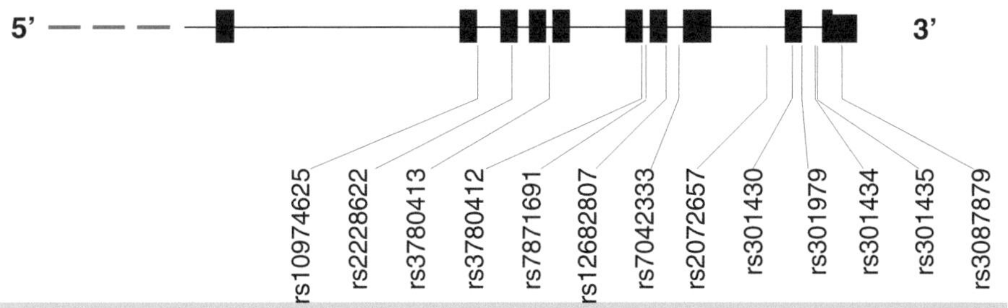

	rs10974625	rs2228622	rs3780413	rs3780412	rs7871691	rs12682807	rs7042333	rs2072657	rs301430	rs301979	rs301434	rs301435	rs3087879
Arnold et al. (2006)													
SNP											+	+	+
Haplotype											○		○
Dickel et al. (2006)													
SNP				+					+				
Haplotype									○	○			
Stewart et al. (2007)													
SNP		+		+									
Haplotype						○		○	○				
Kwon et al. (2009)													
SNP		+[a]		+[a]									
Haplotype		○	○	○									

Fig. 8.3 *SLC1A1* organization and single-nucleotide polymorphism (SNP) locations (from the University of California at Santa Cruz Genome Browser, Mar 2006 Assembly). The horizontal line represents the genomic sequence, and vertical bars represent exons. Plus signs and circles denote SNPs significantly associated with obsessive–compulsive disorder (Arnold et al. 2006; Dickel et al. 2006; Stewart et al. 2007) or second-generation antipsychotic-induced obsessive–compulsive symptoms (Kwon et al. 2009) in single-marker and haplotype analyses. [a]Only trends of association were observed with nominal $P<0.05$

In a succeeding investigation, our group tested another candidate gene involved in the glutamatergic neurotransmission, the discs, large-associated protein 3 gene *(DLGAP3),* also known as SAP90/PSD-95-associated protein 3 gene (*SAPAP3*) (Ryu et al. 2011). In that study, we also explored the interaction effect of *DLGAP3* and *SLC1A1* on SGA-induced OCSs. Among the seven tag SNPs of *DLGAP3*, the only nominally significant association was found in rs7525948 (nominal $P<0.05$). In the logistic regression analysis of gene–gene interaction, a significant interaction effect of rs7525948 of *DLGAP3* and rs2228622 of *SLC1A1* (permutation $P=0.036$) on SGA-induced OCSs was observed.

More recently, Cai et al. (2013) investigated the influence of three genes regulating glutamate transmission, i.e., *SLC1A1*, the glutamate receptor, ionotropic, N-methyl-D-aspartate 2B gene (*GRIN2B*), and the glutamate receptor, ionotropic, kainate 2 gene (*GRIK2*), on clozapine-induced OCSs in the Chinese population. The subjects included 250 clinically stable patients with schizophrenia receiving clozapine treatment, and they were divided into the OC group and the non-OC group based on almost the same criteria used in previous studies by our group (Kwon et al. 2009; Ryu et al. 2011). The authors observed trends of association of rs2228622 of *SLC1A1* and rs890 of *GRIN2B* with clozapine-induced OCSs and a significant interaction effect of *SLC1A1* and *GRIN2B* on this phenotype. They also reported the interaction effect of these two genes on the Y-BOCS score of the OC group.

Another replication trial of the association between *SLC1A1* and SGA-induced OCSs was conducted in a European population mostly of German descent (Schirmbeck et al. 2012). Subjects included 103 schizophrenia patients treated with SGAs. The authors genotyped three SNPs including SNPs composing the risk haplotype identified in the previous study by Kwon et al. (2009). However, the positive finding observed in the previous study could not be reproduced, either in a single-marker analysis or in a haplotype analysis.

The discrepancy between study results might be due to ethnic differences and high vulnerability of these studies with a small sample size to a false-positive or false-negative result. In addition, differences in the phenotype definition, i.e., criteria for the OCS and non-OCS groups, between studies, and confounding effects of the medication type should be carefully considered. In the study by Schirmbeck and colleagues (Schirmbeck et al. 2012), the authors divided the patients into the OCS group and the non-OCS group based on the Y-BOCS score with the cutoff score of 8. Among the 103 subjects, 37.9 % of whom were treated with clozapine, 42.7 % (44/103) of subjects were diagnosed with SGA-induced OCSs (the OCS group). This rate was much higher compared to the rate of OCSs associated with SGAs (12.4 %) defined and identified in the previous study by our group (Lim et al. 2007) where a similar proportion (35.9 %) of the subjects were receiving clozapine. Regarding the medication type, all subjects were receiving clozapine in the study by Cai et al. (2013). In the previous study by Kwon et al. (2009), medication types (clozapine, olanzapine, or risperidone) were almost matched, showing no statistically significant difference between the OC and non-OC groups. However, in the study by Schirmbeck et al. (2012), there was a significant imbalance in medication types between the OCS and non-OCS groups. Thirty-seven out of 44 patients (84.1 %) of the OCS group were receiving clozapine or olanzapine, which are known to have a high OCS-inducing propensity (Schirmbeck et al. 2013). In the non-OCS group, a much smaller proportion of patients (22/59, 37.3 %) were receiving these drugs. In contrast, the rate of receiving amisulpride or aripiprazole, which were reported to have a low or no OCS-inducing propensity, was 4.5 % in the OCS group and 45.8 % in the non-OCS group. Although the authors included the medication type as a covariate in their analysis, it might not be sufficient to control for the strong imbalance effect of the medication type between groups.

So far, independent replication studies for *DLGAP3* and *GRIN2B* have not been conducted. There may be many more functional candidate genes for SGA-induced OCSs, e.g., genes of the dopaminergic and serotonergic systems, and other genes reported to be associated with OCD. In addition to association studies for individual genes, gene–gene interaction analyses are also warranted. Since SGAs are used for the treatment of psychiatric disorders other than schizophrenia, genetic studies in broader range of illness would be helpful for exploring the biological mechanism of SGA-induced OCS. In the future, GWAS or sequencing approaches would also be possible in large-scale pharmacogenomic studies.

For future large-scale multicenter studies, replication studies, and meta-analyses, standardized criteria for antipsychotic (or drug)-induced OCSs that can be reliably applied to various research settings are needed. OCSs occurring in the course of schizophrenia have a heterogeneous clinical presentation (Schirmbeck and Zink 2013). Sometimes, it is difficult to differentiate them from overvalued ideas or delusional thinking (Hwang et al. 2009) (for details on the distinction between delusion and obsession, see Chap. 3). To limit the phenotype to drug-induced OCSs, the inclusion criteria should ensure de novo onset of OCSs during the treatment, an ego-dystonic nature of OCS (to be differentiated from the direct result of delusions), and clear distinction from delusions or other psychotic symptoms. In addition, subjects need to be clinically stable at the time of research assessment to reliably report on the nature of OCSs. Valid inclusion and exclusion criteria for the control (non-OCS) group are also important. The control group should have been treated with the drug for a long enough time period to minimize the possibility of delayed-onset phenotype. Adopting the criteria used in previous studies performed by our group (Kwon et al. 2009; Ryu et al. 2011) as the backbone and reflecting the changes in diagnostic criteria of OCD in DSM-5, we propose minimum research criteria for drug-induced OCSs in schizophrenia (Table 8.2). These criteria focus on the minimization of false-positive diagnosis of the phenotype and would be acceptable in various research settings. For a definite decision on the "causation," i.e., the causal relationship between the drug and OCSs, additional criteria are needed (Table 8.2).

Table 8.2 Research criteria for drug-induced obsessive–compulsive symptoms in schizophrenia: a proposed phenotype definition for genetic studies

Minimum research criteria	1. Meet criteria A of DSM-IV or DSM-5 (definition of obsessions and compulsions) for OCD and criteria C of DSM-IV or criteria B of DSM-5 (distressful and time-consuming nature) for OCD
	2. OCSs are not the direct result of delusions, and their contents are clearly differed from active or residual psychotic symptoms
	3. OCSs were developed de novo while receiving the drug. Patients with a history of transient OCSs in childhood or adolescence were determined to have de novo OCSs if they experienced substantial OCS-free periods before the onset of psychotic illness
Criteria for definite causation	1. Meet all of the above criteria
	2. Discontinuation of the drug with consequent remission of OCSs
	3. Rechallenge of the drug with consequent reappearance of OCSs

OCD obsessive–compulsive disorder, *OCSs* obsessive–compulsive symptoms

8.5 Implications of Pharmacogenetic Studies for the Neurobiological Mechanism

All of the three genes (*SLC1A1*, *DLGAP3*, *GRIN2B*) reported to be associated with SGA-induced OCSs are involved in the glutamatergic neurotransmission. They showed a positive association with OCD in earlier studies. Evidences of dysregulation of the glutamatergic system in OCD have not only been generated by genetic studies but also by neuroimaging, neurochemical, and animal model studies (Pittenger et al. 2011).

The glutamate transporter gene *SLC1A1*, which is located on chromosome 9p24, is considered as a positional and functional candidate gene for vulnerability to OCD (Pauls 2008). *SLC1A1* codes for the excitatory amino acid transporter 3, EAAT3 (also known as excitatory amino acid carrier 1, EAAC1), that maintains extracellular glutamate concentrations by reuptake of synaptically released glutamate (Tzingounis and Wadiche 2007). EAAT3 is highly expressed in the cerebral cortex, striatum, and thalamus, regions that might be involved in the pathogenesis of OCD. Compared to the astrocytic glutamate transporters, EAAT1 and EAAT2, the neuronal EAAT3 plays a more minor role in the glutamate reuptake (Pittenger et al. 2011). However, evidences from an animal study (Aoyama et al. 2006) indicate that EAAT3 is also essential for normal neuronal function and survival, by protecting neurons from oxidative damage. Regarding the relationship between EAAT3 and SGAs, significant downregulation of EAAT3 by chronic treatment with clozapine was observed in the cingulate cortex of the rat brain (Schmitt et al. 2003b). Changes in the transcript expression of excitatory amino acid transporter (EAAT)-interacting protein that modulates subcellular localization and activity of the EAATs including EAAT3 were also reported in clozapine-treated rats (Huerta et al. 2006). In other studies, clozapine treatment enhanced K^+-stimulated glutamate release (Yamamoto and Cooperman 1994) and upregulated *N*-methyl-D-aspartate (NMDA) receptor binding (Schmitt et al. 2003a) in the nucleus accumbens of the rat brain. Increased expression of the vesicular glutamate transporter 2 (VGluT2) mRNA (Moutsimilli et al. 2008) and decreased NMDA binding (Choi et al. 2009) by risperidone treatment were also reported. Based on the evidence of a biological relationship between the glutamatergic system and both OCSs and SGAs, *SLC1A1* is a promising candidate gene for genetic susceptibility to SGA-induced OCSs. Interestingly, the SNPs associated with SGA-induced OCSs in the study by Kwon et al. (2009) (rs2228622 and rs3780412) are identical to the SNPs that showed a significant association with OCD in the investigation by Stewart et al. (2007), and one of them (rs3780412) was associated with OCD in the study by Dickel et al. (2006) (Fig. 8.3). rs2228622 is a synonymous SNP located in exon 4, and rs3780412 is an intronic SNP. As these SNPs and other risk variants of OCD in *SLC1A1* are non-translated DNA sequences or synonymous exonal SNPs, their effects on gene expression or protein function have not yet been well investigated. One study performed by Wendland and colleagues (2009) investigated the functional meaning of risk variants of OCD. Through experiments with lymphoblastoid cell lines and postmortem human brain tissues, the authors demonstrated the functional role of some OCD-related SNPs and haplotypes in the expression of *SLC1A1* (Pittenger et al. 2011).

DLGAP3, also known as *SAPAP3*, is another candidate gene for OCD, and it showed an interaction effect with *SLC1A1*on SGA-induced OCSs (Ryu et al. 2011). The SAPAP family proteins are postsynaptic density (PSD) components that interact with other proteins to form a key scaffolding complex at the glutamatergic synapses (Kim et al. 1997; Takeuchi et al. 1997). *DLGAP3* is highly expressed in the striatum (Kindler et al. 2004; Welch et al. 2004), and mice with a *DLGAP3* genetic deletion developed an OCD-like phenotype, including increased anxiety and compulsive grooming behavior (Welch et al. 2007). In addition, this phenotype of *DLGAP3* knockout mice could be rescued by the administration of fluoxetine, which is widely used as an anti-OCD drug in clinical practice (Welch et al. 2007). In human genetic studies, polymorphisms in the *DLGAP3* were associated with OCD-related phenotypes, grooming disorders (pathological nail biting, pathological skin picking, and trichotillomania) (Bienvenu et al. 2009), and Tourette syndrome (Crane et al. 2011). Another study identified multiple rare missense variants of *DLGAP3* in OCD and/or trichotillomania patients (Zuchner et al. 2009). Interestingly, in a recent GWAS for OCD (Stewart et al. 2013), two SNPs showing the strongest association in the case–control analysis were located in *DLGAP1*, which belongs to the same family as *DLGAP3*. The SNPs rs7525948 of *DLGAP3* which showed an association with SGA-induced OCSs in our study (Ryu et al. 2011) and rs6662980 which showed an association with grooming disorder in the investigation by Bienvenu et al. (2009) lie within the same intron. In addition, rs11264126 and the rs11264126-rs12141243 haplotype block which showed significant associations with Tourette syndrome in the study by Crane et al. (2011) and three short exons in which rare missense variants were identified in either trichotillomania or OCD by a recent study (Zuchner et al. 2009) physically occur within the rs4653112-rs7525948 haplotype block that showed a marginally significant association with SGA-induced OCSs in our study (Ryu et al. 2011).

GRIN2B is the third glutamate-related gene which was associated with SGA-induced OCSs in a previous study (Cai et al. 2013). It encodes the NR2B subunit of NMDA receptors and plays an important role in glutamate synaptic function. Variants of this gene were reported to be associated with OCD (Arnold et al. 2004) and the orbital frontal cortex and anterior cingulate cortex volume of pediatric patients with OCD (Arnold et al. 2009). The SNP associated with SGA-induced OCSs in the study by Cai et al. (2013) (rs890) is located in the 3' untranslated region (3'-UTR). Although variants in the 3'-UTR might be related to messenger RNA processing of the gene, the exact role of rs890 in the function of the protein is not yet known (Cai et al. 2013).

The susceptibility to SGA-induced OCSs might be induced by multiple genes. Considering the hypothetical mechanism of OCD and pharmacodynamic profiles of SGAs, candidate genes involved in serotonergic, dopaminergic, and GABAergic systems as well as more glutamatergic genes should be tested in future studies. The susceptibility might be due to an interactive effect of these genes causing dysregulation of the cortico-striato-thalamo-cortical (CSTC) circuitry, a candidate brain network related to OCD (Milad and Rauch 2012; Pauls et al. 2014). The CSTC circuitry uses both glutamate and GABA as its primary neurotransmitters (Pittenger et al. 2011).

Gene–environment interactions also seemed to play an etiologic role for OCD or OCSs (Monzani et al. 2014). Adverse perinatal events (Geller et al. 2008), psychosocial stressors and traumatic life events (Grisham et al. 2011; Lafleur et al. 2011; Landau et al. 2011), and streptococcal infections (Murphy et al. 2010) have been suggested as environmental triggers for OCD or related phenotypes. These events could trigger the expression of genes involved in the CSTC circuitry through epigenetic mechanisms (Pauls et al. 2014). However, biological mechanisms of gene–environment interactions remain to be elucidated. Furthermore, valid methods for the assessment of environmental factors have not yet been well established (Pauls et al. 2014). Compared to the abovementioned environmental factors, substances and medications including SGAs would be a more straightforward environmental factor that can be reliably measured. Therefore, genetic studies on the SGA-induced OCSs could provide an important early insight into the complete genetic architecture of OCSs or OCD in schizophrenia.

Conclusions

It is well known that a significantly higher rate of OCSs or OCD is demonstrated in schizophrenia patients compared to the general population. As genetic factors play a major role in the development of both schizophrenia and OCD, the mechanism underlying their link and combination could also be elucidated through genetic studies. Until now, only a limited number of genetic studies have been performed on OCSs or comorbid OCD in schizophrenia. Recently, pharmacogenetic studies generated stimulating findings suggesting the role of glutamatergic genes in the development of SGA-induced OCSs. They seem to be a relatively homogeneous phenotype having a unique environmental triggering factor (the drug). Investigation of this phenotype would be an important starting point, which can be extended to further genetic studies targeting a broader range of OCSs in schizophrenia. More clinical attention and research efforts are needed on various types of comorbid OCSs or OCD developing in the course of schizophrenia.

References

Aoyama K, Suh SW, Hamby AM et al (2006) Neuronal glutathione deficiency and age-dependent neurodegeneration in the EAAC1 deficient mouse. Nat Neurosci 9(1):119–126

Arnold PD, Rosenberg DR, Mundo E et al (2004) Association of a glutamate (NMDA) subunit receptor gene (GRIN2B) with obsessive-compulsive disorder: a preliminary study. Psychopharmacology (Berl) 174:530–538

Arnold PD, Sicard T, Burroughs E et al (2006) Glutamate transporter gene SLC1A1 associated with obsessive-compulsive disorder. Arch Gen Psychiatry 63(7):769–776

Arnold PD, MacMaster FP, Hanna GL et al (2009) Glutamate system genes associated with ventral prefrontal and thalamic volume in pediatric obsessive-compulsive disorder. Brain Imaging Behav 3(1):64–76

Arranz MJ, de Leon J (2007) Pharmacogenetics and pharmacogenomics of schizophrenia: a review of last decade of research. Mol Psychiatry 12(8):707–747

Baker RW, Chengappa KN, Baird JW et al (1992) Emergence of obsessive compulsive symptoms during treatment with clozapine. J Clin Psychiatry 53:439–442

Bienvenu OJ, Wang Y, Shugart YY et al (2009) Sapap3 and pathological grooming in humans: results from the OCD collaborative genetics study. Am J Med Genet B Neuropsychiatr Genet 150B:710–720

Bloch MH, Landeros-Weisenberger A, Rosario MC et al (2008) Meta-analysis of the symptom structure of obsessive-compulsive disorder. Am J Psychiatry 165:1532–1542

Bottas A, Cooke RG, Richter MA (2005) Comorbidity and pathophysiology of obsessive-compulsive disorder in schizophrenia: is there evidence for a schizo-obsessive subtype of schizophrenia? J Psychiatry Neurosci 30(3):187–193

Byerly M, Goodman W, Acholonu W et al (2005) Obsessive compulsive symptoms in schizophrenia: frequency and clinical features. Schizophr Res 76:309–316

Cai J, Zhang W, Yi Z et al (2013) Influence of polymorphisms in genes SLC1A1, GRIN2B, and GRIK2 on clozapine-induced obsessive-compulsive symptoms. Psychopharmacology (Berl) 230(1):49–55

Cardno AG, Sham PC, Murray RM et al (2001) Twin study of symptom dimensions in psychoses. Br J Psychiatry 179:39–45

Cardno AG, Sham PC, Farmer AE et al (2002) Heritability of Schneider's first-rank symptoms. Br J Psychiatry 180:35–38

Choi KS, Jeon HO, Lee YS et al (2007) Familial association of schizophrenia symptoms retrospectively measured on a lifetime basis. Psychiatr Genet 17:103–107

Choi YK, Gardner MP, Tarazi FI (2009) Effects of risperidone on glutamate receptor subtypes in developing rat brain. Eur Neuropsychopharmacol 19(2):77–84

Crane J, Fagerness J, Osiecki L et al (2011) Family-based genetic association study of DLGAP3 in Tourette Syndrome. Am J Med Genet B Neuropsychiatr Genet 156B:108–114

Cross-Disorder Group of the Psychiatric Genomics Consortium (2013) Identification of risk loci with shared effects on five major psychiatric disorders: a genome-wide analysis. Lancet 381:1371–1379

de Haan L, Linszen DH, Gorsira R (1999) Clozapine and obsessions in patients with recent-onset schizophrenia and other psychotic disorders. J Clin Psychiatry 60:364–365

Denys D, Zohar J, Westenberg HGM (2004) The role of dopamine in obsessive-compulsive disorder: preclinical and clinical evidence. J Clin Psychiatry 65(Suppl 14):11–17

Dickel DE, Veenstra-VanderWeele J, Cox NJ et al (2006) Association testing of the positional and functional candidate gene SLC1A1/EAAC1 in early-onset obsessive-compulsive disorder. Arch Gen Psychiatry 63(7):778–785

Ertugrul A, Anil Yagcioglu AE, Eni N et al (2005) Obsessive-compulsive symptoms in clozapine-treated schizophrenic patients. Psychiatry Clin Neurosci 59:219–222

Fanous AH, Neale MC, Webb BT et al (2007) A genome-wide scan for modifier loci in schizophrenia. Am J Med Genet B Neuropsychiatr Genet 144B:589–595

Fanous AH, Zhou B, Aggen SH et al (2012) Genome-wide association study of clinical dimensions of schizophrenia: polygenic effect on disorganized symptoms. Am J Psychiatry 169:1309–1317

Faragian S, Pashinian A, Fuchs C et al (2009) Obsessive-compulsive symptom dimensions in schizophrenia patients with comorbid obsessive-compulsive disorder. Prog Neuropsychopharmacol Biol Psychiatry 33:1009–1012

Favalli G, Li J, Belmonte-de-Abreu P et al (2012) The role of BDNF in the pathophysiology and treatment of schizophrenia. J Psychiatr Res 46(1):1–11

Geller DA, Wieland N, Carey K et al (2008) Perinatal factors affecting expression of obsessive compulsive disorder in children and adolescents. J Child Adolesc Psychopharmacol 18(4):373–379

Goodman WK, Price LH, Rasmussen SA et al (1989) The Yale-Brown Obsessive Compulsive Scale. II. Validity. Arch Gen Psychiatry 46:1012–1016

Grisham JR, Fullana MA, Mataix-Cols D et al (2011) Risk factors prospectively associated with adult obsessive-compulsive symptom dimensions and obsessive-compulsive disorder. Psychol Med 41(12):2495–2506

Ha TH, Youn T, Rho KS et al (2004) Symptom dimensions of obsessive-compulsive disorder and their relation to comorbid personality pathology. J Korean Neuropsychiatr Assoc 43:46–53

Hahn OS, Ahn JH, Song SH et al (2000) Development of Korean version of structured clinical interview schedule for DSM-IV axis I disorder: interrater reliability. J Korean Neuropsychiatr Assoc 39:362–372

Hamshere ML, Holmans PA, McCarthy GM et al (2011) Phenotype evaluation and genomewide linkage study of clinical variables in schizophrenia. Am J Med Genet B Neuropsychiatr Genet 156B:929–940

Hanna GL, Himle JA, Curtis GC et al (2005) A family study of obsessive-compulsive disorder with pediatric probands. Am J Med Genet B Neuropsychiatr Genet 134B(1):13–19

Hashim HM, Fawzy N, Fawzi MM et al (2012) Brain-derived neurotrophic factor Val66Met polymorphism and obsessive-compulsive symptoms in Egyptian schizophrenia patients. J Psychiatr Res 46(6):762–766

Hasler G, LaSalle-Ricci VH, Ronquillo JG et al (2005) Obsessive-compulsive disorder symptom dimensions show specific relationships to psychiatric comorbidity. Psychiatry Res 135:121–132

Hasler G, Pinto A, Greenberg BD et al (2007) Familiality of factor analysis-derived YBOCS dimensions in OCD-affected sibling pairs from the OCD Collaborative Genetics Study. Biol Psychiatry 61:617–625

Hettema JM, Meale MC, Kendler KS (2001) A review and meta-analysis of the genetic epidemiology of anxiety disorders. Am J Psychiatry 158(10):1568–1578

Hong KS, Nam HJ, Lim M (2008) Emergence of obsessive-compulsive symptoms during clozapine treatment in a pair of monozygotic twins. Br J Psychiatry eLetter 190:81-a #20594 (http://bjp.rcpsych.org/cgi/eletters/190/1/81-a#20594)

Huerta I, McCullumsmith RE, Haroutunian V et al (2006) Expression of excitatory amino acid transporter interacting protein transcripts in the thalamus in schizophrenia. Synapse 59(7):394–402

Hwang MY, Kim SW, Yum SY et al (2009) Management of schizophrenia with obsessive-compulsive features. Psychiatr Clin North Am 32:835–851

Joo EJ, Joo YH, Hong JP et al (2004) Korean version of the diagnostic interview for genetic studies: validity and reliability. Compr Psychiatry 45:225–229
Kendler KS, Diehl SR (1993) The genetics of schizophrenia: a current, genetic-epidemiologic perspective. Schizophr Bull 19:261–285
Kim E, Naisbitt S, Hsueh YP et al (1997) GKAP, a novel synaptic protein that interacts with the guanylate kinase-like domain of the PSD-95/SAP90 family of channel clustering molecules. J Cell Biol 136:669–678
Kim SJ, Choi NK, Hong HJ et al (2004) Dimensional analyses of the Yale-Brown obsessive-compulsive scale and Yale-Brown obsessive-compulsive scale checklist. Korean J Psychopharmacol 15:339–345
Kim JH, Ryu S, Nam H et al (2012) Symptom structure of antipsychotic-induced obsessive compulsive symptoms in schizophrenia patients. Prog Neuropsychopharmacol Biol Psychiatry 39(1):75–79
Kindler S, Rehbein M, Classen B et al (2004) Distinct spatiotemporal expression of SAPAP transcripts in the developing rat brain: a novel dendritically localized mRNA. Brain Res Mol Brain Res 126:14–21
Kwon JS, Joo YH, Nam HJ et al (2009) Association of glutamate transporter gene SLC1A1 with atypical antipsychotics-induced obsessive compulsive symptoms. Arch Gen Psychiatry 66(11):1233–1241
Lafleur DL, Petty C, Mancuso E et al (2011) Traumatic events and obsessive compulsive disorder in children and adolescents: is there a link? J Anxiety Disord 25(4):513–519
Landau D, Iervolino AC, Pertusa A et al (2011) Stressful life events and material deprivation in hoarding disorder. J Anxiety Disord 25(2):192–202
Leckman JF, Grice DE, Boardman J et al (1997) Symptoms of obsessive-compulsive disorder. Am J Psychiatry 154:911–917
Lim M, Park DY, Kwon JS et al (2007) Prevalence and clinical characteristics of obsessive-compulsive symptoms associated with atypical antipsychotics. J Clin Psychopharmacol 27(6):712–713
López-Gil X, Artigas F, Adell A (2010) Unraveling monoamine receptors involved in the action of typical and atypical antipsychotics on glutamatergic and serotonergic transmission in prefrontal cortex. Curr Pharm Des 16(5):502–515
Lykouras L, Alevizos B, Michalopoulou P et al (2003) Obsessive-compulsive symptoms induced by atypical antipsychotics. A review of the reported cases. Prog Neuropsychopharmacol Biol Psychiatry 27:333–346
Mahendran R, Liew E, Subramaniam M (2007) De novo emergence of obsessive-compulsive symptoms with atypical antipsychotics in Asian patients with schizophrenia or schizoaffective disorder: a retrospective, cross-sectional study. J Clin Psychiatry 68(4):542–545
Malhotra AK (2002) Pharmacogenetics and pharmacogenomics of psychotropic drug response. In: Lerer B (ed) Pharmacogenetics of psychotropic drugs. Cambridge University Press, Cambridge, pp 21–35
Mataix-Cols D, Boman M, Monzani B et al (2013) Population-based, multigenerational family clustering study of obsessive-compulsive disorder. JAMA Psychiatry 70:709–717
Mattheisen M, Samuels JF, Wang Y et al (2014) Genome-wide association study in obsessive-compulsive disorder: results from the OCGAS. Mol Psychiatry. doi:10.1038/mp.2014.43 [Epub ahead of print]
Milad MR, Rauch SL (2012) Obsessive-compulsive disorder: beyond segregated cortico-striatal pathways. Trends Cogn Sci 16:43–51
Monzani B, Rijsdijk F, Harris J et al (2014) The structure of genetic and environmental risk factors for dimensional representations of DSM-5 obsessive-compulsive spectrum disorders. JAMA Psychiatry 71(2):182–189
Moutsimilli L, Farley S, El Khoury MA et al (2008) Antipsychotics increase vesicular glutamate transporter 2 (VGLUT2) expression in thalamolimbic pathways. Neuropharmacology 54(3):497–508

Murphy TK, Kurlan R, Leckman J (2010) The immunobiology of Tourette's disorder, pediatric autoimmune neuropsychiatric disorders associated with Streptococcus, and related disorders: a way forward. J Child Adolesc Psychopharmacol 20(4):317–331

Nestadt G, Samuels J, Riddle M et al (2000) A family study of obsessive-compulsive disorder. Arch Gen Psychiatry 57:358–363

Pauls DL (2008) The genetics of obsessive compulsive disorder: a review of the evidence. Am J Med Genet C Semin Med Genet 148(2):133–139

Pauls DL, Abramovitch A, Rauch SL et al (2014) Obsessive-compulsive disorder: an integrative genetic and neurobiological perspective. Nat Rev Neurosci 15(6):410–424

Pittenger C, Bloch MH, Williams K (2011) Glutamate abnormalities in obsessive compulsive disorder: neurobiology, pathophysiology, and treatment. Pharmacol Ther 132(3):314–332

Poyurovsky M, Kriss V, Weisman G et al (2005a) Familial aggregation of schizophrenia-spectrum disorders and obsessive-compulsive associated disorders in schizophrenia probands with and without OCD. Am J Med Genet B Neuropsychiatr Genet 133B(1):31–36

Poyurovsky M, Michaelovsky E, Frisch A et al (2005b) COMT Val158Met polymorphism in schizophrenia with obsessive-compulsive disorder: a case–control study. Neurosci Lett 389(1):21–24

Ryu S, Oh S, Cho EY et al (2011) Interaction between genetic variants of DLGAP3 and SLC1A1 affecting the risk of atypical antipsychotics-induced obsessive-compulsive symptoms. Am J Med Genet B Neuropsychiatr Genet 156B(8):949–959

Ryu S, Won H-H, Oh S et al (2013) Genome-wide linkage scan of quantitative traits representing symptom dimensions in multiplex schizophrenia families. Psychiatry Res 210(3):756–760

Sadock BJ, Sadock VA (2007) Kaplan & Sadock's synopsis of psychiatry, 10th edn. Lippincott Williams & Wilkins, Philadelphia, p 604

Scheltema Beduin AA, Swets M, Machielsen M et al (2012) Obsessive-compulsive symptoms in patients with schizophrenia: a naturalistic cross-sectional study comparing treatment with clozapine, olanzapine, risperidone, and no antipsychotics in 543 patients. J Clin Psychiatry 73(11):1395–1402

Schirmbeck F, Zink M (2013) Comorbid obsessive-compulsive symptoms in schizophrenia: contributions of pharmacological and genetic factors. Front Pharmacol 4:99

Schirmbeck F, Nieratschker V, Frank J et al (2012) Polymorphisms in the glutamate transporter gene SLC1A1 and obsessive-compulsive symptoms induced by second-generation antipsychotic agents. Psychiatr Genet 22(5):245–252

Schirmbeck F, Rausch F, Englisch S et al (2013) Differential effects of antipsychotic agents on obsessive-compulsive symptoms in schizophrenia: a longitudinal study. J Psychopharmacol 27(4):349–357

Schmitt A, Zink M, Muller B et al (2003a) Effects of long-term antipsychotic treatment on NMDA receptor binding and gene expression of subunits. Neurochem Res 28(2):235–241

Schmitt A, Zink M, Petroianu G (2003b) Decreased gene expression of glial and neuronal glutamate transporters after chronic antipsychotic treatment in rat brain. Neurosci Lett 347(2):81–84

Stewart SE, Fagerness JA, Platko J et al (2007) Association of the SLC1A1 glutamate transporter gene and obsessive-compulsive disorder. Am J Med Genet B Neuropsychiatr Genet 144(8):1027–1033

Stewart SE, Yu D, Scharf JM et al (2013) Genome-wide association study of obsessive-compulsive disorder. Mol Psychiatry 18:788–798

Sullivan PF, Kendler KS, Neale MC (2003) Schizophrenia as a complex trait: evidence from a meta-analysis of twin studies. Arch Gen Psychiatry 60:1187–1192

Takeuchi M, Hata Y, Hirao K et al (1997) SAPAPs. A family of PSD-95/SAP90-associated proteins localized at postsynaptic density. J Biol Chem 272:11943–11951

Taylor S (2011) Etiology of obsessions and compulsions: a meta-analysis and narrative review of twin studies. Clin Psychol Rev 31:1361–1372

The Schizophrenia Psychiatric Genome-Wide Association Study (GWAS) Consortium (2011) Genome-wide association study identifies five new schizophrenia loci. Nat Genet 43(10):969–976

Tzingounis AV, Wadiche JI (2007) Glutamate transporters: confining runaway excitation by shaping synaptic transmission. Nat Rev Neurosci 8(12):935–947

Van Grootheest DS, Cath DC, Beekman AT et al (2005) Twin studies on obsessive-compulsive disorder: a review. Twin Res Hum Genet 8(5):450–458

Vassos E, Sham PC, Cai G et al (2008) Correlation and familial aggregation of dimensions of psychosis in affected sibling pairs from China. Br J Psychiatry 193:305–310

Wang Y, Mathews CA, Li Y et al (2011) Brain-derived neurotrophic factor (BDNF) plasma levels in drug-naïve OCD patients are lower than those in healthy people, but are not lower than those in drug-treated OCD patients. J Affect Disord 133(1–2):305–310

Welch JM, Wang D, Feng G (2004) Differential mRNA expression and protein localization of the SAP90/PSD-95-associated proteins (SAPAPs) in the nervous system of the mouse. J Comp Neurol 472:24–39

Welch JM, Lu J, Rodriguiz RM et al (2007) Cortico-striatal synaptic defects and OCD-like behaviours in Sapap3-mutant mice. Nature 448:894–900

Wendland JR, Moya PR, Timpano KR et al (2009) A haplotype containing quantitative trait loci for SLC1A1 gene expression and its association with obsessive-compulsive disorder. Arch Gen Psychiatry 66(4):408–416

Wickham H, Walsh C, Asherson P et al (2001) Familiality of symptom dimensions in schizophrenia. Schizophr Res 47(2–3):223–232

Yamamoto BK, Cooperman MA (1994) Differential effects of chronic antipsychotic drug treatment on extracellular glutamate and dopamine concentrations. J Neurosci 14(7):4159–4166

Zinkstok J, van Nimwegen L, van Amelsvoort T et al (2008) Catechol-O-methyltransferase gene and obsessive-compulsive symptoms in patients with recent-onset schizophrenia: preliminary results. Psychiatry Res 157(1–3):1–8

Zuchner S, Wendland JR, Ashley-Koch AE et al (2009) Multiple rare SAPAP3 missense variants in trichotillomania and OCD. Mol Psychiatry 14:6–9

9 Obsessive-Compulsive Symptoms in Schizophrenia: Neurophysiological and Neuroimaging Findings

Naren P. Rao and Ganesan Venkatasubramanian

Abbreviations

ACC	Anterior cingulate cortex
CSF	Cerebrospinal fluid
DLPFC	Dorsolateral prefrontal cortex
LSD	Lysergic acid diethylamide
MRI	Magnetic resonance imaging
MRS	Magnetic resonance spectroscopy
NMDA	N-methyl-D-aspartate
OCD	Obsessive-compulsive disorder
OCS	Obsessive-compulsive symptoms
OFC	Orbitofrontal cortex
PET	Positron emission tomography

N.P. Rao
DST-INSPIRE Faculty, Centre for Neuroscience, Indian Institute of Science, Bangalore, Karnataka, India

Department of Psychiatry & Translational Psychiatry Laboratory, The Schizophrenia Clinic, Neurobiology Research Centre, National Institute of Mental Health and Neurosciences (NIMHANS), Bangalore, Karnataka 560029, India

G. Venkatasubramanian, MD, PhD (✉)
Department of Psychiatry & Translational Psychiatry Laboratory, The Schizophrenia Clinic, Neurobiology Research Centre, National Institute of Mental Health and Neurosciences (NIMHANS), Bangalore, Karnataka 560029, India
e-mail: venkat.nimhans@yahoo.com

L. De Haan et al. (eds.), *Obsessive-Compulsive Symptoms in Schizophrenia*,
DOI 10.1007/978-3-319-12952-5_9

9.1 Introduction

Although schizophrenia and obsessive-compulsive disorder (OCD) are distinct nosological entities, obsessive-compulsive symptoms (OCS) and schizophrenia symptoms frequently coexist in a substantial proportion of patients; the prevalence of OCS in schizophrenia has been reported to range from 8 to 46 % (Eisen et al. 1997; Poyurovsky et al. 2004). Considering the lifetime prevalence of these two illnesses [(1–1.5 % for schizophrenia (Bland et al. 1987) and 2–3 % for obsessive-compulsive disorder (OCD) (Karno et al. 1988)], this co-occurrence of OCS and schizophrenia cannot be explained by mere chance (Tibbo and Warneke 1999). However, whether this co-occurrence is a co-morbidity or represents a distinct entity remains controversial. Nonetheless, some researchers have proposed a schizo-obsessive subgroup of schizophrenia as a separate diagnostic entity (Poyurovsky et al. 2012). This controversy is mainly based on clinical findings and only few studies have examined the neurobiology of OCS in schizophrenia. These studies have reported both overlapping and distinct neurobiological findings between schizophrenia patients with OCD and without OCD (Venkatasubramanian et al. 2009). In this chapter we will review the relation between schizophrenia and OCD in the context of neuroanatomical, neurochemical and neurodevelopmental abnormalities. Initially we will review the neuroimaging and neurophysiological findings in OCD and schizophrenia per se and later summarize the current knowledge regarding co-morbid OCS in schizophrenia.

9.2 Neuroimaging and Neurophysiological Findings in OCD and Schizophrenia

9.2.1 Neuroimaging Findings in OCD

Over the past two decades, different studies have indicated abnormalities of cortico-striato-thalamo-cortical circuits in the pathogenesis of OCD. Whereas increased regional grey matter volumes in basal ganglia structures – namely, bilateral lenticular nuclei, caudate nuclei and putamen – are reported in different meta-analyses (Peng et al. 2012; Radua and Mataix-Cols 2009), one meta-analysis did not find volumetric differences within the basal ganglia (Rotge et al. 2009). Increased grey matter volume has also been reported in the parietal lobule (Peng et al. 2012) and thalami (Rotge et al. 2010). On the other hand, a reduced volume of cortical regions – namely, anterior cingulate cortex (ACC), orbitofrontal cortex (OFC) and dorsolateral prefrontal cortex (DLPFC) – has consistently been reported in all meta-analysis (Rotge et al. 2009, 2010; Peng et al. 2012; Radua et al. 2010). It is important to note that these regional differences are observed in the absence of global grey matter volume differences.

In addition to grey matter volume abnormalities, a recent meta-analysis also reported white matter abnormalities in the form of lower fractional anisotropy (FA) in the cingulum bundles, inferior fronto-occipital fasciculus, superior longitudinal fasciculus, corpus callosum and anterior limb of the internal capsule and increased FA in the left uncinate fasciculus in OCD patients, again suggesting abnormality of frontal cortex connections (Peng et al. 2012; Koch et al. 2014). Positron emission tomography (PET) studies reported increased metabolic rates in the orbitofrontal cortex (OFC) and cingulate cortex in patients with OCD (Baxter et al. 1990; Saxena et al. 2001, 2004; Nordahl et al. 1989). Single photon emission computed tomography (SPECT) studies have reported equivocal findings with some reporting hyperactivity (Lacerda et al. 2003; Alptekin et al. 2001), whereas others did not find any changes (Crespo-Facorro et al. 1999; Busatto et al. 2000). Low metabolic rates in the striatum and thalamus have been reported in most (Saxena et al. 1999; Nordahl et al. 1989; Rauch et al. 2001) but not all studies (Perani et al. 1995).

In summary, these studies substantially support assumed abnormalities in the cortico-striato-thalamo-cortical circuitry in patients with OCD. The proposed circuit arises in the frontal cortex and projects sequentially to ventromedial areas of caudate nucleus, globus pallidus and mediodorsal thalamus before projecting back to the cortex (Bonelli and Cummings 2007). Increased excitatory output from the orbitofrontal/cingulate cortex and increased caudate activity are postulated to cause inhibition of the dorsal thalamus which in turn leads to decreased disinhibition and increased cortical activation (Baxter et al. 1992).

9.2.2 Neuroimaging Findings in Schizophrenia

Established concepts about the mechanisms of schizophrenia postulate a disruption in distributed functional circuits rather than an abnormality in a single brain region such as the prefrontal cortex (Keshavan et al. 2008). In addition to the frontal cortex, brain abnormalities in schizophrenia have been demonstrated in the basal ganglia, the thalamus and the cerebellum (Schultz and Andreasen 1999; Konick and Friedman 2001; Heckers 1997; Keshavan et al. 2008; Andreasen and Pierson 2008). Thalamus abnormalities have been reported in both structural and functional imaging studies (Hazlett et al. 1999; Rao et al. 2010); patients with schizophrenia had smaller thalamic volumes compared to healthy controls (Rao et al. 2010). Studies investigating the volume of the caudate nucleus are controversial with some finding enlarged volumes in schizophrenic patients (Swayze et al. 1992; Breier et al. 1992) and others finding decreased volumes (Keshavan et al. 1998; Shihabuddin et al. 1998). No difference in the size of striatal structures has also been reported (DeLisi et al. 1997). While the majority of studies in schizophrenia have focused on the DLPFC, only a few studies have focused on the OFC; both increased (Hoptman et al. 2005) and decreased volumes (Goldstein et al. 1999) have been reported in schizophrenia compared to healthy controls. Similarly findings are inconclusive with respect to anterior cingulate cortex; both decreased (Haznedar et al. 1997) and increased activation (Catafau et al. 1994) have been reported as well as both decreased volume (Noga et al. 1995) and the absence of differences (Nordahl et al. 1996). Andreasen et al. (1998) have hypothesized a prefrontal-thalamic-cerebellar-prefrontal pathway to explain the symptoms of schizophrenia. It is argued that the thalamus filters out unnecessary information and forwards only relevant information, and the deficit of this function may lead to positive symptoms in schizophrenia (Andreasen 1997). This theory of 'input overload' in schizophrenia has similarity to that proposed for OCD (Tibbo and Warneke 1999).

In summary, abnormalities of the frontal lobe, the basal ganglia, the thalamus and the cerebellum have been demonstrated both in schizophrenia and in OCD. Thus, reviewing literature on neuroanatomical circuits in schizophrenia and OCD reveals more similarities than differences. In fact, recent studies implicate comparable abnormalities in both schizophrenia and OCD (Kang et al. 2008; Kwon et al. 2003). Similarities between OCD and schizophrenia also emerge if one considers the gating or filtering of sensory information as playing a role in either illness.

9.3 Neuroimaging Findings of OCS in Schizophrenia

While a number of studies have examined the clinical characteristics and epidemiological features of OCS in schizophrenia, neuroimaging literature is sparse. Few studies have examined structural and functional abnormalities as possible distinct neurobiological underpinnings of a schizo-obsessive disorder. A study by Aoyama et al. revealed significantly reduced volumes of the left hippocampus, frontal lobes and anterior horn of the lateral and third ventricles in schizophrenia patients with OCS compared to those without OCS (Aoyama et al. 2000). The same study also found an inverse correlation between illness duration and frontal lobe size in schizo-obsessive patients but not in schizophrenia patients. These findings were replicated in another study which also demonstrated enlarged anterior horn of the lateral ventricle and the third ventricle in schizo-obsessive patients compared to schizophrenia only (Iida et al. 1998).

Similar to structural magnetic resonance imaging (MRI) studies, one functional MRI study reported the effect of OCS on brain activation; schizo-obsessive patients exhibited a negative correlation between activation of the left dorsolateral prefrontal cortex and OCS severity (Levine et al. 1998). However, a recent study did not report differences between schizo-obsessive and schizophrenia patients; authors examined working memory tasks in schizo-obsessive, schizophrenia and matched healthy volunteers and reported reduced activation in the right DLPFC and right caudate, as well as decreased functional connectivity (FC) in both schizo-obsessives and schizophrenia compared to healthy controls (Bleich-Cohen et al. 2014). Another recent functional MRI study utilized response inhibition and working memory paradigms to elucidate the effects of second-generation antipsychotic medication on the neural systems related to OCS in schizophrenia (Schirmbeck et al. 2014) (see Chap. 10). Altered brain activation (especially increased activation of OFC during response inhibition) related to the antipsychotic treatment might be a pathogenic mechanism in the development of antipsychotic-induced OCS in schizophrenia (Schirmbeck et al. 2014).

9.4 Neuropsychological Profile of OCS in Schizophrenia

Similar to neuroimaging studies, a possible neuropsychological profile of schizo-obsessive disorder has been investigated. The results are inconsistent when comparing findings to schizophrenia and OCD (for details, see Chap. 7). While few studies have reported deficits in different cognitive domains, namely, set shifting (Hwang et al. 2000; Lysaker et al. 2002; Patel et al. 2010), sustained attention (Lysaker et al. 2002), visuospatial perception, visual memory (Schirmbeck et al. 2013) and delayed visual memory (Berman et al. 1998), other studies have reported better performance on attention and psychomotor speed (Borkowska et al. 2003), set shifting (Borkowska et al. 2003), verbal fluency (Lee et al. 2009) and immediate visual recall (Lysaker et al. 2002) in patients with a schizo-obsessive disorder compared to schizophrenia. No difference between schizo-obsessive disorder and schizophrenia is also reported in attention (Berman et al. 1998; Tumkaya et al. 2009), response inhibition (Berman et al. 1998; Tumkaya et al. 2009; Lee et al. 2009; Patel et al. 2010), set shifting (Borkowska et al. 2003; Berman et al. 1998; Hermesh et al. 2003; Tumkaya et al. 2009), verbal fluency (Berman et al. 1998; Borkowska et al. 2003), planning and decision-making (Hermesh et al. 2003; Patel et al. 2010), visual memory (Tumkaya et al. 2009; Lee et al. 2009) and verbal memory (Tumkaya et al. 2009; Lee et al. 2009). In a recent study (Schirmbeck et al. 2013), schizophrenia patients with antipsychotic-associated OCS had greater deficits in visuospatial perception and visual memory, executive functioning and cognitive flexibility compared to schizophrenia patients without OCS. These differences were found to be longitudinally stable over 12 months. A recent meta-analysis found higher impairment in abstract reasoning in schizo-obsessive patients compared to patients with schizophrenia with no difference in performance on other measures of executive function (Cunill et al. 2013). A recent study that attempted to examine whether candidate cognitive endophenotypes may be used to validate a schizo-obsessive subtype found no differential cognitive impairment in this group of patients (Meijer et al. 2013). In the context of these findings, it has been suggested that the majority of previous studies, which investigated the cognitive profile of schizophrenia patients with OCS, might have been confounded by a greater severity of psychosis. Hence, further research examining patients and their unaffected relatives is warranted to clarify the nature of genetic and environmental factors in schizophrenia with co-morbid obsessive-compulsive symptoms (Meijer et al. 2013).

9.5 Neurophysiological Findings in Schizo-Obsessive Disorder

Only one study examined the neurophysiological abnormalities in schizo-obsessive patients using event-related potentials (ERPs) during a discriminative response task. The study reported a distinct ERP pattern, with abnormally increased target activation and reduced P300 amplitudes in a schizo-obsessive group in comparison to a schizophrenia group and an OCD group (Pallanti et al. 2009).

9.6 Neurochemical Circuit Overlap in Schizophrenia and OCD

Several neurochemical systems interact in both OCS and psychotic disorders, most importantly serotonin, glutamate and dopamine.

Serotonin Serotonergic abnormalities are documented in both schizophrenia and OCD; elevated levels of 5-HT_2 receptors are demonstrated in the frontal cortex in schizophrenia, and lysergic acid diethylamide (LSD), a 5-HT_2 agonist, is a well-known psychotomimetic (Busatto and Kerwin 1997). Moreover, serotonergic modulation of dopaminergic function provides a viable mechanism in schizophrenia (Agid et al. 2008). Serotonergic abnormalities play a pivotal role as indicated by the differential efficacy of serotonergic reuptake inhibitors in alleviating OCS (Murphy et al. 1989) over noradrenergic tricyclic antidepressants like desipramine. In addition, serotonin transporter and serotonin receptor (Bengel et al. 1999; Mundo et al. 2002) abnormalities are documented in OCD.

Glutamate Glutamate abnormality, mainly NMDA receptor deficiency, is one of the influential hypotheses for schizophrenia pathogenesis (Sodhi et al. 2008). The phencyclidine model of schizophrenia symptoms and up-regulation of glutamate receptor expression in the frontal cortex after chronic exposure to clozapine or olanzapine (Tascedda et al. 2001) provide further support to glutamate abnormalities in schizophrenia. In OCD, reports from neuroimaging, genetic and cerebrospinal fluid (CSF) studies support involvement of glutamatergic system in the pathogenesis of OCD (Bhattacharyya and Chakraborty 2007): (a) neuroimaging studies using magnetic resonance spectroscopy (MRS) consistently have demonstrated increased glutamate in caudate and frontal cortex (Rosenberg et al. 2000; MacMaster et al. 2008); (b) genes involved in glutamate transmission (SLC1A1) have been implicated in association studies (Dickel et al. 2006); (c) a CSF study examining glutamate levels has reported increased glutamate in OCD patients (Chakrabarty et al. 2005); and (d) the glutamate antagonist riluzole is useful in treatment refractory OCD (Coric et al. 2005).

Dopamine The revised dopaminergic hypothesis of schizophrenia postulates a regional abnormality in the dopaminergic system and dopamine as the final common pathway in the pathophysiology of schizophrenia (Keshavan et al. 2008; Kapur et al. 2005; Meyer-Lindenberg 2010). In its current form, the dopamine hypothesis of schizophrenia postulates a hyperdopaminergic state in the mesolimbic pathway resulting in psychotic symptoms and a hypodopaminergic state in the frontal cortical terminal fields of the mesocortical dopamine neurons as the basis of the 'negative symptoms' of schizophrenia (Duncan et al. 1999).

Dopamine and serotonin abnormalities have been demonstrated in patients with OCD (Marazziti et al. 1992), and several lines of evidence from preclinical and clinical investigations implicate dopamine in the mediation of certain types of repetitive behaviour (Goodman et al. 1990). Antipsychotic augmentation of treatment with serotonin reuptake inhibitors (SRI) suggests that dopamine receptor antagonism may further reduce OCS severity in SSRI-refractory OCD patients (Bloch et al. 2006). In summary, studies show abnormalities of serotonin, glutamate and dopamine in schizophrenia as well as in OCD. However, no study has examined neurochemical abnormalities in schizo-obsessive patients compared to schizophrenia and OCD which would provide further insights into the underlying neurochemical changes.

9.7 Summary

In summary, this review of neurobiological findings points towards significantly shared structural and functional brain abnormalities, namely, frontal lobe dysfunction and basal ganglia dysfunction in both schizophrenia and OCD. The preliminary evidence also suggests a greater deficit in schizo-obsessive patients than schizophrenia patients without OCS on neuroimaging, neuropsychological and neurophysiological measures. However, the number of studies investigating schizo-obsessive patients is limited and inconclusive and warrants further examination in longitudinal studies with bigger samples to delineate the underlying neurobiology.

References

Agid O, Kapur S, Remington G (2008) Emerging drugs for schizophrenia. Expert Opin Emerg Drugs 13(3):479–495. doi:10.1517/14728214.13.3.479

Alptekin K, Degirmenci B, Kivircik B, Durak H, Yemez B, Derebek E, Tunca Z (2001) Tc-99 m HMPAO brain perfusion SPECT in drug-free obsessive-compulsive patients without depression. Psychiatry Res 107(1):51–56, S0925492701000865 [pii]

Andreasen NC (1997) The role of the thalamus in schizophrenia. Can J Psychiatry 42(1):27–33

Andreasen NC, Pierson R (2008) The role of the cerebellum in schizophrenia. Biol Psychiatry 64(2):81–88. doi:10.1016/j.biopsych.2008.01.003, S0006-3223(08)00049-8 [pii]

Andreasen NC, Paradiso S, O'Leary DS (1998) "Cognitive dysmetria" as an integrative theory of schizophrenia: a dysfunction in cortical-subcortical-cerebellar circuitry? Schizophr Bull 24(2):203–218

Aoyama F, Iida J, Inoue M, Iwasaka H, Sakiyama S, Hata K, Kishimoto T (2000) Brain imaging in childhood- and adolescence-onset schizophrenia associated with obsessive-compulsive symptoms. Acta Psychiatr Scand 102(1):32–37

Baxter LR Jr, Schwartz JM, Guze BH, Bergman K, Szuba MP (1990) PET imaging in obsessive compulsive disorder with and without depression. J Clin Psychiatry 51(Suppl):61–69; discussion 70

Baxter LR Jr, Schwartz JM, Bergman KS, Szuba MP, Guze BH, Mazziotta JC, Alazraki A, Selin CE, Ferng HK, Munford P et al (1992) Caudate glucose metabolic rate changes with both drug and behavior therapy for obsessive-compulsive disorder. Arch Gen Psychiatry 49(9):681–689

Bengel D, Greenberg BD, Cora-Locatelli G, Altemus M, Heils A, Li Q, Murphy DL (1999) Association of the serotonin transporter promoter regulatory region polymorphism and obsessive-compulsive disorder. Mol Psychiatry 4(5):463–466

Berman I, Merson A, Viegner B, Losonczy MF, Pappas D, Green AI (1998) Obsessions and compulsions as a distinct cluster of symptoms in schizophrenia: a neuropsychological study. J Nerv Ment Dis 186(3):150–156

Bhattacharyya S, Chakraborty K (2007) Glutamatergic dysfunction–newer targets for anti-obsessional drugs. Recent Pat CNS Drug Discov 2(1):47–55

Bland RC, Newman SC, Orn H (1987) Schizophrenia: lifetime co-morbidity in a community sample. Acta Psychiatr Scand 75(4):383–391

Bleich-Cohen M, Hendler T, Weizman R, Faragian S, Weizman A, Poyurovsky M (2014) Working memory dysfunction in schizophrenia patients with obsessive-compulsive symptoms: an fMRI study. Eur Psychiatry 29(3):160–166. doi:10.1016/j.eurpsy.2013.02.004, S0924-9338(13)00020-5 [pii]

Bloch MH, Landeros-Weisenberger A, Kelmendi B, Coric V, Bracken MB, Leckman JF (2006) A systematic review: antipsychotic augmentation with treatment refractory obsessive-compulsive disorder. Mol Psychiatry 11(7):622–632. doi:10.1038/sj.mp.4001823, 4001823 [pii]

Bonelli RM, Cummings JL (2007) Frontal-subcortical circuitry and behavior. Dialogues Clin Neurosci 9(2):141–151

Borkowska A, Pilaczynska E, Rybakowski JK (2003) The frontal lobe neuropsychological tests in patients with schizophrenia and/or obsessive-compulsive disorder. J Neuropsychiatry Clin Neurosci 15(3):359–362

Breier A, Buchanan RW, Elkashef A, Munson RC, Kirkpatrick B, Gellad F (1992) Brain morphology and schizophrenia. A magnetic resonance imaging study of limbic, prefrontal cortex, and caudate structures. Arch Gen Psychiatry 49(12):921–926

Busatto GF, Kerwin RW (1997) Perspectives on the role of serotonergic mechanisms in the pharmacology of schizophrenia. J Psychopharmacol 11(1):3–12

Busatto GF, Zamignani DR, Buchpiguel CA, Garrido GE, Glabus MF, Rocha ET, Maia AF, Rosario-Campos MC, Campi Castro C, Furuie SS, Gutierrez MA, McGuire PK, Miguel EC (2000) A voxel-based investigation of regional cerebral blood flow abnormalities in obsessive-compulsive disorder using single photon emission computed tomography (SPECT). Psychiatry Res 99(1):15–27, S0925492700000500 [pii]

Catafau AM, Parellada E, Lomena FJ, Bernardo M, Pavia J, Ros D, Setoain J, Gonzalez-Monclus E (1994) Prefrontal and temporal blood flow in schizophrenia: resting and activation technetium-99 m-HMPAO SPECT patterns in young neuroleptic-naive patients with acute disease. J Nucl Med 35(6):935–941

Chakrabarty K, Bhattacharyya S, Christopher R, Khanna S (2005) Glutamatergic dysfunction in OCD. Neuropsychopharmacology 30(9):1735–1740. doi:10.1038/sj.npp.1300733, 1300733 [pii]

Coric V, Taskiran S, Pittenger C, Wasylink S, Mathalon DH, Valentine G, Saksa J, Wu YT, Gueorguieva R, Sanacora G, Malison RT, Krystal JH (2005) Riluzole augmentation in treatment-resistant obsessive-compulsive disorder: an open-label trial. Biol Psychiatry 58(5):424–428. doi:10.1016/j.biopsych.2005.04.043, S0006-3223(05)00563-9 [pii]

Crespo-Facorro B, Cabranes JA, Lopez-Ibor Alcocer MI, Paya B, Fernandez Perez C, Encinas M, Ayuso Mateos JL, Lopez-Ibor JJ Jr (1999) Regional cerebral blood flow in obsessive-compulsive patients with and without a chronic tic disorder. A SPECT study. Eur Arch Psychiatry Clin Neurosci 249(3):156–161

Cunill R, Huerta-Ramos E, Castells X (2013) The effect of obsessive-compulsive symptomatology on executive functions in schizophrenia: a systematic review and meta-analysis. Psychiatry Res. doi:10.1016/j.psychres.2013.05.029

DeLisi LE, Sakuma M, Tew W, Kushner M, Hoff AL, Grimson R (1997) Schizophrenia as a chronic active brain process: a study of progressive brain structural change subsequent to the onset of schizophrenia. Psychiatry Res 74(3):129–140

Dickel DE, Veenstra-VanderWeele J, Cox NJ, Wu X, Fischer DJ, Van Etten-Lee M, Himle JA, Leventhal BL, Cook EH Jr, Hanna GL (2006) Association testing of the positional and functional candidate gene SLC1A1/EAAC1 in early-onset obsessive-compulsive disorder. Arch Gen Psychiatry 63(7):778–785. doi:10.1001/archpsyc.63.7.778, 63/7/778 [pii]

Duncan GE, Sheitman BB, Lieberman JA (1999) An integrated view of pathophysiological models of schizophrenia. Brain Res Brain Res Rev 29(2–3):250–264

Eisen JL, Beer DA, Pato MT, Venditto TA, Rasmussen SA (1997) Obsessive-compulsive disorder in patients with schizophrenia or schizoaffective disorder. Am J Psychiatry 154(2):271–273

Goldstein JM, Goodman JM, Seidman LJ, Kennedy DN, Makris N, Lee H, Tourville J, Caviness VS Jr, Faraone SV, Tsuang MT (1999) Cortical abnormalities in schizophrenia identified by structural magnetic resonance imaging. Arch Gen Psychiatry 56(6):537–547

Goodman WK, McDougle CJ, Price LH, Riddle MA, Pauls DL, Leckman JF (1990) Beyond the serotonin hypothesis: a role for dopamine in some forms of obsessive compulsive disorder? J Clin Psychiatry 51(Suppl):36–43; discussion 55–38

Hazlett EA, Buchsbaum MS, Byne W, Wei TC, Spiegel-Cohen J, Geneve C, Kinderlehrer R, Haznedar MM, Shihabuddin L, Siever LJ (1999) Three-dimensional analysis with MRI and PET of the size, shape, and function of the thalamus in the schizophrenia spectrum. Am J Psychiatry 156(8):1190–1199

Haznedar MM, Buchsbaum MS, Luu C, Hazlett EA, Siegel BV Jr, Lohr J, Wu J, Haier RJ, Bunney WE Jr (1997) Decreased anterior cingulate gyrus metabolic rate in schizophrenia. Am J Psychiatry 154(5):682–684

Heckers S (1997) Neuropathology of schizophrenia: cortex, thalamus, basal ganglia, and neurotransmitter-specific projection systems. Schizophr Bull 23(3):403–421

Hermesh H, Weizman A, Gur S, Zalsman G, Shiloh R, Zohar J, Gross-Isseroff R (2003) Alternation learning in OCD/schizophrenia patients. Eur Neuropsychopharmacol 13(2):87–91

Hoptman MJ, Volavka J, Weiss EM, Czobor P, Szeszko PR, Gerig G, Chakos M, Blocher J, Citrome LL, Lindenmayer JP, Sheitman B, Lieberman JA, Bilder RM (2005) Quantitative MRI measures of orbitofrontal cortex in patients with chronic schizophrenia or schizoaffective disorder. Psychiatry Res 140(2):133–145. doi:10.1016/j.pscychresns.2005.07.004, S0925-4927(05)00109-5 [pii]

Hwang MY, Morgan JE, Losconzcy MF (2000) Clinical and neuropsychological profiles of obsessive-compulsive schizophrenia: a pilot study. J Neuropsychiatry Clin Neurosci 12(1):91–94

Iida J, Matumura K, Aoyama F (1998) Cerebral MRI findings in childhood-onset schizophrenia, comparison of patients with prodromal obsessive-compulsive symptoms and those without symptoms. Recent Prog Child Adolesc Psychiatry 2:75–83

Kang DH, Kim SH, Kim CW, Choi JS, Jang JH, Jung MH, Lee JM, Kim SI, Kwon JS (2008) Thalamus surface shape deformity in obsessive-compulsive disorder and schizophrenia. Neuroreport 19(6):609–613. doi:10.1097/WNR.0b013e3282fa6db9

Kapur S, Mizrahi R, Li M (2005) From dopamine to salience to psychosis–linking biology, pharmacology and phenomenology of psychosis. Schizophr Res 79:59–68

Karno M, Golding JM, Sorenson SB, Burnam MA (1988) The epidemiology of obsessive-compulsive disorder in five US communities. Arch Gen Psychiatry 45(12):1094–1099

Keshavan MS, Rosenberg D, Sweeney JA, Pettegrew JW (1998) Decreased caudate volume in neuroleptic-naive psychotic patients. Am J Psychiatry 155(6):774–778

Keshavan MS, Tandon R, Boutros NN, Nasrallah HA (2008) Schizophrenia, "just the facts": what we know in 2008 Part 3: neurobiology. Schizophr Res 106(2–3):89–107. doi:10.1016/j.schres.2008.07.020, S0920-9964(08)00332-0 [pii]

Koch K, Reess TJ, Rus OG, Zimmer C, Zaudig M (2014) Diffusion tensor imaging (DTI) studies in patients with obsessive-compulsive disorder (OCD): a review. J Psychiatr Res 54C:26–35. doi:10.1016/j.jpsychires.2014.03.006, S0022-3956(14)00079-X [pii]

Konick LC, Friedman L (2001) Meta-analysis of thalamic size in schizophrenia. Biol Psychiatry 49(1):28–38, S0006-3223(00)00974-4 [pii]

Kwon JS, Shin YW, Kim CW, Kim YI, Youn T, Han MH, Chang KH, Kim JJ (2003) Similarity and disparity of obsessive-compulsive disorder and schizophrenia in MR volumetric abnormalities of the hippocampus-amygdala complex. J Neurol Neurosurg Psychiatry 74(7):962–964

Lacerda AL, Dalgalarrondo P, Caetano D, Camargo EE, Etchebehere EC, Soares JC (2003) Elevated thalamic and prefrontal regional cerebral blood flow in obsessive-compulsive disorder: a SPECT study. Psychiatry Res 123(2):125–134, S0925492703000611 [pii]

Lee MJ, Shin YB, Sunwoo YK, Jung SH, Kim WH, Kang MH, Lee JS, Bae JN, Kim CE (2009) Comparative analysis of cognitive function in schizophrenia with and without obsessive compulsive disorder. Psychiatry Invest 6(4):286–293. doi:10.4306/pi.2009.6.4.286

Levine JB, Gruber SA, Baird AA, Yurgelun-Todd D (1998) Obsessive-compulsive disorder among schizophrenic patients: an exploratory study using functional magnetic resonance imaging data. Compr Psychiatry 39(5):308–311

Lysaker PH, Bryson GJ, Marks KA, Greig TC, Bell MD (2002) Association of obsessions and compulsions in schizophrenia with neurocognition and negative symptoms. J Neuropsychiatry Clin Neurosci 14(4):449–453

MacMaster FP, O'Neill J, Rosenberg DR (2008) Brain imaging in pediatric obsessive-compulsive disorder. J Am Acad Child Adolesc Psychiatry 47(11):1262–1272. doi:10.1097/CHI.0b013e318185d2be

Marazziti D, Hollander E, Lensi P, Ravagli S, Cassano GB (1992) Peripheral markers of serotonin and dopamine function in obsessive-compulsive disorder. Psychiatry Res 42(1):41–51, 0165-1781(92)90037-4 [pii]

Meijer JH, Swets M, Keeman S, Nieman DH, Meijer CJ (2013) Is a schizo-obsessive subtype associated with cognitive impairment? Results from a large cross-sectional study in patients with psychosis and their unaffected relatives. J Nerv Ment Dis 201(1):30–35

Meyer-Lindenberg A (2010) From maps to mechanisms through neuroimaging of schizophrenia. Nature 468:194–202

Mundo E, Richter MA, Zai G, Sam F, McBride J, Macciardi F, Kennedy JL (2002) 5HT1Dbeta Receptor gene implicated in the pathogenesis of obsessive-compulsive disorder: further evidence from a family-based association study. Mol Psychiatry 7(7):805–809. doi:10.1038/sj.mp.4001059

Murphy DL, Zohar J, Benkelfat C, Pato MT, Pigott TA, Insel TR (1989) Obsessive-compulsive disorder as a 5-HT subsystem-related behavioural disorder. Br J Psychiatry Suppl 8:15–24

Noga JT, Aylward E, Barta PE, Pearlson GD (1995) Cingulate gyrus in schizophrenic patients and normal volunteers. Psychiatry Res 61(4):201–208

Nordahl TE, Benkelfat C, Semple WE, Gross M, King AC, Cohen RM (1989) Cerebral glucose metabolic rates in obsessive compulsive disorder. Neuropsychopharmacology 2(1):23–28, 0893-133X(89)90003-1 [pii]

Nordahl TE, Kusubov N, Carter C, Salamat S, Cummings AM, O'Shora-Celaya L, Eberling J, Robertson L, Huesman RH, Jagust W, Budinger TF (1996) Temporal lobe metabolic differences in medication-free outpatients with schizophrenia via the PET-600. Neuropsychopharmacology 15(6):541–554. doi:10.1016/S0893-133X(96)00098-X, S0893-133X(96)00098-X [pii]

Pallanti S, Castellini G, Chamberlain SR, Quercioli L, Zaccara G, Fineberg NA (2009) Cognitive event-related potentials differentiate schizophrenia with obsessive-compulsive disorder (schizo-OCD) from OCD and schizophrenia without OC symptoms. Psychiatry Res 170(1):52–60. doi:10.1016/j.psychres.2008.11.002, S0165-1781(08)00401-0 [pii]

Patel DD, Laws KR, Padhi A, Farrow JM, Mukhopadhaya K, Krishnaiah R, Fineberg NA (2010) The neuropsychology of the schizo-obsessive subtype of schizophrenia: a new analysis. Psychol Med 40(6):921–933. doi:10.1017/S0033291709991255

Peng Z, Lui SS, Cheung EF, Jin Z, Miao G, Jing J, Chan RC (2012) Brain structural abnormalities in obsessive-compulsive disorder: converging evidence from white matter and grey matter. Asian J Psychiatry 5(4):290–296. doi:10.1016/j.ajp.2012.07.004, S1876-2018(12)00128-1 [pii]

Perani D, Colombo C, Bressi S, Bonfanti A, Grassi F, Scarone S, Bellodi L, Smeraldi E, Fazio F (1995) [18F]FDG PET study in obsessive-compulsive disorder. A clinical/metabolic correlation study after treatment. Br J Psychiatry 166(2):244–250

Poyurovsky M, Weizman A, Weizman R (2004) Obsessive-compulsive disorder in schizophrenia: clinical characteristics and treatment. CNS Drugs 18(14):989–1010, 18144 [pii]

Poyurovsky M, Zohar J, Glick I, Koran LM, Weizman R, Tandon R, Weizman A (2012) Obsessive-compulsive symptoms in schizophrenia: implications for future psychiatric classifications. Compr Psychiatry 53(5):480–483. doi:10.1016/j.comppsych.2011.08.009

Radua J, Mataix-Cols D (2009) Voxel-wise meta-analysis of grey matter changes in obsessive-compulsive disorder. Br J Psychiatry 195(5):393–402. doi:10.1192/bjp.bp.108.055046, 195/5/393 [pii]

Radua J, van den Heuvel OA, Surguladze S, Mataix-Cols D (2010) Meta-analytical comparison of voxel-based morphometry studies in obsessive-compulsive disorder vs other anxiety disorders. Arch Gen Psychiatry 67(7):701–711. doi:10.1001/archgenpsychiatry.2010.70, 67/7/701 [pii]

Rao NP, Kalmady S, Arasappa R, Venkatasubramanian G (2010) Clinical correlates of thalamus volume deficits in anti-psychotic-naive schizophrenia patients: a 3-Tesla MRI study. Indian J Psychiatry 52(3):229–235. doi:10.4103/0019-5545.70975

Rauch SL, Whalen PJ, Curran T, Shin LM, Coffey BJ, Savage CR, McInerney SC, Baer L, Jenike MA (2001) Probing striato-thalamic function in obsessive-compulsive disorder and Tourette syndrome using neuroimaging methods. Adv Neurol 85:207–224

Rosenberg DR, MacMaster FP, Keshavan MS, Fitzgerald KD, Stewart CM, Moore GJ (2000) Decrease in caudate glutamatergic concentrations in pediatric obsessive-compulsive disorder patients taking paroxetine. J Am Acad Child Adolesc Psychiatry 39(9):1096–1103

Rotge JY, Guehl D, Dilharreguy B, Tignol J, Bioulac B, Allard M, Burbaud P, Aouizerate B (2009) Meta-analysis of brain volume changes in obsessive-compulsive disorder. Biol Psychiatry 65(1):75–83. doi:10.1016/j.biopsych.2008.06.019, S0006-3223(08)00787-7 [pii]

Rotge JY, Langbour N, Guehl D, Bioulac B, Jaafari N, Allard M, Aouizerate B, Burbaud P (2010) Gray matter alterations in obsessive-compulsive disorder: an anatomic likelihood estimation meta-analysis. Neuropsychopharmacology 35(3):686–691. doi:10.1038/npp.2009.175, npp2009175 [pii]

Saxena S, Brody AL, Maidment KM, Dunkin JJ, Colgan M, Alborzian S, Phelps ME, Baxter LR Jr (1999) Localized orbitofrontal and subcortical metabolic changes and predictors of response to paroxetine treatment in obsessive-compulsive disorder. Neuropsychopharmacology 21(6):683–693. doi:10.1016/S0893-133X(99)00082-2, S0893133X99000822 [pii]

Saxena S, Brody AL, Ho ML, Alborzian S, Ho MK, Maidment KM, Huang SC, Wu HM, Au SC, Baxter LR Jr (2001) Cerebral metabolism in major depression and obsessive-compulsive disorder occurring separately and concurrently. Biol Psychiatry 50(3):159–170, S0006322301011234 [pii]

Saxena S, Brody AL, Maidment KM, Smith EC, Zohrabi N, Katz E, Baker SK, Baxter LR Jr (2004) Cerebral glucose metabolism in obsessive-compulsive hoarding. Am J Psychiatry 161(6):1038–1048

Schirmbeck F, Rausch F, Englisch S, Eifler S, Esslinger C, Meyer-Lindenberg A, Zink M (2013) Stable cognitive deficits in schizophrenia patients with comorbid obsessive-compulsive symptoms: a 12-month longitudinal study. Schizophr Bull 39(6):1261–1271. doi:10.1093/schbul/sbs123, sbs123 [pii]

Schirmbeck F, Mier D, Esslinger C, Rausch F, Englisch S, Eifler S, Meyer-Lindenberg A, Kirsch P, Zink M (2014) Increased orbitofrontal cortex activation associated with 'pro-obsessive' antipsychotic treatment in patients with schizophrenia. J Psychiatry Neurosci 39:140021

Schultz SK, Andreasen NC (1999) Schizophrenia. Lancet 353(9162):1425–1430, S0140673698075497 [pii]

Shihabuddin L, Buchsbaum MS, Hazlett EA, Haznedar MM, Harvey PD, Newman A, Schnur DB, Spiegel-Cohen J, Wei T, Machac J, Knesaurek K, Vallabhajosula S, Biren MA, Ciaravolo TM, Luu-Hsia C (1998) Dorsal striatal size, shape, and metabolic rate in never-medicated and previously medicated schizophrenics performing a verbal learning task. Arch Gen Psychiatry 55(3):235–243

Sodhi M, Wood KH, Meador-Woodruff J (2008) Role of glutamate in schizophrenia: integrating excitatory avenues of research. Expert Rev Neurother 8(9):1389–1406. doi:10.1586/14737175.8.9.1389

Swayze VW 2nd, Andreasen NC, Alliger RJ, Yuh WT, Ehrhardt JC (1992) Subcortical and temporal structures in affective disorder and schizophrenia: a magnetic resonance imaging study. Biol Psychiatry 31(3):221–240, 0006-3223(92)90046-3 [pii]

Tascedda F, Blom JM, Brunello N, Zolin K, Gennarelli M, Colzi A, Bravi D, Carra S, Racagni G, Riva MA (2001) Modulation of glutamate receptors in response to the novel antipsychotic olanzapine in rats. Biol Psychiatry 50(2):117–122, S0006322301011350 [pii]

Tibbo P, Warneke L (1999) Obsessive-compulsive disorder in schizophrenia: epidemiologic and biologic overlap. J Psychiatry Neurosci 24(1):15–24

Tumkaya S, Karadag F, Oguzhanoglu NK, Tekkanat C, Varma G, Ozdel O, Atesci F (2009) Schizophrenia with obsessive-compulsive disorder and obsessive-compulsive disorder with poor insight: a neuropsychological comparison. Psychiatry Res 165(1–2):38–46. doi:10.1016/j.psychres.2007.07.031

Venkatasubramanian G, Rao NP, Behere RV (2009) Neuroanatomical, neurochemical, and neurodevelopmental basis of obsessive-compulsive symptoms in schizophrenia. Indian J Psychol Med 31(1):3–10. doi:10.4103/0253-7176.53308

Effects of Antipsychotic Treatment on Obsessive-Compulsive Symptoms

10

Frederike Schirmbeck and Mathias Zink

Abbreviations

AE	Adverse event
AMS	Amisulpride
APZ	Aripiprazole
ARMS	At-risk mental state
BDNF	Brain-derived neurotrophic factor
CBT	Cognitive behavioural therapy
CLZ	Clozapine
CR	Case report
CS	Case series
DLGAP3	Discs large-associated protein 3
ESM	Experienced sampling methods
fMRI	Functional magnetic resonance imaging
GxEI	Gene and environment interaction
OCD	Obsessive-compulsive disorder
OCS	Obsessive-compulsive symptoms
OFC	Orbitofrontal cortex
OLZ	Olanzapine
SGA	Second-generation antipsychotics
SLC1A1	Solute carrier family gene 1A1
SNP	Single-nucleotide polymorphism
SSRI	Selective serotonin reuptake inhibitor

F. Schirmbeck, PhD
Department of Psychiatry, Academic Medical Centre, University of Amsterdam, Meibergdreef 5, Amsterdam 1105 AZ, The Netherlands
e-mail: n.f.schirmbeck@amc.nl

M. Zink, MD (✉)
Department of Psychiatry and Psychotherapy, Central Institute of Mental Health, Medical Faculty Mannheim/Heidelberg University, 12 21 20, Mannheim, D-68072, Germany
e-mail: mathias.zink@zi-mannheim.de

L. De Haan et al. (eds.), *Obsessive-Compulsive Symptoms in Schizophrenia*,
DOI 10.1007/978-3-319-12952-5_10

10.1 Introduction

Research in psychiatry has achieved important progress both in pathogenic concepts and in therapeutic interventions over the past decades. However, compared to other chronic medical conditions, the biological mechanisms of psychiatric disorders are still poorly understood. This fact results in a lack of innovative therapeutic interventions in psychiatry (Insel and Scolnick 2006). As a result of stagnation in treatment innovation and improvement, the stigmatisation of schizophrenia patients did not markedly decrease since 1990 (Angermeyer et al. 2013). Although therapeutic potencies of currently available antipsychotic substances are comparable to drugs used in general medicine (Leucht et al. 2012a), a lack of insight into the neurobiological pathomechanisms of schizophrenia limits the therapeutic benefit for the individual patient. Basic research focusing on molecular targets for innovative interventions is necessary.

10.1.1 Biological Mechanisms Leading to Obsessive-Compulsive Symptoms in Schizophrenia

Elucidating the neurobiological mechanisms is not only necessary for the major psychiatric disorders per se, but also for a better understanding of their comorbidities, such as the co-occurrence of psychotic and obsessive-compulsive symptoms (OCS). The interaction between genetic and environmental factors (GxEIs) displays a general pathomechanism in psychiatry. Applied to schizophrenia, genetic risk constellations dispose to an increased liability and sensitivity for specific stressors, such as migration, other stressful life events or effects of psychotropic substances (van Os et al. 2008, 2010; van Os and Kapur 2009). GxEIs have also been described in the development of depression (Keers and Uher 2012), anxiety disorders (Gregory et al. 2008; Nugent et al. 2011) and OCD (Nicolini et al. 2009; Pauls 2010). Although a remarkable number of studies have investigated these mechanisms for the mentioned major disorders, research focusing on comorbidities, where syndromes or disorders manifest simultaneously in individual patients, is still limited. Preliminary results of studies investigating GxEIs in the development of comorbid OCS in schizophrenia strongly suggest the involvement of genetic and environmental stressors (e.g. pharmacological and/or psychosocial factors) (Schirmbeck and Zink 2013b) (see Chap. 8).

10.1.2 Pathogenic Concepts of the Primary Disorders and Clinical Subgroups Within the Comorbid Sample

The current pathogenic concepts of schizophrenia and OCD constitute the basis for aetiological explanations of their comorbidity. Schizophrenia represents a clinical manifestation of several heterogeneous neurobiological processes (van Os and Kapur

2009). Genetic properties or early environmental disturbances elicit long-lasting effects due to persistent alterations of pre- and perinatal neural plasticity (Jakob and Beckmann 1986, 1989; Readler et al. 1998; Zink 2007). These alterations change brain connectivity and the interaction of neurotransmitter systems, most importantly dopaminergic, serotonergic and amino acid neurotransmissions (Howes et al. 2012; Kantrowitz and Javitt 2013; Stan and Lewis 2012). It has been proposed by T. Insel that effective therapeutic interventions would have to address these neurodevelopmental aspects which precede the actual manifestation of psychosis and referred to this paradigmatic change as "rethinking schizophrenia" (Insel 2010).

Current concepts of OCD define a critical dysfunction within the frontocortical-striato-thalamo-cortical (CSTC) circuitry connecting the orbitofrontal cortex (OFC), the anterior cingulate cortex and the basal ganglia (thalamus and caudate nucleus) (Graybiel and Rauch 2000; Karch and Pogarell 2011; Pogarell et al. 2003; Saxena et al. 1998). Family and twin studies suggested a strong heritability of OCD (Nicolini et al. 2009; Pauls 2010). However, so far association studies of candidate genes showed rather inconsistent results. Only findings regarding single-nucleotide polymorphisms (SNPs) localised in the gene SLC1A1 (solute carrier family) on chromosome 9p24 encoding the neuronal glutamate transporter EAAC1 (excitatory amino acid carrier 1) have repeatedly been linked to the risk for OCD in independent studies (Arnold et al. 2006; Dickel et al. 2006; Shugart et al. 2009; Stewart et al. 2007; Veenstra-VanderWeele et al. 2001; Wendland et al. 2009). The role of dysfunctional serotonergic neurotransmission was based on neuroimaging results, observed treatment effects with serotonin-specific reuptake inhibitors (SSRIs) and changes in neurotransmission after cognitive behavioural therapy (CBT) (Bandelow et al. 2008; Nakao et al. 2005; Saxena et al. 1999; Linden 2006; Saxena et al. 2009).

The summarised concepts of schizophrenia and OCD share common pathogenic mechanisms. This corresponds to the clinical phenomenology of patients presenting with both psychosis and OCS. The complex psychopathology of their co-occurrence might be elucidated if nosological knowledge and research perspectives of schizophrenia and OCD are combined. It is further necessary to define utmost homogeneous subgroups within the broad heterogeneity of comorbid patients (see Chap. 4). According to differences in time of first OCS onset, clinical course and phenotypic presentation, patients might be attributed to (1) OCS as part of the at-risk mental state (ARMS), (2) OCS as a sub-syndrome of schizophrenia or (3) as a co-occurring syndrome and (4) antipsychotic-associated OCS. Regarding evidence on OCS during the ARMS, we refer to Chap. 4. Further research on schizotypal OCD and the concepts of a schizo-obsessive subtype of schizophrenia is discussed in Chaps. 5 and 7.

The current chapter particularly focuses on the association between antipsychotic treatment, in particular clozapine, and OCS occurrence. Within this context, it is essential to differentiate catatonia and treatment-resistant psychotic symptoms from OCS, because clozapine is the antipsychotic of first choice in treatment-resistant schizophrenia but is not indicated in the treatment of OCS.

In summary, pathogenic insight is necessary for any therapeutic progress but may be impossible to achieve, if heterogeneous cases are included in any kind of basic research. As mentioned, the diversity in time of onset, clinical course over time and cross-sectional psychopathology facilitates the definition of homogeneous subgroups within the comorbid sample. Patients with second-onset and stable OCS after initiation of anti-serotonergic SGA treatment constitute one such subgroup and provide an exceptional opportunity to understand the pathogenic processes leading to OCS.

10.2 Main Part

10.2.1 OCS Induced by Second-Generation Antipsychotic Agents (SGA)

One subgroup within the heterogeneous comorbid cohort is characterised by a specific pattern of symptom onset and clinical course over time. Careful assessment of the medical history and application of a rather simple categorisation helps to identify these patients: (1) When did the first psychotic manifestation occur? (2) When was antipsychotic treatment initiated? (3) When did OCS develop or increase in severity? A significant subgroup of patients reports onset or aggravation of OCS subsequent to the manifestation of psychotic symptoms and antipsychotic treatment initiation. Based on this observation in case reports and case series, it has been proposed that the de novo occurrence or marked aggravation of OCS might represent an adverse event (AE) of second-generation antipsychotics (SGAs) (Schirmbeck and Zink 2012).

With respect to the course of comorbid OCS, only few longitudinal studies investigated quantitative changes of OCS severity over time. De Haan et al. found predominantly fluctuating courses of OCS severity in a large sample of comorbid patients. Interestingly, patients who developed de novo OCS or reported persistent OCS over time were more likely treated with olanzapine (OLZ) or CLZ (de Haan et al. 2013). In accordance, a German study, which grouped patients according to their mode of antipsychotic monotherapy, found remarkable persistence of co-occurring OCS in patients treated with CLZ or OLZ over 12 months (Schirmbeck et al. 2012b, 2013).

In conclusion, the diverse clinical course of comorbid OCS suggests an involvement of different aetiological factors. Within a subgroup of patients, pharmacodynamic effects of SGA treatment seem to play a role. Clinicians are often unaware of how many schizophrenia patients experience the de novo development or persistent aggravation of OCS during antipsychotic treatment, although the mentioned simple clinical exploration can help to identify this subgroup.

10.2.2 Empirical Evidence Supporting the Concept of SGA-Induced OCS

During treatment with first-generation antipsychotics (FGA), the described pattern of symptom onset has rarely been observed. The first reports of

SGA-associated OCS were published by Baker et al. (1992) and de Haan et al. (1999). Since then several studies showed a clear link between SGA treatment, most importantly CLZ (Schirmbeck and Zink 2012), and the de novo occurrence of OCS (de Haan et al. 2004; Kwon et al. 2009; Reznik et al. 2004; Schirmbeck et al. 2011). Subsequently, some authors suggested that OCS might represent an AE of specific SGAs and introduced the term "antipsychotic-induced OCS" in their publications (Kwon et al. 2009; Lykouras et al. 2003). Whereas Doyle et al. (2014) proposed that CLZ-induced OCS might be distinguished from classical OCS, other studies did not find phenomenological differences (Kim et al. 2012).

The following paragraphs summarise epidemiological and pharmacological arguments which support the assumption of SGA-induced OCS (for summary see Tables 10.1 and 10.2).

10.2.2.1 Epidemiological Evidence

High Prevalence Rates of OCS in Schizophrenia After Market Approval of SGAs

The co-occurrence of OCS did not gain much clinical awareness in scientific publications as long as treatment with different FGAs was the first-line-therapy in schizophrenia. Only few studies reported observed comorbidities during FGA treatment (Berman et al. 1995a, b; Fenton and McGlashan 1986; Nolfe et al. 2010). With the approval of SGAs, the situation markedly changed. CLZ was introduced for the treatment of schizophrenia in the 1970s in Europe and the late 1980s in the USA (Hippius 1989; Kang and Simpson 2010). After this paradigmatic change in treatment, the prevalence estimations markedly increased. A recent meta-analysis concludes that 13.6 % of patients with schizophrenia fulfil the criteria for comorbid OCD and 30.3 % experience at least mild OCS severity (Swets et al. 2013) (see Fig. 10.1 and Chap. 4). Even if a potential publication bias and an increased general awareness have to be considered, the high numbers may indirectly reflect an interrelation between CLZ treatment and OCS.

Higher OCS Prevalence Rates During Later Stages of the Psychotic Illness

As described in more detail within Chap. 4, prevalence rates of OCS/OCD increase during the course of psychotic illness. During the ARMS only 5.42 % (CI: 4.41–6.43) of investigated patients fulfilled the criteria for OCD and only 12.98 % (CI: 10.63–15.33) reported OCS (Zink et al. 2014a). These rates are considerably lower compared to 7.3 % OCD and 17.1 % OCS prevalence rates in first-episode patients and even lower to the above mentioned rates of 13.6 and 30.3 % in later disease stages (Swets et al. 2013) (see Fig. 10.1). As the disease progresses patients are more likely treated with CLZ and are cumulatively exposed to higher dosage and longer treatment duration. The observed increase in prevalence and severity of OCS over the course of psychotic illness could partly be attributed to the proposed pro-obsessive effects of CLZ.

Table 10.1 Evidence for SGA-induced OCS derived from epidemiological investigations

Observation		References	Number of patients and mode of clinical characterisation	Design of the study	Individual main findings
The prevalence increases from at-risk mental states to first-episode samples to chronic course of schizophrenia	At-risk mental state samples	Summary of previous literature (Zink et al. 2014a)	Review about 11 individual studies including 1,590 patients (regarding OCD) or 553 patients (regarding OCS)	Cross-sectional assessment of OCD or OCS using different diagnostic procedures	Weighted for sample sizes of individual reports, ARMS patients fulfil criteria for OCD in only 5.2 % and for OCS in 13.7 %
		Zink et al. (2014a, b)	233 ARMS patients presenting BS, APS and BLIPS	Cross-sectional assessment of OCS according to SCID I	5.2 % of PREVENT patients, the patients fulfil criteria of OCD and 11.2 % for OCS
	First episode patient	Zink et al. (2014a, b)	Review about 6 individual studies including 630 FEP patients (ad OCD) or 578 FEP patients (ad OCS)	Cross-sectional assessment of OCD or OCS using different diagnostic procedures	Weighted for sample sizes of individual reports, 7.3 % of FEP patients fulfil criteria for OCD and 17.1 for OCS
		Strakowski et al. (1993)	27 FEP	Cross-sectional assessment of comorbid conditions at first hospitalisation using SCID	7.4 % of FEP fulfil criteria of OCD Tendency towards longer duration of hospitalisation
		Strakowski et al. (1995)	18 FEP	Cross-sectional assessment of comorbid conditions at first hospitalisation using SCID	11 % of FEP fulfil criteria of OCD
		Craig et al. (2002)	225 FEP	Cross-sectional assessment of comorbid conditions at first hospitalisation using SCID	4 % of FEP fulfil criteria of OCD and 21 % of OCS
	Schizophrenic patients	Mukhopadhaya et al. (2009)	Review of previous studies including 1972 patients	Cross-sectional assessments of OCS based on SCID, YBOCS, HZI, PADUA and other scales	High variability and mean prevalence of OCS in 22 % of schizophrenia patients
		Buckley et al. (2009)	Review covering 3656 patients	Cross-sectional assessment of OCS in schizophrenia	Mean prevalence rate of 23 %
		Lysaker and Whitney (2009)	Not specified	Review of studies reporting on OCS prevalence in schizophrenia	Amongst schizophrenic patients, more than one-third suffers from clinically significant OCS, 10–25 % meet diagnostic criteria of OCD
		Swets et al. (2013)	Review of 43 individual studies about 3978 patients	Review of studies reporting OCS and OCD prevalence rates in schizophrenia	Mean prevalence for OCD: 12.3 % (13.6 % after adjustment in meta-regression), for OCS 30.7 % (30.3 % adjusted in meta-regression). Higher prevalence rates in studies using DSM IV, YBOCS assessment and including patients with longer duration of illness

Observation of *de novo* onset or exacerbation of OCS during antipsychotic treatment	Case reports and series: Zink et al. (2006, 2007), Englisch et al. (2009)	9 SCH patients	Longitudinal observation of course of illness	First manifestation and start of antipsychotic treatment precede onset of OCS
	De Haan et al. (1999)	121 recent-onset SCH patients	Longitudinal observation of course of illness	Emergence or increase of OCS in 1.3 % of non-clozapine-treated and 20.6 % of clozapine-treated patients
	Lykouras et al. (2003)	55 SCH patients	Systematic review of published case reports	Until 2003, a de novo onset or exacerbation of OCS had been published regarding clozapine ($N=30$), risperidone ($N=16$), olanzapine ($N=8$) and quetiapine ($N=1$)
	De Haan et al. (2004)	200 recent-onset SCH patients	Longitudinal observation of course of illness	Emergence or increase of OCS in 0 % of non-clozapine-treated and 9.8 % of clozapine-treated patients
Proportion of SGA-induced OCS within the complete comorbid sample	Lin et al. (2006)	CLZ: 102	Cross-sectional. Stratification for CLZ treatment with or without OCS	Within 39 clozapine-treated patients with OCS, 29 were classified as clozapine-induced
	Lim et al. (2007)	Total sample: 209, comorbid subsample: 26	Cross-sectional. Stratification for SZ with or without OCS	Within 26 SGA-associated schizophrenics with OCS, only 3 had a history of transient OCS before the onset of psychosis
	Schirmbeck et al. (2011)	CLZ: 26 OLZ: 13	Cross-sectional. Stratification for treatment with SGAs in monotherapy	Within 39 patients, 28 showed OCS, but only 3 reported OCS before or at onset of psychosis

(continued)

Table 10.1 (continued)

Observation	References	Number of patients and mode of clinical characterisation	Design of the study	Individual main findings
Assumption of different clinical features	Doyle et al. (2014)	CLZ: 62 OCD: 35	Qualitative evaluation of OCS using the OCI	Two of fourteen OCS-positive, CLZ-treated patients suffered from OCS before start of CLZ treatment (14 %). OCS prevalence in CLZ group: 22 %. No correlation of CLZ dosage with OCS severity. OCS-positive CLZ-treated patients present pronounced doubting, OCD patients pronounced washing
	Kim et al. (2012)	51 schizophrenia patients with SGA-induced OCS	Comparison of symptom structure to primary OCD patients using the YBOCS	Similar to primary OCD patients, five identical factors (forbidden thoughts, hoarding, cleaning, symmetry, and counting) accounted for 70.7 % of the total variance
	Michalopoulou et al. (2014)	Schizophrenia patients with (N=20) or without (N=20) OCS and 20 matched controls	Comprehensive neurocognitive characterisation	Lower performance in processing speed discriminated patients with or without OCS, but did not correlate with OCS severity. No differences in other neurocognitive domains

Epidemiological studies show an increase of OCS and OCD prevalence, if ARMS, FEP and schizophrenia patients are compared, as well as the observation of de novo onset or aggravation of OCS during antipsychotic treatment. Astonishingly high proportions of comorbid patients were attributed to the subgroup of SGA-induced OCS

Abbreviations: *APS* attenuated psychotic symptoms, *BLIPS* brief limited intermittent psychotic symptoms, *BS* basic symptoms, *DSM IV* Diagnostic and Statistical Manual of Mental Disorders, Fourth Edition, *FEP* first-episode schizophrenic patients, *FGA* first-generation antipsychotics, *OCD* obsessive-compulsive disorder, *OCI* obsessive-compulsive inventory, *OCS* obsessive-compulsive symptoms, *OLZ* olanzapine, *SCH* schizophrenia, *SCID* structured clinical interview for DSM IV, *SGA* second-generation antipsychotics, *SIPS* structured interview for prodromal symptoms, *SZ* schizophrenia and schizophrenia spectrum disorders, *UHR* ultra high risk

Table 10.2 Evidence for SGA-induced OCS derived from pharmacological investigations

Argument	Reference	Number of patients	Design	Main findings
Association of CLZ with comorbid OCS	Lim et al. (2007)	Total sample: $n=209$, comorbid subsample: $n=26$	Cross-sectional. Stratification for SZ with or without OCS	CLZ treatment in 35.9 % of the total sample, but in 76.9 % of the comorbid patients
Association of OCS with OLZ or CLZ	Sa et al. (2009)	CLZ: $n=40$	Cross-sectional. Stratification for treatment with CLZ or HAL	Prevalence of OCS 20 % (CLZ) vs 10 % (HAL). Higher severity of OCS with CLZ
		HAL: $n=20$		
	Ertugrul et al. (2005)	CLZ: $n=50$	Cross-sectional. Stratification of treatment with CLZ	Within 50 patients treated with CLZ, 76 % showed OCS. 20 % reported retrospectively de novo onset and 18 % an exacerbation
	Schirmbeck et al. (2011)	CLZ: $n=26$	Cross-sectional. Stratification for treatment with SGAs in monotherapy	Prevalence of OCS 71.8 % in CLZ or OLZ vs 9.7 % in AMS or APZ. Highest severity of OCS with CLZ
		OLZ: $n=13$		
		AMS: $n=15$		
		APZ:$n=16$		
	Scheltema Beduin et al. (2012)	CLZ: $n=28$	Cross-sectional. Stratification for treatment with SGAs in monotherapy	Significant differences in OCS prevalence between groups stratified for mode of treatment CLZ (prevalence of OCS: 38.9 %), OLZ (20.1 %), RISP (23.2 %) and untreated patients (19.6 %)
		OLZ: $n=41$		
		RISP: $n=36$		
		Untreated: $n=22$		
Correlation of OCS with duration of treatment	Lin et al. (2006)	CLZ: $n=102$	Cross-sectional. Stratification for CLZ treatment with or without OCS	Duration of CLZ treatment significantly longer in CLZ-OCS patients (82 vs 56 months), no difference in duration of illness
	Schirmbeck et al. (2011)	CLZ: $n=26$	Cross-sectional. Stratification for CLZ monotherapy	Duration of CLZ treatment correlates positively with OCS severity (YBOCS, $R=0.59$)
	Scheltema Beduin et al. (2012)	CLZ: $n=72$	Cross-sectional. Stratification for CLZ treatment with or without OCS	Patients treated with CLZ for longer than 6 months suffer from OCS more often than patients recently switched to CLZ (47.3 % vv 11.8 %)

(continued)

Table 10.2 (continued)

Argument	Reference	Number of patients	Design	Main findings
Correlation of OCS with CLZ dosage or plasma concentration	Reznik et al. (2004)	$n=15$	Cross-sectional. Stratification for CLZ therapy	Dosage-related, pro-obsessive influence of CLZ
	Mukhopadhaya et al. (2009)	$n=59$	Cross-sectional. Stratification for CLZ therapy	Higher CLZ dosage in patients with comorbid OCS (432 mg/day) than without (351 mg/day)
	Schirmbeck et al. (2011)	CLZ: $n=26$	Cross-sectional. Stratification for CLZ monotherapy	CLZ dosage correlates positively with OCS severity (YBOCS, $R=0.50$)
	Lin et al. (2006)	CLZ: $n=102$	Cross-sectional. Stratification for CLZ treatment with or without OCS	Higher plasma concentrations in CLZ-treated patients with OCS (595 ng/L) than without OCS (434 ng/L)
Improvement after CLZ dose-reduction in combination with APZ or ZIPR	Rocha and Hara (2006)	$n=3$	Longitudinal observation of OCS severity	Reduction of OCS severity after CLZ down-tapering in combination with APZ
	Zink et al. (2006)	$n=1$	Longitudinal observation of OCS severity	Reduction of OCS severity from YBOCS 24 to 19 after reduction of CLZ from 500 to 250 mg/die and combination with APZ (30 mg)
	Englisch et al. (2009)	$n=7$	Longitudinal observation of OCS severity	Reduction of OCS severity from YBOCS 19 to 12 after reduction of CLZ from 364 to 293 mg/die and combination with APZ (23 mg)
	Villari et al. (2011)	$n=2$	Longitudinal assessment of OCS severity	Improvement of OCS severity in two cases after add-on of APZ
	Eryilmaz et al. (2013)	$n=4$	Longitudinal assessment of OCS severity	Improvement of OCS severity in four cases after add-on of APZ
	Krause et al. (2013)	$n=6$	Longitudinal assessment of OCS severity	Improvement of OCS severity in six cases after add-on of ZIPR

Increase of OCS severity during treatment with CLZ or OLZ	Schirmbeck et al. (2013)	$n=75$	Longitudinal observation of OCS severity	CLZ progressively aggravates OCS. A significant time effect discriminates between groups treated with CLZ/OLZ or AMS/APZ
Modulation of brain activation by SGA treatment	Schirmbeck et al. (2014)	$n=40$	Comparison of brain activation in fMRI	Patients treated with CLZ or OLZ did not differ in brain activation patterns during a working memory task from samples treated with AMS or APZ but showed significantly increased activation in the orbitofrontal cortex (OFC) during response inhibition
Improvement of OCS severity by serotonergic treatment	Poyurovsky et al. (1999)	Interventional clinical trials	Assessment of influences of serotonergic antidepressants on OCS severity	Improvement of obsessions, positive and negative psychotic symptoms by fluvoxamine
	Stryjer et al. (2012)	15 schizophrenia patients with comorbid OCD	Interventional clinical trial with escitalopram 20 mg/die for 12 weeks	Significant improvement in YBOCS total score, obsessions and compulsion, improvement in PANSS positive and negative scores, particularly regarding anxiety, tension, depression and preoccupation

Pharmacological evidence in favour of an association between clozapine treatment and OCS

Abbreviations: *AMS* amisulpride, *APZ* aripiprazole, *CLZ* clozapine, *FGA* first-generation antipsychotics, *fMRI* functional magnetic resonance imaging, *HAL* haloperidol, *OCS* obsessive-compulsive symptoms, *OLZ* olanzapine, *RISP* risperidone, *SGA* second-generation antipsychotics, *SZ* schizophrenia and schizophrenia spectrum disorders, *vs* versus, *YBOCS* Yale-Brown Obsessive-Compulsive Scale, *ZIPR* ziprasidone

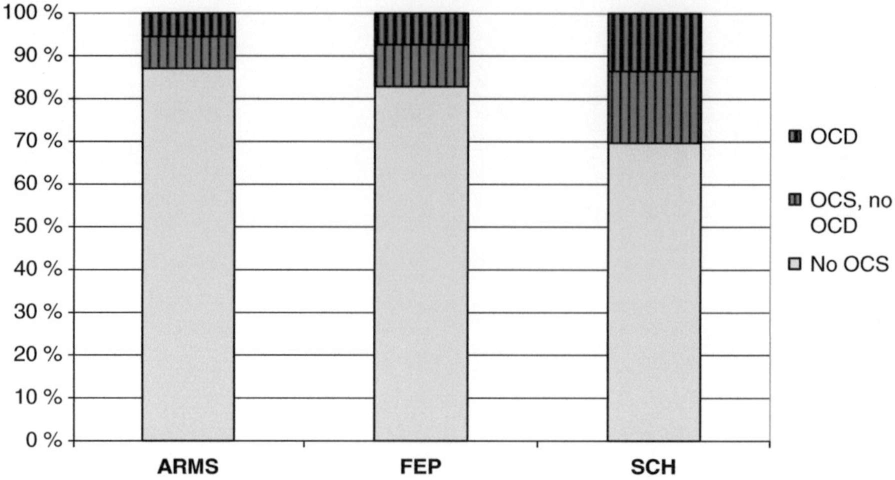

Fig. 10.1 Data on prevalence of OCS and OCD in different stages of psychotic disorders strongly suggest that during progress of illness and its treatment, pro-obsessive factors are active. One of them might be the antipsychotic pharmacotherapy. Data were extracted from epidemiological publications as summarised in (Zink et al. 2014a), the PREVENT trial and the meta-analysis of Swets et al. (2013). From left to right: Prevalence rates in at-risk-mental state studies (*ARMS*). Prevalence rates in first-episode psychotic patients. Prevalence rates in schizophrenia patients

Observation of De Novo OCS or Marked Aggravation During Antipsychotic Treatment

A growing number of case reports and case series report the mentioned sequential order of the events, “onset of psychosis”, “start of antipsychotic treatment” and “onset or aggravation of OCS”, as recently summarised (Schirmbeck and Zink 2012). Most studies describe this pattern during treatment with CLZ; however, the de novo occurrence of OCS has also been reported during other SGAs such as OLZ and risperidone (de Haan et al. 2002; Kulkarni et al. 2012; Lykouras et al. 2003; Poyurovsky et al. 2004). Unfortunately, prospective investigations with randomised assignment to different modes of SGA treatment are still missing, and studies are limited by retrospective assessments (Schirmbeck et al. 2011) or narrative design (Lykouras et al. 2003). Prospective observational studies confirm an increase in OCS severity in patients treated with CLZ or OLZ (de Haan et al. 2002; Schirmbeck et al. 2013) (see Sect. 10.2.2.2).

Estimated Proportions of SGA-Induced OCS Within Comorbid Samples

Several authors have investigated the proportion of SGA-associated OCS within their comorbid samples. In their review Poyurovski et al. concluded that 70 % of investigated cases experienced de novo emergence of OCS during treatment with pro-obsessive SGAs (Poyurovsky et al. 2004). Accordingly, Lykouras et al. reviewed published data and reported de novo OCS in 77 % of CLZ-treated patients (Lykouras et al. 2003). Other investigations resulted in even higher numbers of second-onset OCS within investigated samples: 29 of 39 (74 %) (Lin et al. 2006), 23 of 26 (88 %)

(Lim et al. 2007), 25 of 28 patients (89 %) (Schirmbeck et al. 2011) and 12 of 14 (86 %) (Doyle et al. 2014). These numbers further argue in favour of a potential causal interrelation between SGAs, especially CLZ and OCS occurrence.

10.2.2.2 Pharmacological Evidence

Apart from these epidemiological data, additional pharmacological arguments support the assumption of SGA-induced OCS (see also Table 10.2).

The Differential Effect of Pharmacodynamic Properties on OCS Comorbidity Rates

When comparing schizophrenia patients who have been grouped according to pharmacodynamics properties of their antipsychotic treatment, the risk for comorbid OCS markedly differs. High prevalence rates in CLZ-treated patients contrast with low rates during treatment with FGAs, for instance, haloperidol or other SGAs (Ertugrul et al. 2005; Sa et al. 2009; Scheltema Beduin et al. 2012).

SGAs differ in their specific pharmacodynamic properties, in particular, regarding inherent serotonergic and dopaminergic blockade, monoaminergic reuptake inhibition or even partial serotonergic agonism (Lopez-Gil et al. 2010; Meltzer and Sumiyoshi 2008; Remington 2008; Shapiro et al. 2003). CLZ and OLZ can be described as potent serotonergic antagonists combined with rather weak antidopaminergic effects (Bymaster et al. 1997; Meltzer et al. 2003). Substances such as amisulpride (AMS), a dopamine D3/D2 receptor antagonist (Kim et al. 2008; Pani et al. 2008) with inherent predominantly dopaminergic blocking activities (Scatton et al. 1997) and the partial dopaminergic and serotonergic agonist aripiprazole (APZ) (Sparshatt et al. 2010) have even been proposed to have a potential antiobsessive effect in patients with schizophrenia (Chang et al. 2008; Englisch et al. 2009; Englisch and Zink 2008; Zink et al. 2006).

Consequently, comparing OCS frequency and severity in groups treated with CLZ/OLZ vs AMS/APZ is of particular interest to elucidate pharmacodynamic effects. A recent study found that more than 70 % of patients within the first group reported OCS compared to less than 10 % of patients treated with AMS or APZ (Schirmbeck et al. 2011). Vice versa, if schizophrenia patients were grouped according to the presence or absence of comorbid OCS, 77 % of comorbid individuals, but only 36 % of non-comorbid patients were treated with CLZ (Lim et al. 2007). However, the cross-sectional design of these studies precludes causal conclusions and confounding effects due to the selection of specific SGAs for specific subgroups of patients have to be considered.

Longitudinal Effects of SGAs on OCS Severity

Schirmbeck et al. tried to overcome these limitations by investigating potential differential effects of the abovementioned pharmacodynamically diverse SGA groups over time. Integrating the two factors "group" and "time" into their statistical analysis resulted in a significant interaction effect (completer analysis: $p=0.006$; full sample analysis: $p=0.007$). Whereas the CLZ/OLZ group showed persistently high OCS severity over a 12-month observational period, the AMS/APZ group reported a significant decrease in symptom severity (Schirmbeck et al. 2013).

Treatment Duration and Dose-Related Variation in OCS

Several studies added to the current state of research by investigating associations between OCS severity and duration, as well as dosage and serum levels of CLZ treatment. Findings suggested dosage-related effects.

Lin et al. (2006) compared CLZ-treated patients with vs without comorbid OCS and found significantly longer treatment durations in the comorbid group. Noteworthy, groups did not differ regarding duration of illness. In accordance, Schirmbeck et al. reported a positive correlation between OCS severity and duration of CLZ treatment (Schirmbeck et al. 2011), and Scheltema et al. found increased OCS prevalence rates in patients treated with CLZ for longer than 6 months (Scheltema Beduin et al. 2012). Similar observations were reported by de Haan et al. regarding the closely related SGA OLZ. Again severity of OCS was significantly associated with longer duration of treatment (de Haan et al. 2002).

Several authors further demonstrated that higher levels of OCS severity were correlated with higher dosage and/or blood serum level of CLZ (Lin et al. 2006; Mukhopadhaya et al. 2009; Reznik et al. 2004; Schirmbeck et al. 2011). In addition, the reduction of daily CLZ dosage, for instance, using a combination with APZ or ziprasidone, was accompanied by an alleviation of OCS severity (Englisch et al. 2009; Eryilmaz et al. 2013; Krause et al. 2013; Rocha and Hara 2006; Villari et al. 2011; Zink et al. 2006). This observed improvement in OCS may represent both a reduction of dose-related side effect of CLZ and the proposed favourable effect of APZ. Anti-obsessive effects of APZ were suggested in a *placebo*-controlled randomised trial, which revealed reduced OCS severity after combination with APZ during constant CLZ dosage (Chang et al. 2008).

It has to be acknowledged that contradicting findings have been published: An alleviation of OCS severity has been observed after addition of CLZ (Peters and de 2009), an increase in CLZ dosage (Lykouras et al. 2003) or start with OLZ treatment (Poyurovsky 2013; van Nimwegen et al. 2008). These controversial findings might be explained by differences in sample characteristics.

Due to mentioned diagnostic difficulties (Chap. 3), psychotic symptoms might have been misperceived as OCS. Patients with treatment-resistant schizophrenia or patients who exhibit obsessive ruminations, stereotypic thoughts or repetitive ritualised behaviour clearly related to the content of delusions or hallucinations might indeed benefit from treatment with OLZ or CLZ.

Beneficial effects of SGAs have also been reported in primary OCD, especially in cases with treatment resistance to serotonergic antidepressants (Bandelow et al. 2008; Bloch et al. 2006; Dold et al. 2011; Muscatello et al. 2011). However, CLZ has not been found effective in OCD (McDougle et al. 1995), and no treatment guidelines recommend CLZ as an augmentation strategy in this group of patients (Kordon et al. 2011).

In summary, cumulative evidence and especially the dosage-dependent drug-OCS interaction strongly suggest a causal interrelation. The vast majority of investigations involved CLZ, suggesting that OCS can be considered an AE of SGAs with strong anti-serotonergic mechanisms. To further validate the concept of

SGA-induced OCS, recent investigations tried to elucidate possible underlying mechanisms and focused on genetic risk factors, neural correlates in neuroimaging studies and comprehensive neurocognitive characterisations.

10.2.2.3 Genetic Disposition

As mentioned in Sect. 10.1.1, efforts to elucidate pathomechanisms in psychiatry often focus on the interaction of both genetic and environmental factors. Applied to the co-occurrence of OCS and schizophrenia, SGA treatment can be perceived as an environmental factor possibly acting on the background of a primary genetic predisposition (see Chap. 8) . To investigate this hypothesis, a South Korean research group evaluated association of the glutamate transporter gene *SLC1A1 and* second-onset OCS during treatment with SGAs (Kwon et al. 2009). Within primary OCD, several independent studies have consistently reported disease risk associated with SNPs in this gene (Veenstra-VanderWeele et al. 2001) (Arnold et al. 2006; Dickel et al. 2006; Shugart et al. 2009; Stewart et al. 2007; Wendland et al. 2009). Kwon et al. hypothesised that genetic variations in the candidate gene *SLC1A1* modulate the susceptibility to develop OCS during SGA treatment (Kwon et al. 2009). Accordingly, they found a strong association (odds ratio of 3.96) with the A/C/G dominant haplotype rs2228622/rs3780413/rs37801412. However, a study investigating 103 schizophrenia patients of European descent could not replicate these findings (Schirmbeck et al. 2012a). Meanwhile additional genetic risk factors have been proposed: Kwon et al. described a genetic interaction of the *SLC1A1* polymorphism with variants in the gene *DLGAP3* (discs large-associated protein 3) and an association with SGA-induced OCS (Ryu et al. 2011). In a Chinese sample, an interaction of SNPs in *SLC1A1* and the type 2B subunit of the N-methyl-D-aspartate receptor gene (GRIN2B) was reported (Cai et al. 2013). Based on neurotrophic theories, an association between the Val66Met polymorphism in the gene BDNF (brain-derived neurotrophic factor) and OCS in schizophrenia has been proposed (Hashim et al. 2012). So far, findings regarding *BDNF*, *DLGAP3* and GRIN2B have not been replicated in independent studies. Future studies investigating GxEIs in the development of second-onset OCS should include additional environmental factors such as psychosocial stressors (e.g. critical life events, interpersonal relations, changes of the vocational situation or the present state of general physical health) (Schirmbeck and Zink 2013b).

10.2.2.4 Neurocognitive Correlates of SGA-Induced OCS

A set of neurocognitive deficits have been consistently linked to primary OCD, such as impaired cognitive shifting abilities, inhibitory control and effective planning strategies (Kuelz et al. 2004). In accordance, associations between cognitive impairment and comorbid OCS have been thoroughly investigated in patients with schizophrenia (Cunill et al. 2013; Lysaker and Whitney 2009) (see Chap. 7). Attempts to differentiate between schizophrenia patients with and without OCS resulted in somewhat inconclusive findings. Several authors did not find any significant differences (Achim et al. 2011; Hermesh et al. 2003; Meijer et al. 2013; Öngür and Goff 2005; Tiryaki and Ozkorumak 2010; Tumkaya et al. 2009; Whitney et al. 2004), others even reported better cognitive abilities (Borkowska et al. 2013; Lee et al. 2009), especially during ARMS (Zink et al. 2014a). Most publications, however, documented more pronounced deficits in processing speed (Michalopoulou et al. 2014), executive functioning (Hwang et al. 2000; Lysaker et al. 2002, 2009), cognitive flexibility (Kumbhani et al. 2010; Patel et al. 2010) and also delayed visual memory (Berman et al. 1998; Schirmbeck et al. 2011). The observed heterogeneity may partly be explained by the diverse clinical characteristics of investigated comorbid samples.

Only one study specifically focused on SGA-induced OCS and included a comprehensive set of OCD-related cognitive domains. At baseline (Schirmbeck et al. 2011) and 12 months later (Schirmbeck et al. 2012b), patients with comorbid OCS showed pronounced deficits in cognitive flexibility, visuospatial perception and visual memory, with increased between-group effect sizes over the 12-month assessment period. Performance in these domains correlated with OCS severity.

These findings suggest similarities between neurocognitive correlates of primary OCD and of OCS in schizophrenia. Consequently, subsequent functional magnetic resonance imaging (fMRI) approaches were conducted to further elucidate neuronal correlates of SGA-induced OCS.

10.2.2.5 Neuroimaging and SGA-Induced OCS

As described in Chap. 9, neuroimaging data on comorbid OCS in schizophrenia is still scarce. Of those studies conducted, three based the recruitment only on the clinical phenotype and did not account for possible pathogenic differences, nor for pharmacodynamic mechanisms involved in OCS occurrence. Using structural analyses Aoyama et al. reported a significant volume reduction of the left hippocampus in schizophrenia patients with OCS (Aoyama et al. 2000). Levine et al. applied functional magnetic resonance imaging (fRMI) and a verbal fluency task. They observed negative associations between OCS and the activation of the left dorsolateral prefrontal cortex (Levine et al. 1998). Finally, Bleich-Cohen et al. compared phenotypically defined groups regarding fMRI in a working memory paradigm. Regardless of the presence or absence of comorbid OCS, schizophrenia patients performed worse than healthy controls and showed less activation in dorsolateral prefrontal cortex and right caudate nucleus (Bleich-Cohen et al. 2014). These studies did not particularly assess the frontocortical-striato-thalamo-cortical (CSTC) circuitry connecting the orbitofrontal cortex, anterior cingulate cortex, thalamus and caudate nucleus. This is important to note because these regions are thought to play a crucial role in the pathogenesis of OCD (Graybiel and Rauch 2000; Karch and Pogarell 2011; Saxena et al. 1999). Especially, increased task-specific activation of the orbitofrontal cortex has repeatedly been described in primary OCD (Friedlander and Desrocher 2006; Whiteside et al. 2004). Consequently, Schirmbeck et al. included fMRI tasks which reliably activate the CSTC circuitry in their study design. Patients were stratified according to their antipsychotic monotherapy into two groups (I: CLZ or OLZ; $n=21$; II: AMS or APZ; $n=19$) and performed a Go/NoGo task assessing inhibitory control, an n-back task measuring working memory and a theory of mind (TOM) task. Group I patients showed significantly more severe

OCS and pronounced cognitive deficits in specific domains but showed similar brain activation patterns during the working memory task compared to group II patients. However, during the inhibitory control task, they presented significantly increased activation in the orbitofrontal cortex. The authors concluded that these alterations in brain functioning might reflect a pathogenic mechanism in the development of SGA-induced OCS (Schirmbeck et al. 2014). Analyses of the TOM task revealed reduced amygdala activation during processing of emotionally loaded pictures in group I but increased activation in the temporal cortex compared to group II (unpublished data). Further studies with patients in different stages of psychotic illness and with prospective designs should replicate and validate these findings.

10.2.3 Pathogenesis of OCS Induction by SGAs

As summarised, epidemiological and pharmacological data clearly hint towards a causal interrelation between SGA treatment and OCS occurrence in schizophrenia. Based on the mentioned pharmacodynamic properties, pathogenic mechanisms related to the current serotonergic theories of primary OCD have been proposed. As mentioned above, CLZ (Meltzer 2012; Steingard et al. 1993) and OLZ (Duggan et al. 2000) inherent strong anti-serotonergic properties most importantly at 5-HT1C, 5-HT2A and 5HT2C receptors (Coward 1992; Meltzer 1994; Meltzer and Huang 2008). In combination with low affinities to dopamine receptors, these mechanisms of action result in a very small ratio of dopaminergic/serotonergic receptor blockade, which largely differs from other SGAs such as AMS or APZ (Correll 2008; Scatton et al. 1997; Shapiro et al. 2003). In the case of APZ, a relevant anti-serotonergic profile is accompanied by high affinity to D2 dopamine receptors resulting in a strongly differing ratio of receptor interaction. Thus, in contrast to the therapeutic effects of serotonin-specific reuptake inhibitors (SSRIs) in primary OCD patients, it seems likely that the described effects of CLZ and OLZ result in the de novo development or aggravation of OCS in schizophrenia.

Noteworthy, besides serotonergic mechanisms, other systems have to be considered and analysed in further clinical trials. Alterations in dopaminergic activity (Van der Wee et al. 2004) have been related to OCD, and reciprocal interactions of dopaminergic and serotonergic neurotransmission with glutamatergic and GABAergic functions have been described (Lopez-Gil et al. 2010). The glutamatergic theory of OCD (Grados et al. 2013) is based on evidence derived from animal models (Joel 2006; Porton et al. 2013), findings of human magnetic resonance spectroscopy (Starck et al. 2008; Whiteside et al. 2006), treatment effects of glutamatergic agents (Poyurovsky et al. 2010) and genetic studies (Bienvenu et al. 2009; Nicolini et al. 2009; Pauls 2010). The above reported preliminary results of associations between variants in glutamatergic genes and an increased risk to develop SGA-induced OCS support the involvement of glutamatergic mechanisms. Furthermore, FGAs and SGAs exert differential effects on GABAergic and glutamatergic neurotransmission (Peselmann et al. 2012; Zink et al. 2014b), thus the investigation of this pathway in future studies seems indicated.

10.3 Discussion

10.3.1 Open Questions and Limitations

Several open questions regarding the current concepts of SGA-induced OCS remain unanswered. Although summarised arguments support the assumption that specific SGAs increase the risk for secondary OCS via a pharmacodynamic mechanism, proposed causal interrelations still need verification. According to the general criteria of causality suggested by Bradford Hill, the simple observation of the de novo onset of OCS during SGA treatment is no sufficient proof for a causal interaction (Bradford Hill 2011). Instead it would be necessary to observe a decrease of OCS after tapering off the assumed causative agent, followed by re-exposure and reoccurrence of OCS (see also Table 8.2). However, this procedure is obviously not compatible with guidelines of good clinical practice. In addition, the assumption of CLZ-induced OCS could be validated in randomised controlled trials. Again, legal and ethical considerations constitute relevant restrictions for the execution of such trials.

Exposure to antipsychotic treatment is only one of several environmental factors that might influence the co-occurrence and course of comorbid OCS. Preliminary evidence further suggests that these might interact with a set of genetic risk constellations. However, due to so far inconclusive findings, it remains unclear to which extent the general genetic background plays a role in the pathogenesis of SGA-induced OCS. Furthermore, interactions within a set of genes (SNPs in *SLC1A1*, *BDNF*, DLGAP3 and GRIN2B) need further explorations.

Noteworthy, the sometimes difficult differentiation between catatonic, psychotic, affective or obsessive symptoms adds to the clinical heterogeneity within investigated samples.

10.3.2 Future Research Perspectives

The mentioned limitations and open questions strengthen the need for further research. Advances in pathogenic research of comorbid OCS in schizophrenia will most likely be achieved if studies investigate defined homogeneous subgroups (Zink 2014b). Multimodal and longitudinal approaches should include assessments of several environmental factors and genetic characterisations. Results of translational perspectives will hopefully result in guidelines for adjusted treatment approaches for subgroups within the heterogeneous comorbid sample (see Chaps. 11 and 12).

10.3.2.1 Aiming at Homogeneous Subgroups

For an improved pathogenic insight, the heterogeneity within the comorbid sample is an important problem (see Chap. 4). Well-defined homogeneous clinical cohorts should be defined to reduce the number of possible confounding factors to a minimum. This might be achieved with quite simple clinical methods, such as the exploration of the order of symptom onset, the clinical course, the mode of pharmacological treatment and a set of environmental factors. It appears to be both necessary and promising to focus on these subgroups in order to unravel the specific contribution and interplay of psychosocial, pharmacological and genetic factors. With respect to the latter, much larger cohorts have to be recruited in multicentre studies to investigate possible genetic risk constellations. A necessary sample size of about five thousand participants has, for example, been estimated in order to replicate the pre-described SLC1A1 polymorphism in a European sample (Schirmbeck et al. 2012a).

10.3.2.2 Gene and Environment Interactions

So far, only the most simple environmental factor (mode of antipsychotic treatment) has been investigated and associated with possible genetic risk constellations. Further factors such as psychosocial stress induced by critical life events, interpersonal factors, changes of the vocational situation or the present state of general physical health should be investigated. Finally, the reciprocal interactions between OCS and psychotic positive, negative and cognitive symptoms of schizophrenia have to be elucidated and taken into consideration. Here experience sampling methods (ESMs) could be a useful approach. ESM closely monitors symptom variability in real-life situations on a day-to-day basis through repeated assessments. Thereby, symptom changes can be investigated in the context of daily hassles, perceived stress and individual reactions. ESM data can further be related to relevant factors, such as genetic polymorphisms, pharmacological treatment or the mode and efficacy of therapeutic interventions. These multidimensional approaches will help to define risk and resilience constellations for the development of co-occurring OCS and provide the basis for treatment suggestions.

10.3.3 Implications for Clinical Practice

Current knowledge on pro-obsessive effects of SGAs might influence therapeutic considerations in schizophrenia in general, but definitively in schizophrenia patients with comorbid OCS.

10.3.3.1 Antipsychotic Treatment Decisions in First-Episode Psychotic Patients

Any treatment decision is influenced by anticipated or experienced AEs. Therefore, the potential risk of SGA-induced OCS should be considered when deciding on antipsychotic treatment in general.

10.3.3.2 Informed Consent About SGA-Induced OCS

According to guidelines of good clinical practice, the anticipated frequency of an AE determines whether or not the patient has to be informed about this danger. Because summarised evidence suggests that treatment with predominantly anti-serotonergic SGAs displays a frequent risk constellation for the development of OCS, this information should be provided to the patient prior to treatment initiation.

10.3.3.3 Cases with Treatment-Resistant Schizophrenia

In cases with treatment-resistant psychotic symptoms, currently available guidelines indicate CLZ treatment (Hasan et al. 2012). The general importance of CLZ in schizophrenia treatment needs to be emphasised. This SGA is a highly effective and indispensable part of the antipsychotic armament (Joober and Boksa 2010; Kane 2011; Kang and Simpson 2010; Meltzer 2012) and SGA of first choice in treatment-resistant psychoses (Kane et al. 1988). The CATIE study (McEvoy et al. 2006) and several other investigations demonstrated its superior antipsychotic effects in direct comparison (Gupta and Daniel 1995; Kelly et al. 2003; Still et al. 1996). In contrast to a recent Cochrane review which did not come to this conclusion (Asenjo Lobos et al. 2010), the superior antipsychotic efficacy of CLZ was recently confirmed in a large meta-analysis using a random effect model (Leucht et al. 2012b). CLZ has further been described to exert important antisuicidal effects resulting in relative low mortality rates of treated schizophrenia patients (Tiihonen et al. 2009). These favourable effects have led some authors to suggest CLZ as a first- or at least second-line SGA (Remington et al. 2013).

In clinical practice CLZ treatment is often initiated, although first- and second-choice treatment options are applied in non-sufficient dosages, over too short periods of time, without clinical drug monitoring and reliably excluded concomitant substance abuse. Physicians should consider the broad pattern of CLZ-associated side effects during evaluation of first- and second-line treatment and inform the treatment-resistant patient about the pros and cons of this substance. Before starting CLZ treatment, a careful characterisation of neurocognitive abilities and severity of OCS seems advisable. In addition, longitudinal monitoring should be established to allow for early detection of symptoms and anti-obsessive interventions.

Noteworthy, the evaluation of risks and benefits and final decision on the applied antipsychotic substance should primarily focus on the optimised treatment of psychotic symptoms. In the case of treatment-resistant symptoms, the pure risk of OCS development or actual OCS occurrence does not represent a sufficient reason to refuse CLZ treatment or to switch from CLZ to an alternative antipsychotic. Alternatively, polypharmacy might be considered aiming at a minimally sufficient CLZ dosages and serum levels through the combination with other SGAs or augmentation with antidepressants or mood stabiliser (see Chap. 11).

10.3.3.4 Implementation of Non-pharmacological Interventions

Cognitive behavioural therapy (CBT) has been established as an effective adjunctive treatment approach in patients with schizophrenia. A broader implementation of CBT in this group of patients would help to reduce the frequency of non-adherence to antipsychotic treatment, treatment resistance and the subsequent indications for CLZ. Even during CLZ treatment CBT could be an effective method for the prevention, early detection and treatment of co-occurring OCS. At present, controlled clinical trials which investigate CBT as a treatment approach for OCS in schizophrenia are missing. Evidence in support for its effectiveness are largely based on casuistic publications (Schirmbeck and Zink 2013a; Tundo et al. 2012, 2014) (see Chap. 12).

Conclusions

OCS might occur or aggravate subsequent to anti-serotonergic SGA treatment as a dose-dependent AE. Epidemiological and pharmacological data support this notion but large multimodal and longitudinal trials are necessary to validate preliminary evidence. First insight has been gained into specific cognitive profiles of schizophrenia patients with SGA-induced OCS. Other studies investigated genetic risk factors and neural correlates which seem to play a role in the pathogenesis of SGA-induced OCS. Forthcoming research should focus on the prospective assessment of patients, starting in the ARMS, and will most likely be effective if homogeneous subgroups are investigated. Possible interrelations between a genetic disposition and a broad variety of environmental factors should be analysed in order to develop and optimise methods of prevention, early recognition and therapeutic treatment, including both pharmacological and CBT approaches.

Conflicts of Interest *F. S.* was supported by a fellowship within the Postdoc-Programme of the German Academic Exchange Service (DAAD).

M. Z. received unrestricted scientific grants of the European Research Advisory Board (ERAB), German Research Foundation (DFG), Pfizer Pharma GmbH, Servier and Bristol-Myers Squibb Pharmaceuticals; further speaker and travel grants were provided from Janssen Cilag, Astra Zeneca, Lilly, Pfizer Pharma GmbH, Bristol-Myers Squibb Pharmaceuticals, Roche, Servier, Otsuka and Trommsdorff.

References

Achim AM, Maziade M, Raymond E, Olivier D, Merette C, Roy MA (2011) How prevalent are anxiety disorders in schizophrenia? A meta-analysis and critical review on a significant association. Schizophr Bull 37:811–821

Angermeyer MC, Matschinger H, Schomerus G (2013) Attitudes towards psychiatric treatment and people with mental illness: changes over two decades. Br J Psychiatry 203:146–151

Aoyama F, Iida J, Inoue M, Iwasaka H, Sakiyama S, Hata K, Kishimoto T (2000) Brain imaging in childhood- and adolescence-onset schizophrenia associated with obsessive-compulsive symptoms. Acta Psychiatr Scand 102:32–37

Arnold PD, Sicard T, Burroughs E, Richter MA, Kennedy JL (2006) Glutamate transporter gene SLC1A1 associated with obsessive-compulsive disorder. Arch Gen Psychiatry 63:769–776

Asenjo Lobos C, Komossa K, Rummel-Kluge C, Hunger H, Schmid F, Schwarz S, Leucht S (2010) Clozapine versus other atypical antipsychotics for schizophrenia. Cochrane Database of Syst Rev (11):CD006633

Baker RW, Chengappa KN, Baird JW, Steingard S, Christ MA, Schooler NR (1992) Emergence of obsessive compulsive symptoms during treatment with clozapine. J Clin Psychiatry 53:439–442

Bandelow B, Zohar J, Hollander E, Kasper S, ller HJ; WFSBP Task Force on Treatment Guidelines for Anxiety, Obsessive-Compulsive and Post-Traumatic Stress Disorders, Zohar J, Hollander E, Kasper S, ller HJ, Bandelow B, Allgulander C, yuso-Gutierrez J, Baldwin DS, Buenvicius R, Cassano G, Fineberg N, Gabriels L, Hindmarch I, Kaiya H, Klein DF, Lader M, Lecrubier Y, pine JP, Liebowitz MR, Lopez-Ibor JJ, Marazziti D, Miguel EC, Oh KS, Preter M, Rupprecht R, Sato M, Starcevic V, Stein DJ, van AM, Vega J (2008) World Federation of Societies of Biological Psychiatry (WFSBP) guidelines for the pharmacological treatment of anxiety, obsessive-compulsive and post-traumatic stress disorders – first revision. World J Biol Psychiatry 9:248–312

Berman I, Kalinowski A, Berman SM, Lengua J, Green AI (1995a) Obsessive and compulsive symptoms in chronic schizophrenia. Compr Psychiatry 36:6–10

Berman I, Sapers BL, Chang HH, Losonczy MF, Schmildler J, Green AI (1995b) Treatment of obsessive-compulsive symptoms in schizophrenic patients with clomipramine. J Clin Psychopharmacol 15:206–210

Berman I, Merson A, Viegner B, Losonczy MF, Pappas D, Green AI (1998) Obsessions and compulsions as a distinct cluster of symptoms in schizophrenia: a neuropsychological study. J Nerv Ment Dis 186:150–156

Bienvenu OJ, Wang Y, Shugart YY, Welch JM, Grados MA, Fyer AJ, Rauch SL, McCracken JT, Rasmussen SA, Murphy DL, Cullen B, Valle D, Hoehn-Saric R, Greenberg BD, Pinto A, Knowles JA, Piacentini J, Pauls DL, Liang KY, Willour VL, Riddle M, Samuels JF, Feng G, Nestadt G (2009) Sapap3 and pathological grooming in humans: results from the OCD collaborative genetics study. Am J Med Genet B Neuropsychiatr Genet 150B:710–720

Bleich-Cohen M, Hendler T, Weizman R, Faragian S, Weizman A, Poyurovsky M (2014) Working memory dysfunction in schizophrenia patients with obsessive-compulsive symptoms: An fMRI study. Eur Psychiatry 29(3):160–166

Bloch MH, Landeros-Weisenberger A, Kelmendi B, Coric V, Bracken MB, Leckman JF (2006) A systematic review: antipsychotic augmentation with treatment refractory obsessive-compulsive disorder. Mol Psychiatry 11:622–632

Borkowska A, Pilaczynska E, Rybakowski JK (2013) The frontal lobe neuropsychological tests in patients with schizophrenia and/or obsessive-compulsive disorder. J Neuropsychiatry Clin Neurosci 15:359–362

Bradford Hill A (2011) The environment and disease: association or causation? Bull World Health Organ 83:295–300

Buckley PF, Miller BJ, Lehrer DS, Castle DJ (2009) Psychiatric comorbidities and schizophrenia. Schizophr Bull 35:383–402

Bymaster FP, Rasmussen K, Calligaro DO, Nelson DL, DeLapp NW, Wong DT, Moore NA (1997) In vitro and in vivo biochemistry of olanzapine: a novel, atypical antipsychotic drug. J Clin Psychiatry 58(Suppl 10):28–36

Cai J, Zhang W, Lu W, Wu Z, Chen J, Yu S, Fang Y, Zhang C (2013) Influence of polymorphisms in genes SLC1A1, GRIN2B, and GRIK2 on clozapine-induced obsessive-compulsive symptoms. Psychopharmacology in 230(1):49–55

Chang JS, Ahn Y-M, Park HJ, Lee KY, Kim SH, Kang UG, Kim JS (2008) Aripiprazole augmentation in clozapine-treated patients With refractory schizophrenia: an 8-week, randomized, double-blind, placebo-controlled trial. J Clin Psychiatry 69:720–731

Correll CU (2008) Antipsychotic polypharmacy, part 2: why use 2 antipsychotics when 1 is not good enough? J Clin Psychiatry 69:860–861

Coward DM (1992) General pharmacology of clozapine. Br J Psychiatry Suppl 17:5–11

Craig T, Hwang MY, Bromet EJ (2002) Obsessive-compulsive and panic symptoms in patients with first-admission psychosis. Am J Psychiatry 159:592–598

Cunill R, Huerta-Ramos E, Castells X (2013) The effect of obsessive-compulsive symptomatology on executive functions in schizophrenia: a systematic review and meta-analysis. Psychiatry Res 210:21–28. doi:10.1016/j.psychres.2013.05.029

de Haan L, Linszen DH, Gorsira R (1999) Clozapine and obsessions in patients with recent-onset schizophrenia and other psychotic disorders. J Clin Psychiatry 60:364–365

de Haan L, Beuk N, Hoogenboom B, Dingemans P, Linszen D (2002) Obsessive-compulsive symptoms during treatment with olanzapine and risperidone: a prospective study of 113 patients with recent-onset schizophrenia or related disorders. J Clin Psychiatry 63:104–107

de Haan L, Oekeneva A, van Amelsvoore T, Linszen D (2004) Obsessive-compulsive disorder and treatment with clozapine in 200 patients with recent-onset schizophrenia or related disorders. Eur Psychiatry 19:524

de Haan L, Sterk B, Wouters L, Linszen DH (2013) The 5-Year Course of Obsessive-Compulsive Symptoms and Obsessive-Compulsive Disorder in First-Episode Schizophrenia and Related Disorders. Schizophr Bull 39:151–160

Dickel DE, Veenstra-VanderWeele J, Cox NJ, Wu X, Fischer DJ, Van Etten-Lee M, Himle JA, Leventhal BL, Cook EH Jr, Hanna GL (2006) Association testing of the positional and functional candidate gene SLC1A1/EAAC1 in early-onset obsessive-compulsive disorder. Arch Gen Psychiatry 63:778–785

Dold M, Aigner M, Lanzenberger R, Kasper S (2011) Efficacy of antipsychotic augmentation therapy in treatment-resistant obsessive-compulsive disorder – a meta-analysis of double-blind, randomised, placebo-controlled trials. Fortschr Neurol Psychiatr 79:453–466

Doyle M, Chorcorain AN, Griffith E, Trimble T, OGÇÖCallaghan E (2014) Obsessive compulsive symptoms in patients with schizophrenia on clozapine and with obsessive compulsive disorder: a comparison study. Compr Psychiatry 55:130–136

Duggan L, Fenton M, Dardennes RM, El-Dosoky A, Indran S (2000) Olanzapine for schizophrenia. Cochrane Database Syst Rev [computer file]: CD001359

Englisch S, Zink M (2008) Combined antipsychotic treatment involving clozapine and aripiprazole. Prog Neuropsychopharmacol Biol Psychiatry 32:1386–1392

Englisch S, Esslinger C, Inta D, Weinbrenner A, Peus V, Gutschalk A, Schirmbeck F, Zink M (2009) Clozapine-induced obsessive compulsive syndromes improve in combination with aripiprazole. Clin Neuropharmacol 32:227–229

Ertugrul A, nil Yagcioglu AE, Eni N, Yazici KM (2005) Obsessive-compulsive symptoms in clozapine-treated schizophrenic patients. Psychiatry Clin Neurosci 59:219–222

Eryilmaz G, Sayar GH, Ozten E, Gögcegöz I, Karamustafalioglu O (2013) Aripirazole augmentation in clozapine-associated obsessive-compulsive symptoms in schizophrenia. Ann Gen Psychiatry 12:40

Fenton WS, McGlashan TH (1986) The prognostic significance of obsessive-compulsive symptoms in schizophrenia. Am J Psychiatry 143:437–441

Friedlander L, Desrocher M (2006) Neuroimaging studies of obsessive-compulsive disorder in adults and children. Clin Psychol Rev 26:32–49

Grados MA, Specht MW, Sung HM, Fortune D (2013) Glutamate drugs and pharmacogenetics of OCD: a pathway-based exploratory approach. Expert Opin Drug Discov. doi:10.1517/17460441.2013.845553, 1–13

Graybiel AM, Rauch SL (2000) Toward a neurobiology of obsessive-compulsive disorder. Neuron 28:343–347

Gregory A, Lau J, Eley T (2008) Finding gene-environment interactions for generalised anxiety disorder. Eur Arch Psychiatry Clin Neurosci 258:69–75

Gupta S, Daniel DG (1995) Cautions in the clozapine-to-risperidone switch. Ann Clin Psychiatry 7:149

Hasan A, Falkai P, Wobrock T, Lieberman J, Glenthoj B, Gattaz WF, Thibaut F, M+Âller HJ (2012) World Federation of Societies of Biological Psychiatry (WFSBP) guidelines for biological treatment of schizophrenia, part 2: update 2012 on the long-term treatment of schizophrenia and management of antipsychotic-induced side effects. World J Biol Psychiatry 14:2–44

Hashim HM, Fawzy N, Fawzi MM, Karam RA (2012) Brain-derived neurotrophic factor Val66Met polymorphism and obsessive-compulsive symptoms in Egyptian schizophrenia patients. J Psychiatr Res. http://dx.doi.org/10.1016/j.jpsychires.2012.03.007

Hermesh H, Weizman A, Gur S, Zalsman G, Shiloh R, Zohar J, Gross-Isseroff R (2003) Alternation learning in OCD/schizophrenia patients. Eur Neuropsychopharmacol 13:87–91

Hippius H (1989) The history of clozapine. Psychopharmacology (Berl) 99(Suppl):S3–S5

Howes OD, Kambeitz J, Kim E, Stahl D, Slifstein M, bi-Dargham A, Kapur S (2012) The nature of dopamine dysfunction in schizophrenia and what this means for treatment: a meta-analysis of imaging studies. Arch Gen Psychiatry 69:776–786

Hwang MY, Morgan JE, Losconzcy MF (2000) Clinical and neuropsychological profiles of obsessive-compulsive schizophrenia: a pilot study.[see comment]. J Neuropsychiatry Clin Neurosci 12:91–94

Insel TR (2010) Rethinking schizophrenia. Nature 468:187–193

Insel TR, Scolnick EM (2006) Cure therapeutics and strategic prevention: raising the bar for mental health research. Mol Psychiatry 11:11–17

Jakob H, Beckmann H (1986) Prenatal developmental disturbances in the limbic allocortex in schizophrenics. J Neural Transm 65:303–326
Jakob H, Beckmann H (1989) Gross and histological criteria for developmental disorders in brains of schizophrenics. J R Soc Med 82:466–469
Joel D (2006) Current animal models of obsessive compulsive disorder: a critical review. Prog Neuropsychopharmacol Biol Psychiatry 30:374–388
Joober R, Boksa P (2010) Clozapine: a distinct, poorly understood and under-used molecule. J Psychiatry Neurosci 35:147–149
Kane JM (2011) A user's guide to clozapine. Acta Psychiatr Scand 123:407–408
Kane J, Honigfeld G, Singer J, Meltzer H (1988) Clozapine for the treatment-resistant schizophrenic. A double-blind comparison with chlorpromazine. Arch Gen Psychiatry 45:789–796
Kang X, Simpson GM (2010) Clozapine: more side effects but still the best antipsychotic. J Clin Psychiatry 71:982–983
Kantrowitz J, Javitt DC (2013) Glutamatergic transmission in schizophrenia: from basic research to clinical practice. Curr Opin Psychiatry 25:96–102
Karch S, Pogarell O (2011) Neurobiologie der Zwangsstörung. Nervenarzt 82:299–307
Keers R, Uher R (2012) Gene-environment interaction in major depression and antidepressant treatment response. Curr Psychiatry Rep 14:129–137
Kelly DL, Richardson CM, Tamminga CA, Carpenter WT (2003) The efficacy of high-dose olanzapine versus clozapine in treatment-resistant schizophrenia: a double-blind, crossover study. J Clin Psychopharmacol 23:668–670
Kim SW, Shin IS, Kim JM, Yang SJ, Hwang MY, Yoon JS (2008) Amisulpride improves obsessive-compulsive symptoms in schizophrenia patients taking atypical antipsychotics: an open-label switch study. J Clin Psychopharmacol 28:349–352
Kim JH, Ryu S, Nam HJ, Lim M, Baek JH, Joo YH, Kwon JS, Ha TH, Hong KS (2012) Symptom structure of antipsychotic-induced obsessive compulsive symptoms in schizophrenia patients. Prog Neuropsychopharmacol Biol Psychiatry 39:75–79
Kordon A, Zurowski B, Wahl K, Hohagen F (2011) Evidence-based pharmacotherapy and other somatic treatment approaches for obsessive-compulsive disorder: state of the art. Nervenarzt 82:319–320
Krause DL, Matz J, Schennach R, Mueller N, Dehning S (2013) Ziprasidone for obsessive compulsive disorder in schizophrenia. Ther Adv Psychopharmacol 3:115–116
Kuelz AK, Hohagen F, Voderholzer U (2004) Neuropsychological performance in obsessive-compulsive disorder: a critical review. [Review] [108 refs]. Biol Psychol 65:185–236
Kulkarni G, Narayanaswamy JC, Math SB (2012) Olanzapine induced *de-novo* obsessive compulsive disorder in a patient with schizophrenia. Indian J Pharmacol 44:649–650
Kumbhani SR, Roth RM, Kruck CL, Flashman LA, McAllister TW (2010) Nonclinical obsessive-compulsive symptoms and executive functions in schizophrenia. J Neuropsychiatry Clin Neurosci 22:304–312
Kwon JS, Joo YH, Nam HJ, Lim M, Cho EY, Jung MH, Choi JS, Kim B, Kang DH, Oh S, Park T, Hong KS (2009) Association of the glutamate transporter gene SLC1A1 with atypical antipsychotics-induced obsessive-compulsive symptoms. Arch Gen Psychiatry 66:1233–1241
Lee M-J, Shin Y-B, Sunwoo Y-K, Jung S-H, Kim W-H, Kang M-H, Lee J-S, Bae J-M, Kim C-E (2009) Comparative analysis of cognitive function in schizophrenia with and without obsessive compulsive disorder. Psychiatry Investig 6:286–293
Leucht S, Hierl S, Kissling W, Dold M, Davis JM (2012a) Putting the efficacy of psychiatric and general medicine medication into perspective: review of meta-analyses. Br J Psychiatry 200:97–106
Leucht S, Tardy M, Komossa K, Heres S, Kissling W, Salanti G, Davis JM (2012b) Antipsychotic drugs versus placebo for relapse prevention in schizophrenia: a systematic review and meta-analysis. Lancet 379:2063–2071
Levine JB, Gruber SA, Baird AA, Yurgelun-Todd D (1998) Obsessive-compulsive disorder among schizophrenic patients: an exploratory study using functional magnetic resonance imaging data. Compr Psychiatry 39:308–311

Lim M, Park DY, Kwon JS, Joo YH, Hong KS (2007) Prevalence and clinical characteristics of obsessive-compulsive symptoms associated with atypical antipsychotics. J Clin Psychopharmacol 27:712–713

Lin SK, Su SF, Pan CH (2006) Higher plasma drug concentration in clozapine-treated schizophrenic patients with side effects of obsessive/compulsive symptoms. Ther Drug Monit 28:303–307

Linden DE (2006) How psychotherapy changes the brain – the contribution of functional neuroimaging. Mol Psychiatry 11:528–538

Lopez-Gil X, Artigas F, Adell A (2010) Unraveling monoamine receptors involved in the action of typical and atypical antipsychotics on glutamatergic and serotonergic transmission in prefrontal cortex. Curr Pharm Des 16:502–515

Lykouras L, Alevizos B, Michalopoulou P, Rabavilas A (2003) Obsessive-compulsive symptoms induced by atypical antipsychotics. A review of the reported cases. Prog Neuropsychopharmacol Biol Psychiatry 27:333–346

Lysaker PH, Whitney KA (2009) Obsessive-compulsive symptoms in schizophrenia: prevalence, correlates and treatment. Expert Rev Neurother 9:99–107

Lysaker PH, Bryson GJ, Marks KA, Greig TC, Bell MD (2002) Association of obsessions and compulsions in schizophrenia with neurocognition and negative symptoms. J Neuropsychiatry Clin Neurosci 14:449–453

Lysaker PH, Whitney KA, Davis LW (2009) Associations of executive function with concurrent and prospective reports of obsessive-compulsive symptoms in schizophrenia. J Neuropsychiatry Clin Neurosci 21:38–42

McDougle CJ, Barr LC, Goodman WK, Pelton GH, Aronson SC, Anand A, Price LH (1995) Lack of efficacy of clozapine monotherapy in refractory obsessive-compulsive disorder. Am J Psychiatry 152:1812–1814

McEvoy JP, Lieberman JA, Stroup TS, Davis SM, Meltzer HY, Rosenheck RA, Swartz MS, Perkins DO, Keefe RS, Davis CE, Severe J, Hsiao JK, CATIE I, McEvoy JP, Lieberman JA, Stroup TS, Davis SM, Meltzer HY, Rosenheck RA, Swartz MS, Perkins DO, Keefe RSE, Davis CE, Severe J, Hsiao JK, CATIE I (2006) Effectiveness of clozapine versus olanzapine, quetiapine, and risperidone in patients with chronic schizophrenia who did not respond to prior atypical antipsychotic treatment. [see comment]. Am J Psychiatry 163:600–610

Meijer JHM, Swets MM, Keeman SM, Nieman DHP, Meijer CJP, GROUP Investigators (2013) Is a schizo-obsessive subtype associated with cognitive impairment?: results from a large cross-sectional study in patients with psychosis and their unaffected relatives. J Nerv Ment Dis 201:30–35

Meltzer HY (1994) An overview of the mechanism of action of clozapine. J Clin Psychiatry 55(Suppl B):47–52

Meltzer HY (2012) Clozapine. Clin Schizophr Relat Psychoses 6:134–144

Meltzer HY, Huang M (2008) In vivo actions of atypical antipsychotic drug on serotonergic and dopaminergic systems. Prog Brain Res 172:177–197

Meltzer HY, Sumiyoshi T (2008) Does stimulation of 5-HT(1A) receptors improve cognition in schizophrenia? Behav Brain Res 195:98–102

Meltzer HY, Li Z, Kaneda Y, Ichikawa J (2003) Serotonin receptors: their key role in drugs to treat schizophrenia. Prog Neuropsychopharmacol Biol Psychiatry 27:1159–1172

Michalopoulou PG, Konstantakopoulos G, Typaldou M, Papageorgiou C, Christodoulou GN, Lykouras L, Oulis P (2014) Can cognitive deficits differentiate between schizophrenia with and without obsessive-compulsive symptoms? Compr Psychiatry. doi:10.1016/j.comppsych.2013.12.004

Mukhopadhaya K, Krishnaiah R, Taye T, Nigam A, Bailey AJ, Sivakumaran T, Fineberg NA (2009) Obsessive-compulsive disorder in UK clozapine-treated schizophrenia and schizoaffective disorder: a cause for clinical concern. J Psychopharmacol 23:6–13

Muscatello MR, Bruno A, Pandolfo G, Mico U, Scimeca G, Romeo VM, Santoro V, Settineri S, Spina E, Zoccali RA (2011) Effect of aripiprazole augmentation of serotonin reuptake inhibitors or clomipramine in treatment-resistant obsessive-compulsive disorder: a double-blind, placebo-controlled study. J Clin Psychopharmacol 31:174–179

Nakao T, Nakagawa A, Yoshiura T, Nakatani E, Nabeyama M, Yoshizato C, Kudoh A, Tada K, Yoshioka K, Kawamoto M, Togao O, Kanba S (2005) Brain activation of patients with obsessive – compulsive disorder during neuropsychological and symptom provocation tasks before and after symptom improvement: a functional magnetic resonance imaging study. Biol Psychiatry 57:901–910

Nicolini H, Arnold P, Nestadt G, Lanzagorta N, Kennedy JL (2009) Overview of genetics and obsessive-compulsive disorder. Psychiatry Res 170:7–14

Nolfe G, Milano W, Zontini G, Petrella C, De RM, Rundle-Smith S, Nolfe G (2010) Obsessive-compulsive symptoms in schizophrenia: their relationship with clinical features and pharmacological treatment. J Psychiatr Pract 16:235–242

Nugent N, Tyrka A, Carpenter L, Price L (2011) Gene-environment interactions: early life stress and risk for depressive and anxiety disorders. Psychopharmacology (Berl) 214: 175–196

Öngür D, Goff DC (2005) Obsessive-compulsive symptoms in schizophrenia: associated clinical features, cognitive function and medication status. Schizophr Res 75:349–362

Pani L, Villagran JM, Kontaxakis VP, Alptekin K (2008) Practical issues with amisulpride in the management of patients with schizophrenia. Clin Drug Investig 28:465–477

Patel DD, Laws KR, Padhi A, Farrow JM, Mukhopadhaya K, Krishnaiah R, Fineberg NA (2010) The neuropsychology of the schizo-obsessive subtype of schizophrenia: a new analysis. Psychol Med 40:921–933

Pauls DL (2010) The genetics of obsessive-compulsive disorder: a review. Dialogues Clin Neurosci 12:149–163

Peselmann N, Schmitt A, Gebicke-Haerter P, Zink M (2012) Aripiprazole differentially regulates the expression of Gad67 and ã-amino-butyric acid transporters in rat brain. Eur Arch Psychiatry Clin Neurosci. doi:10.1007/s00406-012-0367-y

Peters B, de Haan L (2009) Remission of schizophrenia psychosis and strong reduction of obsessive-compulsive disorder after adding clozapine to aripiprazole. Prog Neuropsychopharmacol Biol Psychiatry 33:1576–1577

Pogarell O, Hamann C, Poepperl G, Juckel G, Chouker M, Zaudig M, Riedel M, Moeller HJ, Hegerl U, Tatsch K (2003) Elevated brain serotonin transporter availability in patients with obsessive-compulsive disorder. Biol Psychiatry 54:1406–1413

Porton B, Greenberg BD, Askland K, Serra LM, Gesmonde J, Rudnick G, Rasmussen SA, Kao HT (2013) Isoforms of the neuronal glutamate transporter gene, SLC1A1/EAAC1, negatively modulate glutamate uptake: relevance to obsessive-compulsive disorder. Transl Psychiatry. doi:10.1038/tp.2013.35, e259

Poyurovsky M (2013) Schizo-obsessive disorder. Cambridge university press 1:1–245

Poyurovsky M, Isakov V, Hromnikov S, Modai I, Rauchberger B, Schneidman M, Weizman A (1999) Fluvoxamine treatment of obsessive-compulsive symptoms in schizophrenic patients: an add-on open study. Int Clin Psychopharmacol 14:95–100

Poyurovsky M, Weizman A, Weizman R (2004) Obsessive-compulsive disorder in schizophrenia: clinical characteristics and treatment. CNS Drugs 18:989–1010

Poyurovsky M, Glick I, Koran LM (2010) Lamotrigine augmentation in schizophrenia and schizoaffective patients with obsessive-compulsive symptoms. J Psychopharmacol 24:861–866

Readler TJ, Knable MB, Weinberger DR (1998) Schizophrenia as a developmental disorder of the cerebral cortex. Curr Opin Neurobiol 8:157–161

Remington G (2008) Alterations of dopamine and serotonin transmission in schizophrenia. Prog Brain Res 172:117–140

Remington G, Agid O, Foussias G, Hahn M, Rao N, Sinyor M (2013) Clozapines role in the treatment of first-episode schizophrenia. Am J Psychiatry 170:146–151

Reznik I, Yavin I, Stryjer R, Spivak B, Gonen N, Strous R, Mester R, Weizman A, Kotler M (2004) Clozapine in the treatment of obsessive-compulsive symptoms in schizophrenia patients: a case series study. Pharmacopsychiatry 37:52–56

Rocha FL, Hara C (2006) Benefits of combining aripiprazole to clozapine: Three case reports. Prog Neuropsychopharmacol Biol Psychiatry 30:1167–1169

Ryu S, Oh S, Cho EY, Nam HJ, Yoo JH, Park T, Joo YH, Kwon JS, Hong KS (2011) Interaction between genetic variants of DLGAP3 and SLC1A1 affecting the risk of atypical antipsychotics-induced obsessive-compulsive symptoms. Am J Med Genet B Neuropsychiatr Genet 156:949–959

Sa AR, Hounie AG, Sampaio AS, Arrais J, Miguel EC, Elkis H (2009) Obsessive-compulsive symptoms and disorder in patients with schizophrenia treated with clozapine or haloperidol. Compr Psychiatry 50:437–442

Saxena S, BRODY AL, SCHWARTZ JM, Baxter LR (1998) Neuroimaging and frontal-subcortical circuitry in obsessive-compulsive disorder. Br J Psychiatry 173:26–37

Saxena S, Brody AL, Maidment KM, Dunkin JJ, Colgan M, Alborzian S, Phelps ME, Baxter LRJ (1999) Localized orbitofrontal and subcortical metabolic changes and predictors of response to paroxetine treatment in obsessive-compulsive disorder. Neuropsychopharmacology 21:683–693

Saxena S, Gorbis E, O'Neill J, Baker SK, Mandelkern MA, Maidment KM, Chang S, Salamon N, BRODY AL, SCHWARTZ JM, London ED (2009) Rapid effects of brief intensive cognitive-behavioral therapy on brain glucose metabolism in obsessive-compulsive disorder. Mol Psychiatry 14:197

Scatton B, Claustre Y, Cudennec A, Oblin A, Perrault G, Sanger DJ, Schoemaker H (1997) Amisulpride: from animal pharmacology to therapeutic action. Int Clin Psychopharmacol 12(Suppl 2):S29–S36

Scheltema Beduin AA, Sweets M, Machielsen M, Korver N, GROUP Consortium (2012) Obsessive-compulsive symptoms in patients with schizophrenia comparing treatment with clozapine, olanzapine, risperidone and no antipsychotics: a naturalistic cross-sectional study of 543 patients. J Clin Psychiatry 73:1395–1402

Schirmbeck F, Zink M (2012) Clozapine-induced obsessive-compulsive symptoms in schizophrenia: a critical review. Curr Neuropharmacol 10:88–95

Schirmbeck F, Zink M (2013a) The cognitive behavioural therapist. The Cognitive Behaviour Therapist 6:1–13. http://dx.doi.org/10.1017/S1754470X13000123

Schirmbeck F, Zink M (2013b) Frontiers in neuropharmacology. Front Pharmacol 4:1–99. doi:10.3389/fphar.2013.00099

Schirmbeck F, Esslinger C, Rausch F, Englisch S, Meyer-Lindenberg A, Zink M (2011) Antiserotonergic antipsychotics are associated with obsessive-compulsive symptoms in schizophrenia. Psychol Med 41:2361–2374

Schirmbeck F, Nieratschker V, Frank J, Englisch S, Rausch F, Meyer-Lindenberg A, Rietschel M, Zink M (2012a) Polymorphisms in the glutamate transporter gene SLC1A1 and obsessive compulsive symptoms induced by second generation antipsychotic agents. Psychiatr Genet 22:245–252

Schirmbeck F, Rausch F, Englisch S, Eifler S, Esslinger C, Meyer-Lindenberg A, Zink M (2012b) Stable cognitive deficits in schizophrenia patients with comorbid obsessive-compulsive symptoms: a 12 months longitudinal study. Schizophr Bull 6:1261–1271. doi:10.1093/schbul/sbs123

Schirmbeck F, Rausch F, Englisch S, Eifler S, Esslinger C, Meyer-Lindenberg A, Zink M (2013) Differential effects of antipsychotic agents on obsessive-compulsive symptoms in schizophrenia: a longitudinal study. J Psychopharmacol 27:349–357

Schirmbeck F, Mier D, Esslinger C, Rausch F, Englisch S, Eifler S, Meyer-Lindenberg A, Kirsch P, Zink M (2014) Increased orbitofrontal cortex activation during treatment with pro-obsessive antipsychotic drugs. J Psychiatry Neurosci. doi: 10.1503/jpn.140021

Shapiro DA, Renock S, Arrington E, Chiodo LA, Liu LX, Sibley DR, Roth BL, Mailman R (2003) Aripiprazole, a novel atypical antipsychotic drug with a unique and robust pharmacology. Neuropsychopharmacology 28:1400–1411

Shugart YY, Wang Y, Samuels JF, Grados MA, Greenberg BD, Knowles JA, McCracken JT, Rauch SL, Murphy DL, Rasmussen SA, Cullen B, Hoehn-Saric R, Pinto A, Fyer AJ, Piacentini J, Pauls DL, Bienvenu OJ, Riddle MA, Liang KY, Nestadt G (2009) A family-based association study of the glutamate transporter gene SLC1A1 in obsessive-compulsive disorder in 378 families. Am J Med Genet B Neuropsychiatr Genet 150B:886–892

Sparshatt A, Taylor D, Patel MX, Kapur S (2010) A systematic review of aripiprazole–dose, plasma concentration, receptor occupancy, and response: implications for therapeutic drug monitoring. J Clin Psychiatry 71:1447–1456

Stan A, Lewis D (2012) Altered cortical GABA neurotransmission in schizophrenia: insights into novel therapeutic strategies. Curr Pharm Biotechnol 13:1557–1562

Starck G, Ljungberg M, Nilsson M, Jonsson L, Lundberg S, Ivarsson T, Ribbelin S, Ekholm S, Carlsson A, Forssell-Aronsson E, Carlsson ML (2008) A 1H magnetic resonance spectroscopy study in adults with obsessive compulsive disorder: relationship between metabolite concentrations and symptom severity. J Neural Transm 115:1051–1062

Steingard S, Chengappa KNR, Baker R, Schooler NR (1993) Clozapine, obsessive symptoms, and serotonergic mechanisms. Am J Psychiatry 150:1435

Stewart SE, Fagerness JA, Platko J, Smoller JW, Scharf JM, Illmann C, Jenike E, Chabane N, Leboyer M, Delorme R, Jenike MA, Pauls DL (2007) Association of the SLC1A1 glutamate transporter gene and obsessive-compulsive disorder. Am J Med Genet B Neuropsychiatr Genet 144 B:1027–1033

Still DJ, Dorson PG, Crismon ML, Pousson C (1996) Effects of switching inpatients with treatment-resistant schizophrenia from clozapine to risperidone. Psychiatr Serv 47:1382–1384

Strakowski SM, Tohen M, Stoll AL, Faedda GL, Mayer PV, Kolbrener ML, Goodwin DC (1993) Comorbidity in psychosis at first hospitalization. Am J Psychiatry 150:752–757

Strakowski SM, Keck PE Jr, McElroy SL, Lonczak HS, West SA (1995) Chronology of comorbid and principal syndromes in first-episode psychosis. Compr Psychiatry 36:106–112

Stryjer R, Dambinsky Y, Timinsky I, Green T, Kotler M, Weizman A, Spivak B (2012) Escitalopram in the treatment of patients with schizophrenia and obsessive-compulsive disorder: an open-label, prospective study. [Article]. Int Clin Psychopharmacol. doi:10.1097/YIC.0b013e32835bd24e

Swets M, Dekker J, van Emmerik-van Oortmerssen K, Smid GE, Smit F, de Haan L, Schoevers RA (2013) The obsessive compulsive spectrum in schizophrenia, a meta-analysis and meta-regression exploring prevalence rates. Schizophr Res. http://dx.doi.org/10.1016/j.schres.2013.10.033

Tiihonen J, Lonnqvist J, Wahlbeck K, Klaukka T, Niskanen L, Tanskanen A, Haukka J (2009) 11-year follow-up of mortality in patients with schizophrenia: a population-based cohort study (FIN11 study).[see comment]. Lancet 374:620–627

Tiryaki A, Ozkorumak E (2010) Do the obsessive-compulsive symptoms have an effect in schizophrenia? Compr Psychiatry 51:357–362

Tumkaya S, Karadag F, Oguzhanoglu NK, Tekkanat C, Varma G, Ozdel O, Atesci F (2009) Schizophrenia with obsessive-compulsive disorder and obsessive-compulsive disorder with poor insight: a neuropsychological comparison. Psychiatry Res 165:38–46

Tundo A, Salvati L, Di Spigno D, Cieri L, Parena A, Necci R, Sciortino S (2012) Cognitive-behavioral therapy for obsessive-compulsive disorder as a comorbidity with schizophrenia or schizoaffective disorder. Psychother Psychosom 81:58–60

Tundo A, Salvati L, Cieri L, Daniele M, Di Spigno D, Necci R, Parena A (2014) Effectiveness and outcome predictors of cognitive-behavioural therapy for obsessive-compulsive disorder co-occurring with psychosis. J Psychopathol 20:127–133

Van der Wee NJ, Stevens H, Hardeman JA, Mandl RC, Denys DA, van Megen HJ, Kahn RS, Westenberg HM (2004) Enhanced Dopamine Transporter Density in Psychotropic-Naive Patients With Obsessive-Compulsive Disorder Shown by [^{123}I]ß-CIT SPECT. Am J Psych 161:2201–2206.

van Nimwegen L, de Haan L, van Beveren N, Laan W, van den Brink W, Linszen D (2008) Obsessive-compulsive symptoms in a randomized, double-blind study with olanzapine or risperidone in young patients with early psychosis. J Clin Psychopharmacol 28:214–218

van Os J, Kapur S (2009) Schizophrenia. Lancet 374:635–645

van Os J, Rutten BP, Poulton R (2008) Gene-environment interactions in schizophrenia: review of epidemiological findings and future directions. Schizophr Bull 34:1066–1082

van Os J, Kenis G, Rutten BP (2010) The environment and schizophrenia. Nature 468:203–212
Veenstra-VanderWeele J, Kim SJ, Gonen D, Hanna GL, Leventhal BL, Cook EH Jr (2001) Genomic organization of the SLC1A1/EAAC1 gene and mutation screening in early-onset obsessive-compulsive disorder. Mol Psychiatry 6:160–167
Villari V, Frieri T, Fagiolini A (2011) Aripiprazole augmentation in clozapine-associated obsessive-compulsive symptoms. J Clin Psychopharmacol 31:375–376
Wendland JR, Moya PR, Timpano KR, Anavitarte AP, Kruse MR, Wheaton MG, Ren-Patterson RF, Murphy DL (2009) A haplotype containing quantitative trait loci for SLC1A1 gene expression and its association with obsessive-compulsive disorder. Arch Gen Psychiatry 66:408–416
Whiteside SP, Port JD, Abramowitz JS (2004) A meta-analysis of functional neuroimaging in obsessive-compulsive disorder. Psychiatry Res 132:69–79
Whiteside SP, Port JD, Deacon BJ, Abramowitz JS (2006) A magnetic resonance spectroscopy investigation of obsessive-compulsive disorder and anxiety. Psychiatry Res 146:137–147
Whitney KA, Fastenau PS, Evans JD, Lysaker PH (2004) Comparative neuropsychological function in obsessive-compulsive disorder and schizophrenia with and without obsessive-compulsive symptoms. Schizophr Res 69:75–83
Zink M (2007) Plasticity of brain development as a perspective of basic science in psychiatry. Shaker Verlag – Online Publication, doi:10.2370/210_194
Zink M (2014), Comorbid obsessive-compulsive symptoms in schizophrenia: insight into pathomechanisms facilitates treatment. Advances in Medicine, in press
Zink M, Knopf U, Kuwilsky A (2006) Management of clozapine-induced obsessive compulsive symptoms in a man with schizophrenia. Aust N Z J Psychiatry 41:293–294
Zink M, Englisch S, Knopf U, Kuwilsky A, Dressing H (2007) Augmentation of clozapine with valproic acid for clozapine-induced obsessive compulsive symptoms. Pharmacopsychiatry 40:202–203
Zink M, Schirmbeck F, Rausch F, Eifler S, Elkin H, Solojenkina X, Englisch S, Wagner M, Maier W, Lautenschlager M, Heinz A, Gudlowski Y, Janssen B, Gaebel W, Michel TM, Schneider F, Lambert M, Naber D, Juckel G, Krueger-Oezguerdal S, Wobrock T, Hasan A, Riedel M, Müller H, Klosterkotter J, Bechdolf A (2014a) Obsessive-compulsive symptoms in at-risk mental states for psychosis are associated with more severe clinical impairment but less cognitive dysfunctions. Acta Psychiatr Scand 130(3):214–226
Zink M, Englisch S, Schmitt A (2014b) Antipsychotic treatment modulates glutamate transport and NMDA receptor expression. Eur Arc Psychiatry Clin Neurosci Suppl 1:S67–S82

Part IV

Therapy

Polypharmacy for Obsessive-Compulsive Symptoms in Schizophrenia: Augmentation and Combination Strategies

11

Susanne Englisch and Mathias Zink

Abbreviations

5HT	5-Hydroxytryptamine, serotonin
AE	Adverse event
AMS	Amisulpride
APP	Antipsychotic polypharmacy
APZ	Aripiprazole
ARMS	At-risk mental state
BD	Bipolar disorder
BDNF	Brain-derived neurotrophic factor
CBT	Cognitive behavioural therapy
CLZ	Clozapine
CR	Case report
CS	Case series
CSTC	Cortico-striato-thalamo-cortical
DLGAP3	Disks large-associated protein 3
ERP	Exposure and response prevention
FGA	First-generation antipsychotic
fMRI	Functional magnetic resonance imaging
GxEI	Gene and environment interaction

S. Englisch, MD
Department of Psychiatry and Psychotherapy,
Medical Faculty Mannheim, Central Institute of Mental Health, Heidelberg University,
12 21 20, Mannheim D-68072, Germany

M. Zink, MD (✉)
Department of Psychiatry and Psychotherapy, Medical Faculty Mannheim,
Central Institute of Mental Health, Heidelberg University,
P. O. Box 12 21 20, Mannheim D-68072, Germany
e-mail: mathias.zink@zi-mannheim.de

L. De Haan et al. (eds.), *Obsessive-Compulsive Symptoms in Schizophrenia*,
DOI 10.1007/978-3-319-12952-5_11

MS	Mood stabilizers
NS	Negative symptoms
OCD	Obsessive-compulsive disorder
OCS	Obsessive-compulsive symptoms
OLZ	Olanzapine
PS	Positive symptoms
QTP	Quetiapine
SGA	Second-generation antipsychotics
SLC1A1	Solute carrier family gene 1A1
SNP	Single-nucleotide polymorphism
SNRI	Serotonin and noradrenaline reuptake inhibitor
SRI	Serotonin reuptake inhibitor
SSRI	Selective serotonin reuptake inhibitor
ZIPR	Ziprasidone

11.1 Introduction

11.1.1 Polypharmacy in Treatment-Resistant Schizophrenia

Polypharmaceutical treatment approaches are common in everyday clinical practice. Multimodal treatment, however, has not yet been implemented on a large scale in schizophrenia, and despite all efforts, only a minority of patients regain their levels of premorbid psychosocial and vocational functioning (Insel 2010). Clozapine (CLZ) has been established as the substance of choice for treatment-refractory schizophrenia (Nielsen et al. 2011). Nevertheless, up to 40 % of patients experience only partial remission of psychotic symptoms in spite of CLZ treatment, and even more do not reach a level of full functional recovery. There are several reasons for insufficient treatment response: (1) Pharmaceutical research in the field of schizophrenia usually puts the focus on core psychotic positive symptoms (PS) while other symptom domains are being neglected or addressed as secondary parameters only. Thus, substances entering the market usually cover a small set of symptoms only within the broad spectrum of schizophrenic psychopathological features. (2) While PS are more striking to the observer, subtler symptoms such as negative symptoms (NS), cognitive deficits, affective dysregulation, substance abuse, post-traumatic stress disorder, anxiety and, finally, obsessive-compulsive symptoms (OCS) account for the major part of treatment-refractory impairments. (3) While their efficacy has been proven in well-designed clinical trials, several therapeutic methods are only insufficiently applied in clinical routine. This is particularly true for cognitive behavioural therapy (CBT), which is highly recommended by international guidelines but hardly ever implemented in everyday practice.

Clinicians are often tempted to respond to treatment resistance with polypharmaceutical approaches. These may comprise the 'combination' of equal-class substances (e.g. parallel use of different antipsychotic agents) and the 'augmentation' with substances of different groups (e.g. add-on of mood stabilizers to pre-existing antipsychotic treatment). Generally, add-on attempts frequently occur and usually result in escalating cumulative doses (Centorrino et al. 2010). Patients with longer courses of illness, lower levels of psychosocial functioning and high levels of treatment adherence are particularly likely to be prescribed more than one drug. Recent investigations have shown that a minimum of 40 % of schizophrenia outpatients worldwide receive two or more antipsychotic agents, and up to 70 % are co-medicated with other psychotropic drugs (Pickar et al. 2008). This trend of antipsychotic polypharmacy (APP) has been stable over the last decades, with higher prevalence rates in Asia and Europe and lower rates in North America. Some characteristics seem to be particularly associated with APP treatment, with inpatient status, use of first-generation antipsychotics (FGAs) and a diagnosis of schizophrenia being the most important predictors (Gallego et al. 2012a).

11.1.2 Substances and Indications for Add-On Strategies

Polypharmacy is usually applied in a symptom-oriented manner (see Sect. 11.1.1) and comprises multiple classes of substances. Aside from FGAs and SGAs that are frequently combined in order to extend the range of receptor profiles, also antidepressants, mood stabilizers, cognitive enhancers and experimental substances are prescribed. This bears the risk of additive side effects, and both pharmacokinetic and pharmacodynamic interactions need to be considered.

In addition to alleviating long-term treatment-refractory symptoms within the psychopathology of schizophrenia, some agents are applied over short periods only in order to manage acute symptoms. In particular, anticholinergic drugs are employed for treatment-emergent extrapyramidal symptoms, and benzodiazepines are administered to arrest psychomotor agitation and anxiety (Zink et al. 2010).

11.1.3 Problems Associated with Simultaneous Use of Multiple Substances

APP is associated with ambiguous results regarding efficacy and tolerability: There may be psychopathological improvement to some extent; the risk of cumulative adverse events (AEs) such as parkinsonism, hyperprolactinaemia, sexual dysfunction, hypersalivation, sedation and somnolence, however, is increased. Some of these conditions require additional treatment (see Sect. 11.1.2), which, in turn, aggravates the liability to pharmacokinetic interactions, a potential loss of 'atypicity' and rising treatment costs. Thus, APP should remain a measure of last resort when monotherapy, a switch in the antipsychotic treatment regimen and combination strategies with non-antipsychotic agents have failed (Gallego et al. 2012b). This is particularly true as one recent meta-analysis found polypharmacy associated with increased mortality rates (Weinmann et al. 2009). This finding, however, was not replicated in two large-scale Scandinavian epidemiological studies (Baandrup et al. 2010; Tiihonen et al. 2009a).

11.1.4 Heterogeneity of Schizophrenia Patients with OCS: Implications for Treatment

Aiming at individualized treatment modalities of OCS in schizophrenia, heterogeneous clinical subgroups (see Chap. 4) can be differentiated by several determinants (Zink 2014a): Primarily, the time and conditions under which the OCS developed (pre/post schizophrenia) have to be elucidated. In addition, factors aggravating or relieving OCS over time as well as the degree of variability need to be considered. Finally, neurogenetic and neurochemical properties appear to be of pivotal importance as they may hint to differential pathogenic factors: There is wide agreement on a dysbalance within the serotonergic neurotransmission in the cortico-striato-thalamo-cortical (CSTC) network (Linden 2006; Pogarell et al. 2003; Saxena et al. 2009), but also alterations within dopaminergic (Van der Wee et al. 2004) and glutamatergic (Grados et al. 2013) structures have been proposed (see Chap. 9). So far, no universal and integrative pathogenic model has been established which would imply for individualized pharmacological or psychotherapeutic treatment approaches. The current state of knowledge derived from clinical trials is clearly limited and indicates a major limitation to the subsequent summary of treatment interventions. Based on several case reports, case series as well as open and sparse controlled clinical trials, therapeutic strategies for the management of comorbid OCS in schizophrenia may be classified as (1) an optimization of antipsychotic monotherapy, (2) CBT interventions, (3) augmentation approaches and (4) combinations of SGAs. Nevertheless, the considerable lack of evidence substantiates the need for further research.

11.2 Treatment Strategies

11.2.1 Monotherapy with Antipsychotic Agents

Antipsychotic agents differ significantly with regard to their pharmacodynamic profiles (Correll 2012). For the pathogenesis of OCS, the affinity to serotonergic $5HT_{2A}$ receptors (Kim et al. 2009) is of major importance. Moreover, partial agonistic effects at the serotonergic system [aripiprazole (APZ) and ziprasidone (ZIPR)] and differences between GABAergic and glutamatergic properties have to be considered as they may have modulatory impact on OCS-related brain regions. A recent pharmacoimaging study comparing patients during CLZ or olanzapine (OLZ) monotherapy with patients treated with amisulpride (AMS) or APZ provided insight into substance-dependent alterations within the CSTC network. During a response-inhibition task, patients treated with CLZ and OLZ monotherapy showed significantly more activation in the orbitofrontal cortex when compared to patients with AMS and APZ treatment (Schirmbeck et al. 2014). Differential effects of FGAs and SGAs on OCS-related brain functions became apparent in primary obsessive-compulsive disorder (OCD) when selective serotonin reuptake inhibitors (SSRIs) – the current treatment of choice – remained ineffective (Bloch et al. 2006; Dold et al. 2011; Fineberg et al. 2006; Gao et al. 2006). It was shown that favourable effects can be expected from haloperidol, risperidone (RISP) (Saxena et al. 2014), AMS,

ZIPR and APZ: APZ has been used successfully in primary OCD both as a first-line therapy (Connor et al. 2005) and when SSRI treatment proved to be inefficient (le Chiaie et al. 2011; Muscatello et al. 2011; Yang et al. 2008). AMS was successfully applied in primary OCD resistant to SSRI treatment (Metin et al. 2003), with an overall favourable range of side effects. AEs included weight gain, mild sedation, asthenia and acute akathisia (Ersche et al. 2012). One small study found quetiapine (QTP) to be superior to ZIPR in treating OCD refractory to SSRIs (Savas et al. 2008). In contrast to positive effects of these SGAs, CLZ monotherapy lacked efficacy in the treatment of refractory OCD (McDougle et al. 1995).

For the treatment of OCS in schizophrenia, APZ and AMS proved particularly important: APZ monotherapy in schizophrenia was associated with lower prevalence rates of OCS (Schirmbeck et al. 2011; Yang et al. 2008) than other SGAs such as CLZ (Coward 1992; Meltzer and Huang 2008; Meltzer 2012) and OLZ (Duggan et al. 2005). This suggests that APZ may carry stand-alone anti-obsessive properties; at least, it seems to have no pro-obsessive effects as has been described for agents with lower antidopaminergic/antiserotonergic ratios.

ZIPR was recently tested in a sample of 29 schizophrenia patients with comorbid OCS. Doses of 80–200 mg/day resulted in a bimodal distribution (Juven-Wetzler et al. 2014): In this open-prospective trial, YBOCS-related symptoms remained unchanged or even worsened in 13 (45 %) patients, while they improved in 16 (55 %) patients, strongly suggesting a differential response of heterogeneous subgroups.

AMS, an SGA lacking $5HT_{2A}$ receptor affinity, was equally effective in schizophrenia samples suffering from comorbid OCS as in primary OCD: Kim et al. found most distinct anti-obsessive effects when the antipsychotic treatment regimen was switched from RISP (13 cases) or APZ (3 cases) to AMS (Kim et al. 2008). These favourable effects were corroborated by Schirmbeck et al. who assessed clinical and neurocognitive parameters (Schirmbeck et al. 2011) in schizophrenia patients stratified according to their mode of antipsychotic treatment in a longitudinal perspective (Schirmbeck et al. 2012, 2013).

Yet, there is no consensus whether an established antipsychotic treatment regimen should be modified in schizophrenia patients suffering from comorbid OCS: Despite the reported favourable effects of AMS (Kim et al. 2008, 2009), dose reductions of OLZ or the attempt of replacing it by APZ previously resulted in psychotic exacerbations (Kulkarni et al. 2012).

As summarized in Chap. 10, several SGAs bear the ris of inducing or aggravating OCS. This is particularly true for CLZ, which is why a switch in pharmacotherapy may be considered. While this appears to be the obvious choice at first glance, the following aspects urge caution in the light of limited evidence: (1) There is a substantial lack of reports on an improvement of OCS after switching from CLZ to other substances. This may be either due to publication biases of positive results or it may result from negative outcomes. (2) In the decision-making process of evaluating the pros and cons for or a particular antipsychotic agent, the management of the psychotic disorder itself should be given priority, whereas AEs in general or OCS in particular should be of subordinate importance. To date, CLZ is considered to be of superior antipsychotic efficacy (Gupta and Daniel 1995; Kelly et al. 2003; Leucht et al. 2012; McEvoy et al. 2006; Still et al. 1996; Tiihonen et al. 2009a) and remains the first-line antipsychotic in otherwise treatment-resistant schizophrenia.

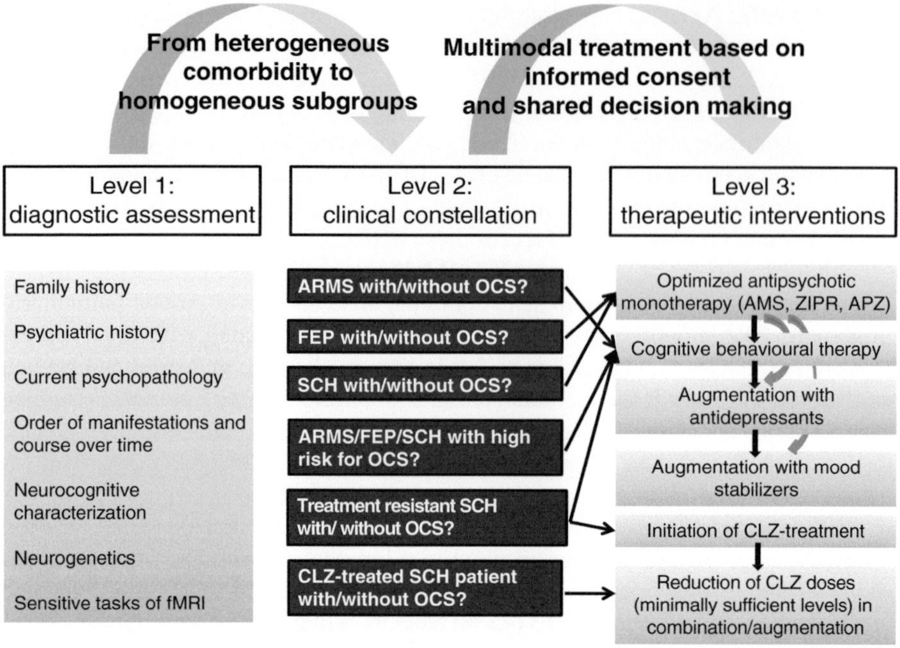

Fig. 11.1 Assessment and treatment of OCS in schizophrenia. Imminent or existing comorbidity with secondary OCS should be integrated into clinical management of all stages of schizophrenia, already beginning at the at-risk mental states (*ARMS*) for psychosis. Methods of level 1 (diagnostic assessment) may be helpful to differentiate between different clinical constellations and to define more or less homogeneous subgroups within the entire sample of patients with comorbid OCS (summarized at level 2). Therapeutic interventions (level 3) should fit each patient's individual needs and be based on informed consent and shared decision-making. Every patient within the schizophrenia spectrum should receive an optimized antipsychotic treatment and CBT. Treatment-resistant psychotic symptoms always require CLZ treatment. Imminent or prevalent comorbid OCS lead to further steps of intervention as the arrows suggest, but individual conditions might change the order of steps (*rounded headline arrows*). *Abbreviations*: *AMS* amisulpride, *APZ* aripiprazole, *ARMS* at-risk mental state, *FEP* first episode of psychosis, *fMRI* functional magnetic resonance imaging, *OCS* obsessive compulsive symptoms, *SCH* schizophrenia, *ZIPR* ziprasidone

Thus, optimizing the antipsychotic monotherapy by implementing agents with low antiserotonergic properties may be an important step in treating manifest or imminent OCS in schizophrenia. However, lacking evidence-based consensus guidelines, the focus should be laid on heightened awareness and early detection by means of psychometric screening and neurocognitive testing. Finally, the patient should be involved in the decision-making process so the individual therapy can be tailored to each patient's particular needs (see also Sect. 11.3.4 and Fig. 11.1).

11.2.2 Cognitive Behavioural Therapy

Aside from efforts to optimize the antipsychotic monotherapy, cognitive behavioural therapy (CBT) should be considered as a core approach in the management of OCS in schizophrenia. With remarkably high effect sizes (Gava et al. 2007; CBT including exposure and response prevention (ERP) is the gold standard for treating primary OCD, with remarkably high effect sizes (Gava et al. 2007; Koran et al. 2007; Kuelz and Voderholzer 2011; Rosa-Akcazar et al. 2008). Based on these results and preliminary evidence from studies evaluating the effectiveness of CBT in comorbid schizophrenia patients it seems to be the appropriate treatment of first choice for some cases (for more details, see Chap. 12).

11.2.3 Polypharmacy

In the case of insufficient response to optimized monotherapy and/or CBT, polypharmacy may be considered as a last-resort option. Both augmentation and combination strategies adding additional psychotropic substances to the basic treatment regimen may be applied.

11.2.3.1 Augmentation Strategies

Antidepressive Substances

The observed responsivity of primary OCD to serotonergic antidepressants largely contributed to the serotonin hypothesis of OCD (Bandelow et al. 2008; Barr et al. 1992; Linden 2006; Nakao et al. 2005; Saxena et al. 1999, 2009). In consequence, SSRIs and SNRIs (serotonin and noradrenaline reuptake inhibitor) have become an integral part of international treatment guidelines for OCD (Koran et al. 2007; Kordon et al. 2011). Based on the assumption of a pathophysiological overlap between primary OCD and secondary comorbid OCS observed in other psychiatric conditions, it seems plausible to modulate the serotonergic neurotransmission in order to attain symptom relief. The cumulative evidence for this approach (Hwang et al. 2009) within schizophrenia-spectrum disorders over the past decades is summarized in Table 11.1. Overall, augmentation strategies with antidepressants have been evaluated in $N=132$ patients with schizophrenia and co-occurring OCS. However, the comparability is restricted by methodological reasons: While there are numerous single and multiple case reports, some trials also employed active (Reznik and Sirota 2000b; Sayeed Khan et al. 2004) or placebo (Berman et al. 1995) controlled conditions. In a three-armed trial, adding anti-obsessive antidepressants to FGA treatment was superior to the treatment with FGAs or SGAs alone (Sayeed Khan et al. 2004). In detail, the tricyclic antidepressant clomipramine (Bark and Lindenmayer 1992; Berman et al. 1995; Kurokawa and Tanino 1997; Margetic et al. 2008; Poyurovsky and Weizman 1998; Zohar et al. 1993) and the following SSRIs have been examined: fluvoxamine (Gahr et al. 2014; Poyurovsky et al. 1999; Reznik and Sirota 2000a, b), sertraline (Hoehns et al. 2001; Poyurovsky et al. 2003), escitalopram (Stryjer et al. 2012) and fluoxetine (Kulkarni et al. 2012). Recently, beneficial effects of the SNRI milnacipran were reported (Hung and Hung 2014). The results of these trials were not entirely homogeneous but showed some overall positive tendencies despite the possibility of a publication bias. Several descriptive observations (de Haan et al. 1999) are also considered.

Adding antidepressants in bipolar disorder (BD) (see also Sect. 11.2.3.2) bears the risk of inducing manic switches. In contrast, the risk of aggravating the primary

Table 11.1 Polypharmacy for OCS in schizophrenia: augmentation with antidepressants

Augmentation	Reference	Diagnosis/patient or sample characteristics	Procedures	Main findings/conclusions
Clomipramine	Bark and Lindenmayer (1992)	1 SCH	Case report	No effect on OCS
	Zohar et al. (1993)	3 SCH 2 SAD	3 patients: off-on-off design 2 patients: off-on-off-on design	Improvement of OCS, psychotic exacerbation ($n = 1$)
	Kurokawa and Tanino (1997)	2 male SCH	Case report (augmentation of haloperidol with clomipramine 30 or 75 mg/die)	Improvements of YBOCS from 16 to 8 and 20 to 9, respectively, in parallel with reduced BPRS
	Poyurovsky and Weizman (1998)	1 SCH	Case report, intravenous application of clomipramine	Improvement of OCS
	Berman et al. (1995)	6 SCH with OCS	Double-blind, randomized cross-over design with placebo	Significantly more improvement of PANSS and YBOCS scores during clomipramine treatment
	Margetic et al. (2008)	1 SCH	Add-on of clomipramine to fluphenazine, levomepromazine and clozapine	Psychotic exacerbation

Fluvoxamine	Poyurovsky et al. (1999)	10 (5 males) SCH patients with YBOCS ≥7	Open-label add-on of 150 mg/die fluvoxamine to antipsychotic agents	Significant improvement of obsessions, but not compulsions
	Reznik and Sirota (2000a)	16 SCH	Open-label add-on of 100–200 mg/die fluvoxamine for 8 weeks	Significant improvement of psychotic symptoms (BPRS by −39.4 %) and OCS (Y-BOCS by −32.9 %) scores; no psychotic exacerbation, no relevant side effects
	Reznik and Sirota (2000b)	30 SCH (14: add-on of fluvoxamine, 16: no add-on)	RCT (8 weeks); add-on of 100–200 mg/die fluvoxamine to antipsychotic agents	Significant improvement of psychotic symptoms (PANSS: −34.3 %) and OCS (Y-BOCS: −29.4 %), no psychotic exacerbations, moderate decrease of CGI scores in both groups; mild and well-tolerated side effects
	Gahr et al. (2014)	1 SCH (female)	Case report, add-on of fluvoxamine to CLZ	Increase of CLZ serum levels via inhibition of CYP 1A2 und 2C19, induction of OCS/need for regular therapeutic drug monitoring
Sertraline	Hoehns et al. (2001)	1 SCH (26-year-old male) without previous history of cardiovascular disease	Medication: CLZ 100 mg twice daily (started 4 y prior to his death), risperidone 3 mg twice daily, sertraline 200 mg once daily, atenolol 50 mg twice daily and lorazepam 0.5 mg four times daily	Sudden cardiac death because of acute cardiac arrhythmia. Autopsy and toxicology studies revealed single-vessel coronary artery disease and cardiomegaly suggestive of idiopathic cardiomyopathy. Sertraline and CLZ blood concentrations within the therapeutic range
	Poyurovsky et al. (2003)	2 SCH (son treated with OLZ 20 mg/die, father with OLZ 7.5 mg/die)	After insufficient response to SRI or SSRIs, sertraline was added with 150 mg/die	Improvement of OCS in both patients/OLZ and sertraline seem to be a well-tolerated combination

(continued)

Table 11.1 (continued)

Augmentation	Reference	Diagnosis/patient or sample characteristics	Procedures	Main findings/conclusions
Escitalopram	Stryjer et al. (2012)	15 SCH	Open-label add-on of escitalopram 20 mg/die for 12 weeks	Significant improvement in YBOCS total score (obsessions and compulsions), improvement in PANSS positive and negative scores with particular improvements of the anxiety, tension, depression and preoccupation subitems
Fluoxetine	Kulkarni et al. (2012)	1 female SCH with OLZ-induced OCS	Add-on of fluoxetine 60 mg/die	Improvement of OCS, psychotic symptoms stably remitted
Milnacipran	Hung and Hung (2014)	1 male SCH with comorbid OCS	Switch from 30 mg escitalopram to 150 mg milnacipran (augmented to 15 mg aripiprazole)	Stable improvement of OCS from YBOCS total score 24–13
Broad classification of anti-obsessive substances	Sayeed Khan et al. (2004)	39 SCH with comorbid OCD	Comparison of FGA plus 'anti-obsessional substances' versus FGA and SGA alone (comparison of three cohorts)	Better improvement of psychotic symptoms (PANSS) and OCS (Padua Inventory) during FGAs in combination with 'anti-obsessional drugs' compared with FGAs or SGAs alone

Abbreviations: *BPRS* brief psychiatric rating scale, *CGI-S* clinical global impression - severity scale, *CLZ* clozapine, *FGA* first-generation antipsychotics, *OCS* obsessive-compulsive symptoms, *OLZ* olanzapine, *PANSS* positive and negative syndrome scale, *RCT* randomized controlled trial, *SAD* schizoaffective disorder, *SCH* schizophrenia, *SGA* second-generation antipsychotics, *SRI* serotonin reuptake inhibitor, *SSRI* selective serotonin reuptake inhibitor, *YBOCS* Yale-Brown obsessive-compulsive scale psychotic symptoms in schizophrenia seems negligible: To date, there are only two publications reporting deteriorations of psychotic symptoms after the add-on of clomipramine (Margetic et al. 2008; Zohar et al. 1993). This is in line with the current perception that antidepressants and even pro-dopaminergic substances such as bupropion (Englisch et al. 2010a, b, 2013) may be applied for the treatment of NS in schizophrenia without jeopardizing the patients' mental state, given they are on stable antipsychotic treatment.

Specific non-psychiatric safety concerns that need to be considered: One patient died from sudden cardiac arrest during polypharmacy with CLZ, RISP, sertraline and lorazepam (Hoehns et al. 2001). Adding pro-serotonergic antidepressants for OCS in schizophrenia renders some additional issues: (1) Clomipramine extends the anticholinergic profile of agents such as CLZ or OLZ and therefore may increase the risk of cardiovascular AEs. (2) SSRIs such as fluoxetine or fluvoxamine bear the potential of marked pharmacokinetic interactions within the cytochrome P450 system. This may result in a rise of antipsychotic serum levels which, in turn, might increase the antiserotonergic effects of CLZ and OLZ in particular and thus aggravate OCS.

Except for milnacipran, for SNRIs such as venlafaxine, duloxetine or vortioxetine, no systematic evaluations have been performed to date. As these agents bear the additional potential of enhancing neurocognition while the risk of pharmacokinetic interactions appears to be low, it will be important to systematically assess these multimodal antidepressants in order to improve the pharmacological treatment of OCS in schizophrenia.

Mood Stabilizers

Mood stabilizers (MS) such as lithium, valproic acid, carbamazepine, lamotrigine and topiramate are the treatment of choice for bipolar disorder and were also effective in reducing OCS secondary to BD (Abdel-Ahad and Kazour 2013). As recently summarized, they have also been used in primary OCD, both as a monotherapy or as an augmentation of non-selective and selective SRIs. The underlying neurobiological mechanisms remain speculative; however, they reach far beyond the serotonergic system. Lamotrigine, for instance, exerts its effects by modulating the glutamatergic neurotransmission (Poyurovsky et al. 2010).

Within the schizophrenia spectrum, the available data on MS is less conclusive (Citrome 2009; Tiihonen et al. 2009b; Zink et al. 2010): Recent meta-analyses on lithium (Leucht et al. 2007), valproic acid (Schwarz et al. 2008), carbamazepine (Leucht et al. 2014) and lamotrigine (Tiihonen et al. 2009b) were unable to confirm their therapeutic effects in schizophrenia. While they may be suited to treat specific conditions such as agitation, aggression or tardive dyskinesia, they are generally considered an off-label treatment for psychotic disorders. Further research is required in order to define their therapeutic effects in schizophrenia on a syndromal level which might also embrace comorbid OCS.

While there are no reports on pregabalin, lithium, topiramate and carbamazepine, descriptions of a small number of patients ($N=18$) with low level of evidence suggest a relief of OCS in schizophrenia when SGAs are augmented with valproic acid (Aukst-Margetic et al. 2011; Bisol and Lara 2009; Canas et al. 2012; Suppes and Rush 1996; Zink et al. 2007) or lamotrigine (Poyurovsky et al. 2010; Rodriguez et al. 2010) (see Table 11.2). In addition to the small number of published cases, their narrative design and a putative publication bias pose further limitations. To date, no controlled trials have been performed to evaluate the efficacy and tolerability of augmentation strategies with mood stabilizers for comorbid OCS in schizophrenia. In addition to investigating changes in psychopathological features, further research should also focus on pharmacokinetic interactions as well as additive AEs which may arise from polypharmacy.

11.2.3.2 Combination Strategies

The combination of different antipsychotic agents aims at two major targets: (1) On a molecular level, combining substances with different modes of action can result in an amplification of both receptor profile and occupancy. This may facilitate a more complete response of hitherto treatment-resistant symptoms. (2) Instead of administering antipsychotic monotherapy in escalating doses and hence increasing the risk of substance-specific AEs, it may prove helpful to introduce a second agent. This strategy will help limit each substance's maintenance dose and will thus reduce the burden of non-additive, substance-specific AEs. While both strategies primarily aim at a relief of otherwise treatment-refractory psychotic symptoms, they may also prove helpful for the treatment of OCS in schizophrenia.

Clozapine Combined with Other Antipsychotics

While there have been recent efforts to implement CLZ therapy earlier in the course of schizophrenia (Leucht et al. 2012; Remington et al. 2013), it is still considered a substance of last resort when other treatment options fail. Thus, patients receiving CLZ are usually the most severely affected, and they also carry the highest risk of developing second-onset OCS (see Chap. 10).

CLZ-treated patients have been in the focus of extensive research, and the evidence for an optimized CLZ treatment employing means of polypharmacy has been summarized in several recent reviews (Kane 2011; Nielsen et al. 2011; Zink et al. 2010). While switching to other SGAs in monotherapy could not be corroborated in clinical trials, it has been shown that CLZ-treated patients with second-onset OCS may benefit from combination strategies with other SGAs (see also Sect. 11.2.1).

As CLZ is a substance with weak antidopaminergic but prominent antiserotonergic properties, it has been proposed to add agents with mainly dopaminergic modes of action in order to counteract pro-obsessive effects inherent to CLZ. In particular, there is some evidence supporting the add-on of APZ (Chang et al. 2008; Englisch et al. 2009; Englisch and Zink 2008; Eryilmaz et al. 2013; Glick et al. 2009; Peters and de Haan 2009; Rocha and Hara 2006; Villari et al. 2011; Zink et al. 2006) and ZIPR (Krause et al. 2013). Based on theoretical considerations, the combination with AMS might also be beneficial (Kim et al. 2008) (see Table 11.3). With respect to these substances, the highest level of evidence exists for APZ, where positive effects have been reported in a number of cases and in one RCT (Chang et al. 2008). However, in general and as previously mentioned (compare sections "Antidepressive substances" and "Mood stabilizers"), the number of cases is limited and may be subject to publication biases. Therefore, conclusions should be drawn with caution.

Table 11.2 Polypharmacy for OCS: augmentation with mood stabilizers

Augmentation with:	Reference	Patient or sample characteristics	Procedure	Main findings
Valproic acid	Suppes and Rush (1996)	27-year-old male SAD patient, CLZ-induced OCS; treatment resistant to sertraline 200 mg/die	Add-on of valproic acid; titration to trough serum levels ≥70 μg/L	Improvement of ritualistic and impulsive behaviour
	Zink et al. (2007)	32-year-old male SCH patient, CLZ-aggravated OCS resistant to CBT and SSRI treatment	Add-on of 1,300 mg valproic acid and reduction of CLZ	Improvement of OCS severity from YBOCS total score 24 (at treatment initiation) to 6 (after 20 weeks of treatment)
	Bisol and Lara (2009)	36-year-old female and 31-year-old male with bipolar disorder	Combination of lamotrigine 100 mg/die + valproic acid 500 mg/die (female), monotherapy with valproic acid 1,000 mg/die (male)	Improvement of OCS [YBOCS improved from 46 to 4 (female) and 23 to 4 (male)]
	Aukst-Margetic et al. (2011)	Male with bipolar disorder	Report on CLZ-induced suicidal obsessions due to increase of dosage from 150 to 300 mg	Improvement after change to CLZ (100 mg/die), quetiapine (600 mg/die) and sodium valproate (900 mg/die)
	Canas et al. (2012)	51-year-old male SCH patient, CLZ-induced OCS	Add-on of 1,000 mg valproic acid to 500 mg CLZ	Improvement of OCS
Lamotrigine	Poyurovsky et al. (2010)	5 SCH/6 SAD patients with YBOCS ≥16	Add-on of lamotrigine (200 mg/day) to antipsychotic agents	Improvement of OCS severity (decrease of YBOCS total score from 22.9 to 17.4), five responders (i.e. decrease in YBOCS scores by at least 35 %)
	Rodriguez et al. (2010)	19-year-old SCH patient, coincident psychotic symptoms and OCS, treatment with CLZ	Resistance to clomipramine, SSRI, dropout from CBT. Add-on of lamotrigine 200 mg/day to CLZ 300 mg/day	Remission of psychosis and improvement of OCS (YBOCS) by about 40 %

Abbreviations: *CBT* cognitive behavioural therapy, *CLZ* clozapine, *OCS* obsessive-compulsive symptoms, *PANSS* positive and negative syndrome scale, *SAD* schizoaffective disorder, *SCH* schizophrenia, *SSRI* selective serotonin reuptake inhibitor, *YBOCS* Yale-Brown obsessive-compulsive scale

Table 11.3 Polypharmacy for OCS in schizophrenia: combination strategies involving different antipsychotic agents

Combinations	Reference	Patient or sample characteristics	Procedure	Main findings
CLZ and APZ	Rocha and Hara (2006)	3 male SCH patients	Add-on of 15 mg APZ to CLZ	Improvement of OCS and dose reduction of CLZ
	Zink et al. (2006)	1 male SCH patient (30 y), treated with 500 mg CLZ	Add-on of 30 mg APZ	Decrease of YBOCS total score from 24 to 16, dose reduction of CLZ to 250 mg/die
	Glick et al. (2009)	7 (6 male) SCH patients with YBOCS ≥16	Add-on of APZ to pre-existing FGA or SGA treatment	Decrease of YBOCS total score by an average of 13 points
	Chang et al. (2008)	29 (22 male) SCH patients (RCT) in CLZ monotherapy	Add-on of 15.5 ± 7.1 mg APZ to 304.3 ± 104.8 CLZ	Decrease of YBOCS total scores from 14.5 to 12.0 points
	Englisch et al. (2009)	7 (6 male) SCH patients	Add-on of 22.9 mg APZ to CLZ	Decrease of YBOCS total scores from 18.7 to 12.4, overall CLZ dose reduction by 19.6 %
	Peters and de Haan (2009)	1 male SCH patient	Add-on of CLZ to APZ	Remission of psychotic symptoms and improvement of OCS
	Villari et al. (2011)	2 male SCH patients	Add-on of APZ to CLZ	Improvement of OCS
	Eryilmaz et al. (2013)	4 SCH with CLZ-associated OCS	Add-on of APZ	Improvement of OCS
CLZ and ZIPR	Krause et al. (2013)	5 SCH (1 female, 44 y/4 males, 27–33 y)	Add-on of a mean dosage of 240 mg/die ZIPR to stable monotherapy with QTP up to 800 mg, clozapine up to 425 mg or flupentixol 15 mg	Improvement of OCS without marked side effects, no abnormal QTc prolongation
OLZ and APZ	Schönfelder et al. (2011)	1 female SCH patient (58 y)	Add-on of 20 mg APZ to OLZ	Improvement of OCS

Abbreviations: *APZ* aripiprazole, *CLZ* clozapine, *FGA* first-generation antipsychotics, *OCS* obsessive-compulsive symptoms, *OLZ* olanzapine, *PANSS* positive and negative syndrome scale, *QTP* quetiapine, *RCT* randomized controlled trial, *SCH* schizophrenia, *SGA* second-generation antipsychotics, *y* years, *YBOCS* Yale-Brown obsessive-compulsive scale, *ZIPR* ziprasidone

While the above-mentioned combination strategies primarily aim to provide a basis for reducing CLZ doses, an improvement of OCS was also observed during constant CLZ doses and co-medication with APZ (Chang et al. 2008). This might be explained by an amplification of the receptor profile within the dopaminergic spectrum and a relative decrease of 5HT receptor blockade. In addition, partial agonistic effects of SGAs such as ZIPR or APZ at monoaminergic receptors constitute another relevant molecular mechanism in the treatment of secondary-onset OCS. APZ (Sparshatt et al. 2010), a partial agonist at dopaminergic D2 receptors, also exerts partial agonistic effects at $5HT_{1A}$ receptors (Bruins Slot et al. 2005; Lopez-Gil et al. 2009, 2010; Nagai et al. 2009) and thereby modulates glutamatergic neurotransmission as could be shown in various animal models (Bontron and Steimle 1997; Cosi et al. 2005; Hollister et al. 1997; Leite et al. 2008; Nagai et al. 2009; Nordquist et al. 2008; Varmeh-Ziaie and Wimann 1997). Interactions between antipsychotic agents and glutamatergic neurotransmission have been summarized in a recent review (Zink et al. 2014b). Accordingly, the serotonergic $5HT_{1A}$ receptor subtype is predominantly expressed on inhibitory GABAergic interneurons (de Almeida and Mengod 2008), and the stimulation of $5HT_{1A}$ receptors results in both reduced discharge rates of GABAergic interneurons and increased pyramidal firing (Llado-Pelfort et al. 2012). In parallel to antagonists at $5HT_6$ and $5HT_7$ receptors (Meltzer and Massey 2011), these findings suggest pro-cognitive downstream effects exerted by partial dopamine and serotonin agonists, which may be additionally helpful in the treatment of comorbid OCS.

Further SGA Combinations

In analogy to CLZ treatment where combination strategies allowed for dose reductions and consequently resulted in an alleviation of comorbid OCS (Englisch et al. 2009; Rocha and Hara 2006; Villari et al. 2011; Zink et al. 2006), similar approaches appear reasonable for other serotonergic SGAs such as QTP or OLZ (Schönfelder et al. 2011) (see Table 11.3). Again, the level of evidence is insufficient and substantiates the need for further research. In particular, forthcoming studies should separately address the effectiveness of treatment strategies for different clinical constellation of imminent, emerging or manifest OCS.

11.3 Open Questions and Further Research

Based on the current evidence, some preliminary treatment guidelines for OCS in schizophrenia can be outlined (see Sect. 11.3.3).

11.3.1 Differential Modes of Treatment for Heterogeneous Subgroups?

OCS in schizophrenia is caused by a broad variety of interacting factors such as genetic disposition, psychosocial stressors and pharmacological effects (Schirmbeck and Zink 2013; Zink 2014a). According to the clinical manifestation and the course of symptoms over time, heterogeneous subgroups can be defined. It can be assumed that distinct subgroups respond differently to therapeutic interventions, and it seems plausible to involve different treatment strategies depending on the putative cause of second-onset OCS. To date, however, no interventional trial has ever employed a consequent stratification of comorbid OCS patients into homogeneous subgroups, leaving it entirely unanswered whether specific groups of patients benefit from distinct treatment interventions. Up to now, only patients with SGA-induced OCS have received clearly defined modes of treatment (i.e. add-on strategies with APZ (Chang et al. 2008; Englisch et al. 2009)), yet studies lack control conditions. Other interventions such as CBT (Tundo et al. 2012) or randomization to add-on treatment with clomipramine or fluvoxamine (Berman et al. 1995; Reznik and Sirota 2000b) were applied within comorbid OCS cohorts irrespective of the underlying aetiology. Thus, further research will have to disentangle which mode of treatment is the most suitable for the different subtypes of OCS in schizophrenia.

11.3.2 Polypharmacy or Stepwise Escalation?

As pointed out previously, there is a considerable lack of evidence regarding the treatment of comorbid OCS in schizophrenia. While different strategies have been applied, no standards have been determined which would permit for an evidence-based escalation of treatment options. In the face of treatment-refractory symptoms, clinicians often choose polypragmatic approaches, with polypharmacy being their most frequent choice. In contrast, CBT including ERP is largely underrepresented in the naturalistic course of schizophrenia treatment. It remains unclear to which extent polypharmacy and CBT approaches prove to be beneficial in schizophrenia patients with OCS, and it must be elucidated whether there is a certain threshold during the development of secondary OCS when the implementation of both pharmacological and non-pharmacological interventions might be useful. In addition and quite in analogy to stepwise plans within other fields of medicine, an algorithm should be defined that clearly elaborates in which way the pharmacological regimen should be escalated. To achieve this, further well-designed clinical trials are mandatory.

11.3.3 Switching Between SGAs?

Optimizing the antipsychotic regimen pursuing monotherapeutic approaches should constitute the basis for the treatment of OCS in schizophrenia. However, as summarized in Sect. 11.2.1, evidence for switching strategies is limited. Largely based on theoretical considerations and lacking appropriate head-to-head trials, SGAs with low antiserotonergic properties such as ZIPR, AMS or APZ should be implemented as first-line treatment for the prevention or alleviation of comorbid OCS in schizophrenia. Attempts to switch from CLZ to another SGA in order to improve second-onset OCS lack any empirical basis and cannot be recommended. This is particularly true as CLZ has proven superior to other antipsychotic agents for the maintenance treatment of schizophrenia in numerous trials and meta-analyses (Gupta and Daniel 1995; Joober and Boksa 2010; Kane et al. 1988; Kane 2011; Kang and Simpson 2010; Kelly et al. 2003; McEvoy et al. 2006; Meltzer 2012; Still et al. 1996; Tiihonen et al. 2009a). Weighing risks and benefits of distinct treatment strategies, the alleviation of psychotic symptoms (positive, negative as well as cognitive dimensions) must remain of paramount importance for the management of schizophrenia.

11.3.4 Consequences for Treatment Guidelines of Comorbid OCS in Schizophrenia?

Recommendations made in this chapter were derived from the data currently available, which - however - did not embrace multimodal characterizations or account for the heterogeneity of clinical subgroups (Hwang et al. 2009; Poyurovsky 2013). Implementing these dimensions in an integrative model (Fig. 11.1), we suggest that schizophrenia patients in all stages of illness will benefit from careful psychometric and neurocognitive evaluation of OCS (level 1). Individual results from such characterizations will help to define risk factors as well as pathogenic and clinical constellations on a descriptive level. This could result in an attribution of comorbid patients to more or less homogeneous subgroups (level 2). Based on these findings, a set of therapeutic interventions could be tailored to the patient's need in a process of informed consent and shared decision-making (level 3). Generally, every patient within the schizophrenia spectrum should receive an optimized antipsychotic treatment and have access to CBT. Imminent or prevalent comorbid OCS then require further decisions on adequate interventions (PLURAL). In the case of treatment failure, an escalation of steps is recommended. First steps should include adapted CBT approaches for comorbid OCS (see Chap. 12) and/or augmentation with antidepressants. Augmentation with mood stabilizers should remain an option of second line because of lower levels of evidence. As a final step, combination with 'anti-obsessive' SGAs (APZ, ZIPR, AMS) is suggested. Noteworthy, the order of steps should be a matter of individual discussion.

Irrespective of comorbid OCS, treatment-resistant psychotic symptoms always warrant the initiation of CLZ treatment. Because of its pro-obsessive properties, CLZ should be titrated to minimal sufficient maintenance doses. This can be achieved by combination with other SGAs or, as a second-line option, with mood stabilizers. While these suggestions may be helpful in order to define future treatment guidelines for OCS in schizophrenia, we strengthen that further research is essential to elucidate pathogenic mechanisms, evaluate treatment options and substantiate proposed pathways.

11.4 Conclusions and Further Perspectives

OCS in schizophrenia may be caused by numerous factors, and their clinical presentation is quite as diverse as their pathogenesis. To date, the gene-environment interaction is only incompletely understood, and a more profound understanding of the aetiology of OCS in schizophrenia will be helpful for an individualized risk assessment as well as for the development of early recognition and monitoring instruments. In addition to descriptive psychopathology, basic research should focus on defining mechanisms and molecular targets for innovative pharmacological interventions. Moreover, further clinical trials will have to deliver evidence for CBT interventions including ERP as well as pharmacological combination and augmentation strategies before guidelines for the treatment of OCS in schizophrenia can be provided.

Conflicts of Interest *S.E.* received travel research grants Lundbeck and Servier Pharmaceuticals. *M. Z.* received unrestricted scientific grants of the European Research Advisory Board (ERAB), German Research Foundation (DFG), Pfizer Pharma GmbH, Servier and Bristol Myers Squibb Pharmaceuticals; further speaker and travel grants were provided from Astra Zeneca, Lilly, Pfizer Pharma GmbH, Bristol Myers Squibb Pharmaceuticals, Roche, Servier, Otsuka, Janssen Cilag and Trommsdorff.

References

Abdel-Ahad P, Kazour F (2013) Non-antidepressant pharmacological treatment of obsessive compulsive disorder: a comprehensive review. Curr Clin Pharmacol

Aukst-Margetic B, Margetic B, Marsanic VB (2011) Suicidal obsessions as dose dependent side-effect of clozapine. Psychopharmacol Bull 44:65–69

Baandrup L, Gasse C, Jensen VD, Glenthoj BY, Nordentoft M, Lublin H, Fink-Jensen A, Lindhardt A, Mortensen PB (2010) Antipsychotic polypharmacy and risk of death from natural causes in patients with schizophrenia: a population-based nested case-control study. J Clin Psychiatry 71:103–108

Bandelow B, Zohar J, Hollander E, Kasper S, Möller HJ; WFSBP Task Force on Treatment Guidelines for Anxiety, Obsessive-Compulsive and Post-Traumatic Stress Disoders, Zohar J, Hollander E, Kasper S, Möller HJ, Bandelow B, Allgulander C, Ayuso-Gutierrez J, Baldwin DS, Buenvicius R, Cassano G, Fineberg N, Gabriels L, Hindmarch I, Kaiya H, Klein DF, Lader M, Lecrubier Y, Lépine JP, Liebowitz MR, Lopez-Ibor JJ, Marazziti D, Miguel EC, Oh KS, Preter M, Rupprecht R, Sato M, Starcevic V, Stein DJ, van Ameringen M, Vega J (2008) World Federation of Societies of Biological Psychiatry (WFSBP) guidelines for the pharmacological treatment of anxiety, obsessive-compulsive and post-traumatic stress disorders - first revision. World J Biol Psychiatry 9:248–312

Bark N, Lindenmayer JP (1992) Ineffectiveness of clomipramine for obsessive-compulsive symptoms in a patient with schizophrenia. Am J Psychiatry 149:136–137

Barr LC, Goodman WK, Price LH, McDougle CJ, Charney DS (1992) The serotonin hypothesis of obsessive compulsive disorder: implications of pharmacologic challenge studies. J Clin Psychiatry 53(Suppl):17–28

Berman I, Sapers BL, Chang HH, Losonczy MF, Schmildler J, Green AI (1995) Treatment of obsessive-compulsive symptoms in schizophrenic patients with clomipramine. J Clin Psychopharmacol 15:206–210

Bisol LW, Lara DR (2009) Improvement of obsessive-compulsive disorder with divalproex and lamotrigine in two patients with bipolar II disorder. Pharmacopsychiatry 42:37–39

Bloch MH, Landeros-Weisenberger A, Kelmendi B, Coric V, Bracken MB, Leckman JF (2006) A systematic review: antipsychotic augmentation with treatment refractory obsessive-compulsive disorder. Mol Psychiatry 11:622–632

Bontron S, Steimle V (1997) Efficient repression of endogenous major histocompatibility complex class II expression through dominant negative CIITA mutants isolated by a functional selection strategy. Mol Cell Biol 17:4249–4258

Bruins Slot LA, Kleven MS, Newman-Tancredi A (2005) Effects of novel antipsychotics with mixed D(2) antagonist/5-HT(1A) agonist properties on PCP-induced social interaction deficits in the rat. Neuropharmacology 49:996–1006

Canas F, Aydinoglu U, Sinani G (2012) Valproic acid augmentation in clozapine-associated hand-washing compulsion. Psychiatry Clin Neurosci 66:463–464

Centorrino F, Ventriglio A, Vincenti A, Talamo A, Baldessarini RJ (2010) Changes in medication practices for hospitalized psychiatric patients: 2009 versus 2004. Hum Psychopharmacol 25:179–186

Chang JS, Ahn Y-M, Park HJ, Lee KY, Kim SH, Kang UG, Kim JS (2008) Aripiprazole augmentation in clozapine-treated patients with refractory schizophrenia: an 8-week, randomized, double-blind, placebo-controlled trial. J Clin Psychiatry 69:720–731

Citrome L (2009) Adjunctive lithium and anticonvulsants for the treatment of schizophrenia: what is the evidence? Expert Rev Neurother 9:55–71

Connor KM, Payne VM, Gadde KM, Zhang W, Davidson JR (2005) The use of aripiprazole in obsessive-compulsive disorder: preliminary observations in 8 patients. J Clin Psychiatry 66:49–51

Correll CU (2012) Assessing and maximizing the safety and tolerability of antipsychotics used in the treatment of children and adolescent. J Clin Psychiatry 69:26–36

Cosi C, Waget A, Rollet K, Tesori V, Newman-Tancredi A (2005) Clozapine, ziprasidone and aripiprazole but not haloperidol protect against kainic acid-induced lesion of the striatum in mice, in vivo: role of 5-HT1A receptor activation. Brain Res 1043:32–41

Coward DM (1992) General pharmacology of clozapine. Br J Psychiatry 17;5–11

de Almeida J, Mengod G (2008) Serotonin 1A receptors in human and monkey prefrontal cortex are mainly expressed in pyramidal neurons and in a GABAergic interneuron subpopulation: implications for schizophrenia and its treatment. J Neurochem 107:488–496

de Haan L, Linszen DH, Gorsira R (1999) Clozapine and obsessions in patients with recent-onset schizophrenia and other psychotic disorders. J Clin Psychiatry 60:364–365

Dold M, Aigner M, Lanzenberger R, Kasper S (2011) Efficacy of antipsychotic augmentation therapy in treatment-resistant obsessive-compulsive disorder – a meta-analysis of double-blind, randomised, placebo-controlled trials. Fortschr Neurol Psychiatr 79:453–466

Duggan L, Fenton M, Dardennes RM, El-Dosoky A, Indran S (2005) Olanzapine for schizophrenia. Cochrane Database Syst Rev (3):CD001359

Englisch S, Zink M (2008) Combined antipsychotic treatment involving clozapine and aripiprazole. Prog Neuropsychopharmacol Biol Psychiatry 32:1386–1392

Englisch S, Esslinger C, Inta D, Weinbrenner A, Peus V, Gutschalk A, Schirmbeck F, Zink M (2009) Clozapine-induced obsessive compulsive syndromes improve in combination with aripiprazole. Clin Neuropharmacol 32:227–229

Englisch S, Esser A, Inta D, Zink M (2010a) Bupropion for depression in schizophrenia. Clin Neuropharmacol 33:257–259

Englisch S, Esser A, Zink M (2010b) Bupropion for depression in schizophrenia: a case report. Pharmacopsychiatry 43:38–39

Englisch S, Morgen K, Meyer-Lindenberg A, Zink M (2013) Risks and benefits of bupropion treatment in schizophrenia: a systematic review of the current literature. Clin Neuropharmacol 36:203–215

Ersche KD, Cumming P, Craig KJ, Muller U, Fineberg NA, Bullmore ET, Robbins TW (2012) Amisulpride-induced acute akathisia in OCD: an example of dysfunctional dopamine-serotonin interactions? J Psychopharmacol 26:887–890
Eryilmaz G, Sayar GH, Ozten E, Gögcegöz I, Karamustafalioglu O (2013) Aripiprazole augmentation in clozapine-associated obsessive-compulsive symptoms in schizophrenia. Ann Gen Psychiatry 12:40
Fineberg NA, Gale TM, Sivakumaran T (2006) A review of antipsychotics in the treatment of obsessive compulsive disorder. J Psychopharmacol 20:97–103
Gahr M, Rehbaum K, Connemann BJ (2014) Clozapine-associated development of second-onset obsessive compulsive symptoms in schizophrenia: impact of clozapine serum levels and fluvoxamine add-on. Pharmacopsychiatry 47:118–120
Gallego JA, Bonetti J, Zhang J, Kane JM, Correll CU (2012a) Prevalence and correlates of antipsychotic polypharmacy: a systematic review and meta-regression of global and regional trends from the 1970s to 2009. Schizophr Res 138:18–28
Gallego JA, Nielsen J, de Hert M, Kane JM, Correll CU (2012b) Safety and tolerability of antipsychotic polypharmacy. Expert Opin Drug Saf 11:527–542
Gao K, Muzina D, Gajwani P, Calabrese JR (2006) Efficacy of typical and atypical antipsychotics for primary and comorbid anxiety symptoms or disorders: a review. J Clin Psychiatry 67:1327–1340
Gava I, Barbui C, Aguglia E, Carlino D, Churchill R, De Vanna M, McGuire, HF (2007) Psychological treatments versus treatment as usual for obsessive compulsive disorder (OCD). Cochrane Database Syst Rev (2):CD005333
Glick ID, Poyurovsky M, Ivanova O, Koran LM (2009) Aripiprazole in schizophrenia patients with comorbid obsessive-compulsive symptoms: an open-label study of 15 patients. J Clin Psychiatry 69:1856–1859
Grados MA, Specht MW, Sung HM, Fortune D (2013) Glutamate drugs and pharmacogenetics of OCD: a pathway-based exploratory approach. Expert Opin Drug Discov 8;1515–27. doi:10.1517/17460441.2013.845553
Gupta S, Daniel DG (1995) Cautions in the clozapine-to-risperidone switch. Ann Clin Psychiatry 7:149
Hoehns JD, Fouts MM, Kelly MW, Tu KB (2001) Sudden cardiac death with clozapine and sertraline combination. Ann Pharmacother 35:862–866
Hollister RD, Xia M, McNamara MJ, Hyman BT (1997) Neuronal expression of class II major histocompatibility complex (HLA-DR) in 2 cases of pick disease. Arch Neurol 54:243–248
Hung S, Hung GCL (2014) A rapid improvement in obsessive-compulsive disorder with milnacipran in a patient with schizophrenia. J Clin Psychopharmacol 34:653–654
Hwang MY, Kim SW, Yum SY, Opler LA (2009) Management of schizophrenia with obsessive-compulsive features. Psychiatr Clin North Am 32:835–851
Insel TR (2010) Rethinking schizophrenia. Nature 468:187–193
Joober R, Boksa P (2010) Clozapine: a distinct, poorly understood and under-used molecule. J Psychiatry Neurosci 35:147–149
Juven-Wetzler A, Fostick L, Cwikel-Hamzany S, Balaban E, Zohar J (2014) Treatment with Ziprasidone for schizophrenia patients with OCD. Eur Neuropsychopharmacol. doi:10.1016/j.euroneuro.2014.06.014
Kane JM (2011) A user's guide to clozapine. Acta Psychiatr Scand 123:407–408
Kane J, Honigfeld G, Singer J, Meltzer H (1988) Clozapine for the treatment-resistant schizophrenic. A double-blind comparison with chlorpromazine. Arch Gen Psychiatry 45:789–796
Kang X, Simpson GM (2010) Clozapine: more side effects but still the best antipsychotic. J Clin Psychiatry 71:982–983
Kelly DL, Richardson CM, Tamminga CA, Carpenter WT (2003) The efficacy of high-dose olanzapine versus clozapine in treatment-resistant schizophrenia: a double-blind, crossover study. J Clin Psychopharmacol 23:668–670

Kim SW, Shin IS, Kim JM, Yang SJ, Hwang MY, Yoon JS (2008) Amisulpride improves obsessive-compulsive symptoms in schizophrenia patients taking atypical antipsychotics: an open-label switch study. J Clin Psychopharmacol 28:349–352

Kim SW, Shin IS, Kim JM, Youn T, Yang SJ, Hwang MY, Yoon JS (2009) The 5-HT2 receptor profiles of antipsychotics in the pathogenesis of obsessive-compulsive symptoms in schizophrenia. Clin Neuropharmacol 32:224–226

Koran LM, Hanna GL, Hollander E, Nestadt G, Simpson HB, American Psychiatric Association (2007) Practice guideline for the treatment of patients with obsessive-compulsive disorder. Am J Psychiatry 164:5–53

Kordon A, Zurowski B, Wahl K, Hohagen F (2011) Evidence-based pharmacotherapy and other somatic treatment approaches for obsessive-compulsive disorder: state of the art. Nervenarzt 82:319–320

Krause DL, Matz J, Schennach R, Mueller N, Dehning S (2013) Ziprasidone for obsessive compulsive disorder in schizophrenia. Ther Adv Psychopharmacol 3:115–116

Kuelz AK, Voderholzer U (2011) Psychotherapie der Zwangsstörung. Nervenarzt 82:308–318

Kulkarni G, Narayanaswamy JC, Math SB (2012) Olanzapine induced *de-novo* obsessive compulsive disorder in a patient with schizophrenia. Indian J Pharmacol 44:649–650

Kurokawa K, Tanino R (1997) Effectiveness of clomipramine for obsessive-compulsive symptoms and chronic pain in two patients with schizophrenia. J Clin Psychopharmacol 17:329–330

Delle Chiaie R, Scarciglia P, Pasquini M, Caredda M, Biondi M (2011) Aripiprazole augmentation in patients with resistant obsessive compulsive disorder: a pilot study. Clin Pract Epidemiol Ment Health 7:107–111

Leite JV, Guimaraes FS, Moreira FA (2008) Aripiprazole, an atypical antipsychotic, prevents the motor hyperactivity induced by psychotomimetics and psychostimulants in mice. Eur J Pharmacol 578:222–227

Leucht S, Kissling W, McGrath J (2007) Lithium for schizophrenia. Cochrane Database Syst Rev (3):CD003834

Leucht S, Kissling W, McGrath J, White P (2014) Carbamazepine for schizophrenia. Cochrane Database Syst Rev (4):CD001258

Leucht S, Tardy M, Komossa K, Heres S, Kissling W, Salanti G, Davis JM (2012) Antipsychotic drugs versus placebo for relapse prevention in schizophrenia: a systematic review and meta-analysis. Lancet 379:2063–2071

Linden DE (2006) How psychotherapy changes the brain – the contribution of functional neuroimaging. Mol Psychiatry 11:528–538

Llado-Pelfort L, Santana N, Ghisi V, Artigas F, Celada P (2012) 5-HT1A receptor agonists enhance pyramidal cell firing in prefrontal cortex through a preferential action on GABA interneurons. Cereb Cortex 22:1487–1497

Lopez-Gil X, Artigas F, Adell A (2009) Role of different monoamine receptors controlling MK-801-induced release of serotonin and glutamate in the medial prefrontal cortex: relevance for antipsychotic action. Int J Neuropsychopharmacol 12:487–499

Lopez-Gil X, Artigas F, Adell A (2010) Unraveling monoamine receptors involved in the action of typical and atypical antipsychotics on glutamatergic and serotonergic transmission in prefrontal cortex. Curr Pharm Des 16:502–515

Margetic B, Aukst-Margetic B, Jakovljevic M (2008) Aggravation of schizophrenia by clomipramine in a patient with comorbid obsessive-compulsive disorder. Psychopharmacol Bull 41:9–11

McDougle CJ, Barr LC, Goodman WK, Pelton GH, Aronson SC, Anand A, Price LH (1995) Lack of efficacy of clozapine monotherapy in refractory obsessive-compulsive disorder. Am J Psychiatry 152:1812–1814

McEvoy JP, Lieberman JA, Stroup TS, Davis SM, Meltzer HY, Rosenheck RA, Swartz MS, Perkins DO, Keefe RS, Davis CE, Severe J, Hsiao JK, CATIE I, McEvoy JP, Lieberman JA, Stroup TS, Davis SM, Meltzer HY, Rosenheck RA, Swartz MS, Perkins DO, Keefe RSE, Davis CE, Severe J, Hsiao JK, CATIE Investigators (2006) Effectiveness of clozapine versus

olanzapine, quetiapine, and risperidone in patients with chronic schizophrenia who did not respond to prior atypical antipsychotic treatment. [see comment]. Am J Psychiatry 163:600–610
Meltzer HY (2012) Clozapine. Clin Schizophr Relat Psychoses 6:134–144
Meltzer HY, Huang M (2008) In vivo actions of atypical antipsychotic drug on serotonergic and dopaminergic systems. Prog Brain Res 172:177–197
Meltzer HY, Massey BW (2011) The role of serotonin receptors in the action of atypical antipsychotic drugs. Curr Opin Pharmacol 11:59–67
Metin O, Yazici K, Tot S, Yazici AE (2003) Amisulpiride augmentation in treatment resistant obsessive-compulsive disorder: an open trial. Hum Psychopharmacol 18:463–467
Muscatello MR, Bruno A, Pandolfo G, Mico U, Scimeca G, Romeo VM, Santoro V, Settineri S, Spina E, Zoccali RA (2011) Effect of aripiprazole augmentation of serotonin reuptake inhibitors or clomipramine in treatment-resistant obsessive-compulsive disorder: a double-blind, placebo-controlled study. J Clin Psychopharmacol 31:174–179
Nagai T, Murai R, Matsui K, Kamei H, Noda Y, Furukawa H, Nabeshima T (2009) Aripiprazole ameliorates phencyclidine-induced impairment of recognition memory through dopamine D1 and serotonin 5-HT1A receptors. Psychopharmacology (Berl) 202:315–328
Nakao T, Nakagawa A, Yoshiura T, Nakatani E, Nabeyama M, Yoshizato C, Kudoh A, Tada K, Yoshioka K, Kawamoto M, Togao O, Kanba S (2005) Brain activation of patients with obsessive- compulsive disorder during neuropsychological and symptom provocation tasks before and after symptom improvement: a functional magnetic resonance imaging study. Biol Psychiatry 57:901–910
Nielsen J, Damkier P, Lublin H, Taylor D (2011) Optimizing clozapine treatment. Acta Psychiatr Scand 123:411–422
Nordquist RE, Risterucci C, Moreau JL, von Kienlin M, Kunnecke B, Maco M, Freichel C, Riemer C, Spooren W (2008) Effects of aripiprazole/OPC-14597 on motor activity, pharmacological models of psychosis, and brain activity in rats. Neuropharmacology 54:405–416
Peters B, de Haan L (2009) Remission of schizophrenia psychosis and strong reduction of obsessive-compulsive disorder after adding clozapine to aripiprazole. Prog Neuro-psychopharmacol Biol Psychiatry 33:1576–1577
Pickar D, Vinik J, Bartko JJ (2008) Pharmacotherapy of schizophrenic patients: preponderance of off-label drug use. PLoS One 3:e3150
Pogarell O, Hamann C, Poepperl G, Juckel G, Chouker M, Zaudig M, Riedel M, Moeller HJ, Hegerl U, Tatsch K (2003) Elevated brain serotonin transporter availability in patients with obsessive-compulsive disorder. Biol Psychiatry 54:1406–1413
Poyurovsky M (2013) Schizo-obsessive disorder. Cambridge University Press, New York, pp 1–245
Poyurovsky M, Weizman A (1998) Intravenous clomipramine for a schizophrenic patient with obsessive-compulsive symptoms. Am J Psychiatry 155:993
Poyurovsky M, Isakov V, Hromnikov S, Modai I, Rauchberger B, Schneidman M, Weizman A (1999) Fluvoxamine treatment of obsessive-compulsive symptoms in schizophrenic patients: an add-on open study. Int Clin Psychopharmacol 14:95–100
Poyurovsky M, Kurs R, Weizman A (2003) Olanzapine-sertraline combination in schizophrenia with obsessive-compulsive disorder. J Clin Psychiatry 64:611
Poyurovsky M, Glick I, Koran LM (2010) Lamotrigine augmentation in schizophrenia and schizoaffective patients with obsessive-compulsive symptoms. J Psychopharmacol 24:861–866
Remington G, Agid O, Foussias G, Hahn M, Rao N, Sinyor M (2013) Clozapine's role in the treatment of first-episode schizophrenia. Am J Psychiatry 170:146–151
Reznik I, Sirota P (2000a) An open study of fluvoxamine augmentation of neuroleptics in schizophrenia with obsessive and compulsive symptoms. Clin Neuropharmacol 23:157–160
Reznik IM, Sirota PMMP (2000b) Obsessive and compulsive symptoms in schizophrenia: a randomized controlled trial with fluvoxamine and neuroleptics. J Clin Psychopharmacol 20:410–416

Rocha FL, Hara C (2006) Benefits of combining aripiprazole to clozapine: three case reports. Prog Neuropsychopharmacol Biol Psychiatry 30:1167–1169

Rodriguez CI, Corcoran C, Simpson HB (2010) Diagnosis and treatment of a patient with both psychotic and obsessive-compulsive symptoms. Am J Psychiatry 167:754–761

Rosa-Alcazar AI, Sanchez-Meca J, Gomez-Conesa A, Marin-Martinez F (2008) Psychological treatment of obsessive-compulsive disorder: a meta-analysis. Clin Psychol Rev 28:1310–1325

Savas HA, Yumru M, Ozen ME (2008) Quetiapine and ziprasidone as adjuncts in treatment-resistant obsessive-compulsive disorder: a retrospective comparative study. Clin Drug Investig 28:439–442

Saxena S, Brody AL, Maidment KM, Dunkin JJ, Colgan M, Alborzian S, Phelps ME, Baxter LRJ (1999) Localized orbitofrontal and subcortical metabolic changes and predictors of response to paroxetine treatment in obsessive-compulsive disorder. Neuropsychopharmacology 21:683–693

Saxena S, Gorbis E, O'Neill J, Baker SK, Mandelkern MA, Maidment KM, Chang S, Salamon N, Brody AL, Sschwartz JM, London ED (2009) Rapid effects of brief intensive cognitive-behavioral therapy on brain glucose metabolism in obsessive-compulsive disorder. Mol Psychiatry 14:197

Saxena S, Wang D, Bystritsky A, Baxter LR (2014) Risperidone augmentation of SRI treatment for refractory obsessive-compulsive disorder. J Clin Psychiatry 57:303–306

Sayeed Khan MN, Arshad N, Ullah N (2004) Treatment outcome of schizophrenia co-morbid with obsessive-compulsive disorder. J Coll Physicians Surg Pak 14:234–236

Schirmbeck F, Zink M (2013) Comorbid obsessive-compulsive symptoms in schizophrenia: contributions of pharmacological and genetic factors. Front Neuropharmacol. doi:10.3389/fphar.2013.00099

Schirmbeck F, Esslinger C, Rausch F, Englisch S, Meyer-Lindenberg A, Zink M (2011) Antiserotonergic antipsychotics are associated with obsessive-compulsive symptoms in schizophrenia. Psychol Med 41:2361–2374

Schirmbeck F, Rausch F, Englisch S, Eifler S, Esslinger C, Meyer-Lindenberg A, Zink M (2012) Stable cognitive deficits in schizophrenia patients with comorbid obsessive-compulsive symptoms: a 12 months longitudinal study. Schizophr Bull. doi:10.1093/schbul/sbs123

Schirmbeck F, Rausch F, Englisch S, Eifler S, Esslinger C, Meyer-Lindenberg A, Zink M (2013) Differential effects of antipsychotic agents on obsessive-compulsive symptoms in schizophrenia: a longitudinal study. J Psychopharmacol 27:349–357

Schirmbeck F, Mier D, Esslinger C, Rausch F, Englisch S, Eifler S, Meyer-Lindenberg A, Kirsch P, Zink M (2014) Increased orbitofrontal cortex activation during treatment with pro-obsessive antipsychotic drugs. J Psychiatry Neurosci. 39(5);140021 [Epub ahead of print]

Schönfelder S, Schirmbeck F, Waltereit R, Englisch S, Zink M (2011) Aripiprazole improves olanzapine-associated obsessive compulsive symptoms in schizophrenia. Clin Neuropharmacol 34:256–257

Schwarz C, Volz A, Li C, Leucht S (2008) Valproate for schizophrenia. Cochrane Database Syst Rev (3):CD004028

Sparshatt A, Taylor D, Patel MX, Kapur S (2010) A systematic review of aripiprazole–dose, plasma concentration, receptor occupancy, and response: implications for therapeutic drug monitoring. J Clin Psychiatry 71:1447–1456

Still DJ, Dorson PG, Crismon ML, Pousson C (1996) Effects of switching inpatients with treatment-resistant schizophrenia from clozapine to risperidone. Psychiatr Serv 47:1382–1384

Stryjer R, Dambinsky Y, Timinsky I, Green T, Kotler M, Weizman A, Spivak B (2012) Escitalopram in the treatment of patients with schizophrenia and obsessive-compulsive disorder: an open-label, prospective study. [Article]. Int Clin Psychopharmacol. doi:10.1097/YIC.0b013e32835bd24e

Suppes T, Rush AJ (1996) Medication optimization during clozapine treatment. J Clin Psychiatry 57:307–308

Tiihonen J, Lonnqvist J, Wahlbeck K, Klaukka T, Niskanen L, Tanskanen A, Haukka J (2009a) 11-year follow-up of mortality in patients with schizophrenia: a population-based cohort study (FIN11 study). [see comment]. Lancet 374:620–627
Tiihonen J, Wahlbeck K, Kiviniemi V (2009b) The efficacy of lamotrigine in clozapine-resistant schizophrenia: a systematic review and meta-analysis. Schizophr Res 109:10–14
Tundo A, Salvati L, Di Spigno D, Cieri L, Parena A, Necci R, Sciortino S (2012) Cognitive-behavioral therapy for obsessive-compulsive disorder as a comorbidity with schizophrenia or schizoaffective disorder. Psychother Psychosom 81:58–60
Van der Wee NJ, Stevens H, Hardeman JA, Mandl RC, Denys DA, van Megen HJ, Kahn RS, Westenberg HM (2004) Enhanced dopamine transporter density in psychotropic-naive patients with obsessive-compulsive disorder shown by [123I]{beta}-CIT SPECT. Am J Psychiatry 161:2201–2206
Varmeh-Ziaie S, Wimann KG (1997) Wig-1, a new p53-induced gene encoding a zinc finger protein. Oncogene 15:2699–2704
Villari V, Frieri T, Fagiolini A (2011) Aripiprazole augmentation in clozapine-associated obsessive-compulsive symptoms. J Clin Psychopharmacol 31:375–376
Weinmann S, Read J, Aderhold V (2009) Influence of antipsychotics on mortality in schizophrenia: systematic review. Schizophr Res 113:1–11
Yang KC, Su TP, Chou YH (2008) Effectiveness of aripiprazole in treating obsessive compulsive symptoms. Prog Neuropsychopharmacol Biol Psychiatry 32:585–586
Zink M (2014a) Comorbid obsessive-compulsive symptoms in schizophrenia: insight into pathomechanisms facilitates treatment. Adv Med 2014(2):1–18
Zink M, Knopf U, Kuwilsky A (2006) Management of clozapine-induced obsessive compulsive symptoms in a man with schizophrenia. Aust N Z J Psychiatry 41:293–294
Zink M, Englisch S, Knopf U, Kuwilsky A, Dressing H (2007) Augmentation of clozapine with valproic acid for clozapine-induced obsessive compulsive symptoms. Pharmacopsychiatry 40:202–203
Zink M, Englisch S, Meyer-Lindenberg A (2010) Polypharmacy in schizophrenia. Curr Opin Psychiatry 23:103–111
Zink M, Englisch S, Schmitt A (2014b) Antipsychotic treatment modulates glutamate transport and NMDA receptor expression. Eur Arch Psychiatry Clin Neurosci 264(Suppl 1):S67–82
Zohar J, Kaplan Z, Benjamin J (1993) Clomipramine treatment of obsessive compulsive symptomatology in schizophrenic patients. J Clin Psychiatry 54:385–388

Cognitive Behavioural Therapy for Co-occurring Obsessive-Compulsive Symptoms

12

Frederike Schirmbeck and Antonio Tundo

12.1 Cognitive Behavioural Therapy for Primary OCD and Schizophrenia

Cognitive behavioural therapy (CBT) refers to a class of interventions that share the basic premise that maladaptive cognition and behaviour contribute to the development and maintenance of mental disorders (Beck and Rector 2005). Randomized clinical trials as well as naturalistic studies widely established that it is an effective treatment approach for a range of mental conditions, including severe psychiatric illnesses (Butler et al. 2006; Hofmann et al. 2012). The goals of CBT is very broad, ranging from specific symptom reduction and increased insight and understanding of illness to distress reduction and the development of adaptive coping skills (Elis et al. 2013).

12.1.1 CBT in the Treatment of Primary OCD

Several reviews and meta-analyses have been conducted to investigate the effectiveness of CBT in primary obsessive-compulsive disorder (OCD). Findings have shown large effect sizes for CBT compared to control groups (Gava et al. 2007; Rosa-Alcazar et al. 2008) and at least comparable efficacy compared to treatment with serotonin reuptake inhibitors (SRIs) (Romanelli et al. 2014). Follow-up studies

F. Schirmbeck, PhD (✉)
Department of Psychiatry, Academic Medical Centre, University of Amsterdam, Meibergdreef 5, Amsterdam 1105 AZ, The Netherlands
e-mail: n.f.schirmbeck@amc.nl

A. Tundo
Cognitive Behavioral Therapy, Direttore Istituto di Psicopatologia, Rome, Italy

L. De Haan et al. (eds.), *Obsessive-Compulsive Symptoms in Schizophrenia*, DOI 10.1007/978-3-319-12952-5_12 with catamnestic assessments indicate that beneficial effects of CBT last for several years (Rufer et al. 2005; van Oppen et al. 2005). CBT is also an effective adjunctive treatment for partial responders to SRI (approximately 40–50 % of treated sample) (Albert et al. 2012; Kampman et al. 2002; Tundo et al. 2007). In a recent randomized clinical trial, CBT augmentation for SRI-resistant OCD shows to be superior to augmentation with risperidone (Simpson et al. 2013).

The principal behavioural approaches, supported by excellent empirical results in randomized controlled trials, are exposure for obsessions and response prevention for rituals (ERP). Of the various modes of exposure, massive vs. graded approaches have not been compared so far, but empirical evidence shows higher effectiveness of the therapist-guided exposure when compared to the self-application of ERP (Rosa-Alcazar et al. 2008).

Based on this empirical support, several guidelines recommend CBT as a safe and effective first-line treatment for primary OCD (Franklin and Foa 2011; Koran et al. 2007). The German guidelines suggest that a disorder-specific CBT, including exposure and response management, should be offered as therapy of first choice. Monotherapy with drugs is indicated only if CBT is rejected, cannot be performed because of the severity of symptoms or is not available due to lack of resources or long waiting times (Kordon et al. 2013).

12.1.2 CBT in the Treatment of Schizophrenia

Antipsychotic medication is the first-line treatment for schizophrenia to reduce psychotic symptoms as well as the risk of relapse during the maintenance phase (Elis et al. 2013; Kreyenbuhl et al. 2010). Unfortunately, pharmacological treatments have limited effects, especially on negative symptoms (Leucht et al. 2013; Leucht et al. 2009). Thus, recommendations and treatment guidelines suggest adjunctive CBT to improve symptom severity (Kreyenbuhl et al. 2010). Several controlled clinical trials and recent meta-analysis have demonstrated positive effects of CBT to reduce resistant positive and negative symptoms, as well as comorbid depressive symptoms (Elis et al. 2013; Grant et al. 2012; Sarin et al. 2011; Wykes et al. 2008). Consequently, international consensus guidelines declared CBT as a core component in the treatment of schizophrenia (Berry and Haddock 2012; Gaebel et al. 2011; Lehman et al. 2004). Regarding comorbid conditions in schizophrenia, integrated CBT approaches have been proven effective especially in the treatment of co-occurring substance use disorders (Barrowclough et al. 2010; Bellack et al. 2006; Ziedonis et al. 2005) and post-traumatic stress disorder. For the latter Frueh et al. developed an exposure-based treatment program demonstrating good tolerability and effectiveness (Frueh et al. 2009).

Based on above-mentioned evidence (clinical trials applying CBT for primary OCD and for core syndromes within schizophrenia), it is compelling to consider CBT as a treatment option for comorbid OCD in patients with schizophrenia.

12.2 Conceptual and Empirical Evidence

12.2.1 Clinical Impact of Co-occurring Obsessive-Compulsive Symptoms

Earlier conceptualizations considered obsessive-compulsive symptoms (OCS) to have a protective effect against psychotic disintegration, and they were thought to be an indicator for good prognosis (Rosen 1957; Stengel 1945). However, this does not appear to be the case. Subsequent research results showed that the comorbid obsessions and related compulsions have a severe impact on the patient's emotional and psychosocial functioning. Schizophrenia patients with OCS reported lower subjective well-being and lower subjective quality of life compared to patients without comorbid OCS (de Haan et al. 2013). Lysaker et al. reported greater levels of hopelessness (Lysaker and Whitney 2006), and several studies found significant associations between the presence of comorbid OCS and more severe depressive symptoms (Bottas et al. 2005; de Haan et al. 2005; Lysaker and Whitney 2009) even resulting in higher suicidal ideation (Sevincok et al. 2007). The majority of studies comparing cognitive performance in schizophrenia patients with and without comorbid OCS reported larger deficits in specific domains, such as executive functioning, cognitive flexibility and visuo-spatial memory in comorbid samples (Patel et al. 2010; Schirmbeck et al. 2012; for details see Chap. 7). Studies investigating the interrelation between obsessive-compulsive and psychotic symptoms reported controversial results. However, contrary to earlier assumptions, the majority of studies found more severe positive and negative symptoms in the comorbid group (Cunill et al. 2009; for details see Chap. 6).

Taken together, co-occurring OCS are associated with higher impairment resulting in social dysfunction (Fenton and McGlashan 1986) and have a negative effect on treatment response (Jaeger et al. 2008) and on the overall prognosis (Lysaker et al. 2004; Öngür and Goff 2005). These results strengthen the clinical relevance of OCS comorbidity in schizophrenia and related disorders and the need for effective treatment strategies.

12.2.2 Effectiveness of Pharmacological Interventions

Differential pharmacological treatment approaches for heterogeneous subgroups within the comorbid sample have been suggested. The American Psychiatric Association (APA) practice guidelines (Koran et al. 2007) suggest treating OCD co-occurring with schizophrenia by combining either typical or atypical antipsychotics with SRIs or by dose adjustment and augmentation strategies for antipsychotic-induced OCS.

However, data on the efficacy and safety of these therapeutic strategies are limited (see Chap. 11). Preliminary results suggest beneficial effects of pharmacological approaches (Hwang et al. 2009; Schirmbeck and Zink 2012), but findings have been heterogeneous with some studies failing to achieve the intended effects of OCS reduction (Bark and Lindenmayer 1992; Margetic et al. 2008). The majority of studies report remaining clinically relevant symptom severity.

Furthermore, additive side effects and pharmacokinetic interactions have to be considered when using combination or augmentation strategies (Andrade 2013). Consequently, the APA states that when OCS in patients with schizophrenia do not respond to treatment options such as adding an SRI or switching to another second-generation antipsychotic, a CBT trial could be an attempt (Koran et al. 2007).

12.2.3 Evaluation of Published Cases of CBT for Comorbid OCD

12.2.3.1 Effectiveness

Despite recommendations to apply CBT for comorbid OCS in patients with schizophrenia, it has not been evaluated in controlled clinical trials. Nevertheless, several important assumptions and suggestions can be derived from published cases. We recently reviewed and summarized results from case reports and one case series (Schirmbeck and Zink 2013a). Including additional cases published before February 2014, we will report results of 31 comorbid patients receiving CBT, in most cases with ERP (see Table 12.1).

Table 12.1 Case reports and case series of cognitive behavioural therapy for OCD in schizophrenia

Reference	Case characteristics	Number of cases	CBT method	Results
Case reports				
Ganesan et al. (2001)	Male, 33 y, since 12 y OCD	3	CBT with ERP+SSRI	8 weeks follow-up:
	Female, 25 y, since 1 y OCD			100 % remission
	Male, 31 y, since 11 y OCD			25–50 % improvement
				60 % improvement
				Significant improvement of psychosis
Mac Cabe et al. (2002)	Male, 50 y, since 5 y OCD	1	4 months of CBT with ERP	11 months follow-up:
				YBOCS 12 $\geq$ 4
				Stabil remitted psychosis
Ekers et al. (2004)	Male, 31 y, since 15 y OCD	1	20 h of CBT with ERP	6 months follow-up:
				YBOCS: 31 $\geq$ 9
				Stabil remitted psychosis

Table 12.1 (continued)

Reference	Case characteristics	Number of cases	CBT method	Results
Peasley-Miklus et al. (2005)	Male, 22 y, since 12 y OCD	1	6 months of CBT with ERP	3 years follow-up:
				35 % symptom reduction
				Washing several hours per day
				≥45–60 min 2× per week
				Significant improvement of psychosis
Rufer and Watzke (2006)	Female	1	45 h of CBT with ERP + SSRI	15 months follow-up:
				HZI: 'washing': Stanine 9 ≥ 6
				'Checking': Stanine 7 ≥ 5
				Stabil remitted psychosis
Kobori et al. (2008)	Male, 26 y, since 6 y OCD	1	19 h of CBT + SSRI	24 months follow-up:
				YBOCS 31 ≥ 11
				Stabil remitted psychosis
Rodriguez et al. (2010)	male 19 y, since ~6 months OCD	1	Few hours of CBT with ERP + SSRI	Initial reduction of OCS after start of CBT, but subsequent dropout
Hagen et al. (2014)	Male, late 20s, OCD for several y	1	9 h of CBT + ERP over 3 weeks	6 months follow-up:
				YBOCS: 24 ≥ 5
Case serie				
Tundo et al. (2012)	13 male, 8 female, ~ 29.3 y, ~ duration of OCD 6.8 y	21	~32 h of CBT with ERP	12 months follow-up:
				YBOCS: SCH: 31,6 ≥26,6
				SCH-A: 30,2 ≥22,7

Abbreviations: *CBT* cognitive behavioural therapy, *ERP* exposure and response prevention, *HZI* hamburger zwangsinventar, *OCD* obsessive-compulsive disorder, *SCH-A* schizoaffective disorder, *SCH* schizophrenia, *SSRI* selective serotonin reuptake inhibitor, *y* years, *YBOCS* Yale-Brown obsessive-compulsive scale

Regarding the demographic and clinical characteristics of treated individuals, 21 (68 %) were male and the mean age was 29 years (range 18–50). All patients reported clinically meaningful symptom severity and were diagnosed with co-occurring OCD. The majority experienced OCS over several years with a mean duration of 6.7 years before start of CBT treatment. With respect to the time course of symptom manifestation, the majority of patients reported first onset of OCD concurrent with or subsequent to the first psychotic episode. Ongoing clozapine treatment was reported in 36 % of these cases. Due to a lack of information, it is impossible to state on causal interrelations; however, this rate would stand in line with previously reported numbers of antipsychotic-induced OCS (Schirmbeck et al. 2011).

At the end of CBT treatment, 15 of 31 (48 %) patients showed a clinically relevant decrease of symptom severity, i.e. a reduction of ≥35 % in the Yale-Brown Obsessive-Compulsive Scale (YBOCS) total score. This percentage of improvement has been defined to represent successful therapy outcome according to the OCD therapy response criteria by Pallanti et al. (Pallanti and Quercioli 2006). Some studies reported follow-up assessments after several months or even years, suggesting stable treatment effects (Table 12.1).

Unfortunately, summarizing case reports is not only limited by the small sample size but also by relevant heterogeneity in patient characteristics and treatment design. While some patients only received few hours of CBT, others were treated for several months. Furthermore, six cases were treated with adjunctive selective serotonin reuptake inhibitors (SSRIs). Although most studies reported limited effectiveness of SSRI treatment prior to CBT initiation (Kobori et al. 2008; Peasley-Miklus et al. 2005; Rodriguez et al. 2010), final conclusions on symptom reduction due to CBT or medication effects cannot be drawn.

More homogeneous information can be derived from the subgroup included in the study by Tundo et al. This investigation in a naturalistic setting evaluated the effectiveness of CBT without concomitant SRI treatment in 21 patients with schizophrenia or schizoaffective disorder and severe, comorbid OCD (mean YBOCS total score = 31.6) (Tundo et al. 2012). Results showed statistically significant OCS reduction over 12 months, as well as improvements in general illness severity and global assessment of functioning. At the end of the trial, the authors classified 52 % of treated patients as 'much or very much' improved, 33 % as responders and 19 % as remitters. With a mean pre- to 1-year follow-up change score in the YBOCS of 8.1 (95 % confidence interval: 5.4–10.8), symptom reduction of comorbid OCS was only slightly less than the overall benchmarks observed in pre- to post-treatment comparisons of ERP (11.4; 10.5–12.2) and CBT studies (10.6; 8.5–12.8) in primary OCD (Houghton et al. 2010). Furthermore, insight into the illness significantly increased (Tundo et al. 2012).

12.2.3.2 Predictors of Response

Recently, Tundo et al. carried out secondary analyses to identify outcome predictors of CBT effectiveness on co-occurring OCS (Tundo et al. 2014). Their findings show that patients with alcohol/substance abuse disorder and those with OCD onset preceding psychosis onset were less likely to improve. No differences were found comparing patients with OCD onset primary or secondary to antipsychotic treatment. These preliminary findings suggest that CBT could also be a useful adjunctive treatment for OCS induced by second-generation antipsychotic agents. Accordingly, one case report shows successful reduction of clozapine-induced obsessions and compulsions after 4 months of CBT (MacCabe et al. 2002).

12.2.3.3 Treatment Tolerability and Adherence

High attention has been raised on possible negative effects of CBT with ERP on schizophrenia symptoms. In fact, one reason why CBT as a treatment modality for comorbid OCS in schizophrenia has been so scarcely investigated can be related to safety and tolerability concerns. Accordingly, in clinical ERP trials for OCD, patients experiencing psychotic symptoms or being diagnosed with a psychotic disorder have been excluded. A study evaluating clinician's perceptions on exposure-based CBT among patients with severe mental illness reported a number of concerns including the fear that ERP and accompanied intervention-related arousal would result in severe exacerbation of psychiatric symptoms (Frueh et al. 2006). Positive results from recent studies which applied CBT with exposure and EMDR for posttraumatic stress disorder (PTSD) in subjects with a psychotic disorder counter these concerns. Studies not only revealed significant PTSD symptom improvement but also positive outcomes for other targeted domains, including auditory hallucinations, delusions, anxiety symptoms, depression symptoms and self-esteem (de Bont et al. 2013; Frueh et al. 2009; van den Berg and van der Gaag 2012).

Accordingly, mentioned cases suggest that CBT with ERP results in significant decrease of OCS severity, while ensuring stable remitted psychosis or even improvement of psychotic symptoms during treatment. In fact, the main reasons for treatment discontinuation were not tolerability concerns but the patient's disbelief that CBT would be helpful. An increase of psychotic positive symptoms was reported in 2 of 31 cases. In one of these cases, the patient showed reluctance to commit to exposure elements and interfering psychotic symptoms. The therapist therefore decided to suspend exposure-based treatment and focused on cognitive techniques (Peasley-Miklus et al. 2005). Tundo et al. reported CBT discontinuation in another case because of psychotic exacerbation and subsequent hospitalization after more than 6 months of psychotherapy (Tundo et al. 2012). In the opinion of the authors, in this case, the worsening of psychotic symptoms represented a natural course of schizophrenia more than symptom intensification related to the involvement in ERP.

In conclusion, reported evidence is certainly limited by the small sample size and the lack of controlled clinical trials. However, preliminary results suggest good adherence to CBT. The drop-out rate of 24 % in the case series is comparable to those reported for patients with primary OCD (13–36 %) (Abramowitz et al. 2002; Tundo et al. 2012). CBT adherence resulted in meaningful or marked reduction of OCS severity in the majority of reported cases.

12.3 Implementation of CBT for Comorbid OCS

What needs to be considered….

(a) Assessing the patient's symptoms
(b) Enhancing safety and treatment adherence
(c) Adapting CBT approaches
(d) Treatment needs for specific subgroups

12.3.1 Assessing the Patient's Symptoms

An early and correct detection of OCS in patients with schizophrenia is the first step for an effective treatment. Therefore an increased clinical awareness for the comorbid condition is certainly necessary, especially because of an often substantially high number of undetected cases (Mukhopadhaya et al. 2009). Detailed symptom exploration and careful diagnostic considerations will help to identify comorbid affected cases and provide pivotal evaluations for subsequent treatment approaches.

Differentiating between delusions and obsessions is often possible on the basis of their content. Whereas delusions commonly revolve around persecutory, grandiose, referential, erotomanic and somatic themes, obsessions refer to contamination, symmetry, exactness or forbidden thoughts and are usually associated with corresponding compulsions (cleaning, ordering and arranging, checking and hoarding) performed to reduce distress or prevent a dreaded event. Repetitive psychotic behaviours on the other hand are mainly independent of specific thought contents.

However, the differentiation between delusions and obsessions can become especially difficult if patients show poor insight into the irrational nature of their obsessions or if delusional thoughts resolve around typical OCD topics such as contamination or infection. Similarly, careful exploration of symptoms is needed to differentiate between compulsions and stereotypic reactions to delusions and hallucinations.

Based on the diagnostic criteria for primary OCD, several guidelines have been proposed, to enable consistent and valid diagnostic decisions on the comorbid condition (Bottas et al. 2005; Pallanti et al. 2011; Schirmbeck and Zink 2013b). Patients should attribute their obsessions, impulsive symptoms and compulsions to their own thinking; they should acknowledge that they are unreasonable or excessive and should show at least some degree of resistance against them. Thus, obsessive ruminations or stereotypic thoughts during acute psychosis or repetitive ritualized behaviour clearly related to the patient's primary psychotic condition should not be rated as OCS. For a final decision on a valid comorbid condition, symptoms should be re-evaluated after the remission of psychotic symptoms (Schirmbeck and Zink 2013b). In cases where a careful differentiation of symptoms was guided by these criteria, reliable assessment of symptom severity of comorbid OCS in patients with schizophrenia has been demonstrated using the Yale-Brown Obsessive-Compulsive Scale (YBOCS) (Boyette et al. 2011).

12.3.2 Enhancing Safety and Treatment Adherence

12.3.2.1 Stable Remitted Psychosis

In patients with schizophrenia and co-occurring OCS, it is imperative to ensure stabilization (remission, if possible) of psychotic symptoms prior and throughout CBT, while challenging OCS. Furthermore, in order to ensure that patients have a good understanding of the development and course of their psychotic disorder, psychoeducational elements focusing on early signs of psychotic exacerbation, individual coping mechanisms and interventions in case of deterioration of schizophrenia should be implemented at the beginning of CBT (Bauml et al. 2006). In addition, the psychotherapist should routinely explore psychotic symptoms throughout sessions and prioritize any signs of exacerbation. By this means, treatment will most likely foster and stabilize remission of the psychotic disorder. In accordance, several case reports not only reported significant improvement of comorbid OCS but also a relevant decrease of psychotic symptoms throughout CBT (Ganesan et al. 2001; Peasley-Miklus et al. 2005).

12.3.2.2 Functional Analysis: Exploring Development and Maintenance of Co-occurring OCS

The analysis of functional interrelations will help to understand the mechanism by which OCS developed and are maintained (Salkovskis 2007; Veale 2007a). Thus, conditional analyses of co-occurring OCS should not only explore the content and frequency, degree of insight and feared consequences but also capture the reactivity to environmental factors and possible interrelations between psychotic symptoms and OCS. Here, assessing possible interrelations between symptom onset or aggravation and antipsychotic medication seems crucial (Schirmbeck et al. 2013; Schirmbeck and Zink 2013b). In addition to possible pharmacologic effects, the impact of other environmental factors on the course of symptoms, such as exposure to critical life events or chronic stress, should also be explored.

The aim of these detailed evaluations is to reach a consensus understanding of symptom development and course, formulate treatment goals, explain treatment rationales and increase adherence to subsequent interventions.

12.3.3 Adapting CBT Approaches

Psychological treatment can be tailored to each patient after careful consideration of their level of insight, treatment adherence and the presence of another comorbid Axis I or alcohol/substance use disorder. Established CBT manuals originally designed to treat primary OCD should be adapted to the unique issues that arise in the comorbid population. Based on successfully treated cases, different authors provided such treatment recommendations including sequencing of treatment elements and adjustment of ERP (Kobori et al. 2008; Rufer and Watzke 2006; Tundo et al. 2014).

As mentioned above, ERP has been shown to be one of the most effective elements in treating primary OCD (Rosa-Alcazar et al. 2008) and has successfully been applied in the mentioned cases. Accordingly, patients are systematically exposed in both imaginary and in vivo ways. Therefore, together with the patient, a hierarchy of most relevant situations with regard to OCS is formulated. Subsequent gradual exposure starts with the least distressing of feared situations (Ekers et al. 2004; Hagen et al. 2014; Rufer and Watzke 2006). With the primary goal not to worsen psychotic symptoms, patients should never be forced into ERP but encouraged to follow the rational of habituation and resist the urge to carry out a particular compulsion. A conjoint goal may be defined in gradually reducing compulsions or delaying them for as long as possible.

Further behavioural and cognitive techniques (relaxation training, modelling, normalization, cognitive restructuring) could supplement exposure and ritual-prevention strategies (Andrews et al. 2003; Hayes et al. 2006; Veale 2007b). At the start of treatment, especially normalization technique could be useful to clarify to patients that the content of the intrusive thoughts and urges are part of the human condition. So, the problem does not lie in the intrusions but in the meaning that they attach to those thoughts and the various strategies that they adopt to try to control or suppress them. Because unreasonable assumptions and cognitive biases play a particularly important role not only in the pathogenesis and maintenance of OCS but also in the formation of psychotic symptoms, cognitive interventions challenging these beliefs represent an indispensable part of treatment (Moritz et al. 2010; Veale 2007b).

12.3.4 Treatment Needs for Specific Subgroups

Due to the diverse clinical presentation of OCS in schizophrenia and the involvement of multiple pathogenic pathways, interventions have to be adapted to different treatment needs. Patients, who show a fluctuating course of symptoms, might already profit from psychoeducation and from detailed functional analyses identifying variables that contribute to the occurrence and remission of comorbid OCS. In contrast, patients with severe and persistent symptoms will need more extensive CBT treatment. In addition, within this subgroup an association between symptom onset/aggravation and the antipsychotic treatment should be explored and pharmacological interventions considered.

12.3.4.1 Combination with Pharmacological Interventions

As mentioned in Chap. 11, in cases with de novo development or marked aggravation of OCS in association with antipsychotic treatment, pharmacological interventions with dose adjustment and/or changes of antipsychotic drug seem primarily indicated. In cases with pre-existing OCS, when symptoms persist over time and develop independently of the course of psychotic illness, additional SRI treatment should be considered (Hwang et al. 2009). However, individuals with antipsychotic-induced OCS could also benefit from adjunctive CBT. Interventions aiming to improve patients' insight into their symptoms will foster better treatment adherence and help to prevent relapse. CBT allows early detection of symptom aggravation and timely interventions. Therefore, a combination of pharmacological and psychotherapeutic approaches seems indicated.

12.3.4.2 Addressing More General Areas of Impairment

Recent research results suggest that normal personality traits in particular high levels of neuroticism (Schirmbeck et al. 2014) and associated avoidant-focused coping strategies (Lysaker and Whitney 2006) might play an important role in the development and maintenance of both sets of disorders. Furthermore, specific neurocognitive deficits seem to be associated with co-occurring OCS (see Chap. 7). Thus more general areas of impairment such as improved coping skills or cognitive remediation might become specifically important to address in specific comorbid cases. Kobori et al., for example, accounted for a so-called lack of real world knowledge due to long hospitalizations and withdrawal from daily routine of their patients. The therapist included practical information and demonstrations about day-to-day living in cognitive restructuring. Behavioural experiments and additional information led to alternative explanations of intrusive thoughts and OCS reduction (Kobori et al. 2008).

12.4 Conclusion and Future Perspectives

Patients with psychotic disorders often suffer from co-occurring OCS, which are associated with additional impairments. Good efficacy of CBT for primary OCD led to its recommendation as a treatment approach for comorbid OCS. The review of the published literature shows promising effects. In the vast majority of cases, CBT results in significant decrease of OCS severity, while ensuring stable remitted psychosis or even improvement of psychotic symptoms during treatment. Results further show good adherence to CBT and suggest that it would add to currently available treatment modes for OCS in schizophrenia. Based on described cases, we outline specific aspects that seem crucial to enhance tolerability and efficacy of CBT in this group of patients. However, as the strength of this evidence is still weak, further research and evaluations in controlled clinical trials are highly desirable.

Because the optimal 'treatment' approach is certainly the primary prevention or early detection of OCS, an increase in clinical awareness for the co-occurring conditions is warranted.

Acknowledgements *F.S.* was supported by a fellowship within the Postdoc-Programme of the German Academic Exchange Service (DAAD).

References

Abramowitz JS, Franklin ME, Foa EB (2002) Empirical status of cognitive-behavioral therapy for obsessive-compulsive disorder: a meta-analytic review. Rom J Cogn Behav Psychother 2:89–104

Albert U, Aguglia A, Bogetto F, Cieri L, Daniele M, Maina G, Necci R, Parena A, Salvati L, Tundo A (2012) Effectiveness of cognitive-behavioral therapy addition to pharmacotherapy in resistant obsessive-compulsive disorder: a multicenter study. Psychother Psychosom 81:383–385

Andrade C (2013) Serotonin reuptake inhibitor treatment of obsessive-compulsive symptoms in clozapine-medicated schizophrenia. J Clin Psychiatry 73:e1362–e1364

Andrews G, Creamer M, Crino R, Hunt C, Lampe L, Page A (2003) The treatment of anxiety disorders: clinician guides and patient manuals, 2nd edn. Cambridge University Press, New York

Bark N, Lindenmayer JP (1992) Ineffectiveness of clomipramine for obsessive-compulsive symptoms in a patient with schizophrenia. Am J Psychiatry 149:136–137

Barrowclough C, Haddock G, Wykes T, Beardmore R, Conrod P, Craig T, Davies L, Dunn G, Eisner E, Lewis S, Moring J, Steel C, Tarrier N (2010) Integrated motivational interviewing and cognitive behavioural therapy for people with psychosis and comorbid substance misuse: randomised controlled trial. BMJ 341

Bauml J, Frobose T, Kraemer S, Rentrop M, Pitschel-Walz G (2006) Psychoeducation: a basic psychotherapeutic intervention for patients with schizophrenia and their families. Schizophr Bull 32(Suppl 1):1–9

Beck AT, Rector NA (2005) Cognitive approaches to schizophrenia: theory and therapy. Annu Rev Clin Psychol 1:577–606

Bellack AS, Bennett ME, Gearon JS (2006) Behavioral treatment for substance abuse in people with serious and persistent mental illness: a handbook for mental health professionals. Routledge, New York

Berry K, Haddock G (2012) The implementation of the NICE guidelines for schizophrenia: barriers to the implementation of psychological interventions and recommendations for the future. Psychol Psychother 81:419–436

Bottas A, Cooke RG, Richter MA (2005) Comorbidity and pathophysiology of obsessive-compulsive disorder in schizophrenia: is there evidence for a schizo-obsessive subtype of schizophrenia? [Review] [90 refs]. J Psychiatry Neurosci 30:187–193

Boyette L, Swets M, Meijer C, Wouters L, G R O U P Authors (2011) Factor structure of the Yale-Brown Obsessive-Compulsive Scale (Y-BOCS) in a large sample of patients with schizophrenia or related disorders and comorbid obsessive-compulsive symptoms. Psychiatry Res 186:409–413

Butler AC, Chapman JE, Forman EM, Beck AT (2006) The empirical status of cognitive-behavioral therapy: a review of meta-analyses. Clin Psychol Rev 26:17–31

Cunill R, Castells X, Simeon D (2009) Relationships between obsessive-compulsive symptomatology and severity of psychosis in schizophrenia: a systematic review and meta-analysis. J Clin Psychiatry 70:70–82

de Bont PAJM, van Minnen A, de Jongh A (2013) Treating PTSD in patients with psychosis: a within-group controlled feasibility study examining the efficacy and safety of evidence-based PE and EMDR protocols. Behav Ther 44:717–730

de Haan L, Hoogenboom B, Beuk N, van Amelsvoort T, Linszen D (2005) Obsessive-compulsive symptoms and positive, negative, and depressive symptoms in patients with recent-onset schizophrenic disorders. Can J Psychiatry 50:519–524

de Haan L, Sterk B, van der Valk R (2013) Presence of obsessive compulsive symptoms in first-episode schizophrenia or related disorders is associated with subjective well-being and quality of life. Early Interv Psychiatry 7:285–290

Ekers D, Carman S, Schlich T (2004) Successful outcome of exposure and response prevention in the treatment of obsessive compulsive disorder in a patient with schizophrenia. Behav Cogn Psychother 32:375–378

Elis O, Caponigro JM, Kring AM (2013) Psychosocial treatments for negative symptoms in schizophrenia: current practices and future directions. Clin Psychol Rev 33:914–928

Fenton WS, McGlashan TH (1986) The prognostic significance of obsessive-compulsive symptoms in schizophrenia. Am J Psychiatry 143:437–441

Franklin ME, Foa EB (2011) Treatment of obsessive compulsive disorder. Annu Rev Clin Psychol 7:229–243

Frueh BC, Cusack KJ, Grubaugh AL, Sauvageot JA, Wells C (2006) Clinicians' perspectives on cognitive-behavioral treatment for PTSD among persons with severe mental illness. Psychiatr Serv 57:1027–1031

Frueh BC, Grubaugh AL, Cusack KJ, Kimble MO, Elhai JD, Knapp RG (2009) Exposure-based cognitive-behavioral treatment of PTSD in adults with schizophrenia or schizoaffective disorder: a pilot study. J Anxiety Disord 23:665–675

Gaebel W, Riesbeck M, Wobrock T (2011) Schizophrenia guidelines across the world: a selective review and comparison. Int Rev Psychiatry 23:379–387

Ganesan V, Kumar TCR, Khanna S (2001) Obsessive-compulsive disorder and psychosis. Can J Psychiatry 46:750–754

Gava I, Barbui C, Aguglia E, Carlino D, Churchill R, De VM, McGuire HF (2007) Psychological treatments versus treatment as usual for obsessive compulsive disorder (OCD). Cochrane Database of Systematic Reviews 18 (2):CD005333

Grant PM, Huh GA, Perivoliotis D, Stolar NM, Beck AT (2012) Randomized trial to evaluate the efficacy of cognitive therapy for low-functioning patients with schizophrenia. Arch Gen Psychiatry 69:121–127

Hagen K, Solem S, Hansen B (2014) Cognitive behavioural therapy for obsessive-compulsive disorder with comorbid schizophrenia: a case report with repetitive measurements. Behav Cogn Psychother 42:374–378

Hayes SC, Luoma JB, Bond FW, Masuda A, Lillis J (2006) Acceptance and commitment therapy: model, processes and outcomes. Behav Res Ther 44:1–25

Hofmann S, Asnaani A, Vonk IJ, Sawyer A, Fang A (2012) The efficacy of cognitive behavioral therapy: a review of meta-analyses. Cognit Ther Res 36:427–440

Houghton S, Saxon D, Bradburn M, Ricketts T, Hardy G (2010) The effectiveness of routinely delivered cognitive behavioural therapy for obsessive-compulsive disorder: a benchmarking study. Br J Clin Psychol 49:473–489

Hwang MY, Kim SW, Yum SY, Opler LA (2009) Management of schizophrenia with obsessive-compulsive features. Psychiatr Clin North Am 32:835–851

Jaeger M, Messer T, Laux G, Pfeiffer H, Naber D, Schmidt LG, Gaebel W, Klosterk+Âtter J, Heuse I, Maier W, Lemke MR, Ruether E, Buckkremer G, Gastpar M, Riedel M, Bottlander R, Strauss A, Moeller H-J (2008) Standardized remission criteria in schizophrenia: descriptive validity and comparability with previously used outcome measures. Pharmacopsychiatry 41:190–195

Kampman M, Keijsers GPJ, Hoogduin CAL, Verbraak MJPM (2002) Addition of cognitive-behaviour therapy for obsessive-compulsive disorder patients non-responding to fluoxetine. Acta Psychiatr Scand 106:314–319

Kobori O, Sato H, Katsukura R, Harada S (2008) Cognitive behavioural therapy for obsessive compulsive symptoms affected by past psychotic experience of schizophrenia: a case report. Behav Cogn Psychother 36:365–369

Koran LM, Hanna GL, Hollander E, Nestadt G, Simpson HB, Association AP (2007) Practice guideline for the treatment of patients with obsessive-compulsive disorder. Am J Psychiatry 164:5–53

Kordon A, Lotz-Rambaldi W, Muche-Borowski C, Hohagen F (2013) S3-Leitlinie Zwangsstörungen. Arbeitsgemeinschaft der Wissenschaftlichen Medizinischen Fachgesellschaften (AWMF). Im Auftrag der Deutschen GEsellschaft für Psychiatrie und Psychotherapie, Psychosomatik und Nervenheilkunde (DGPPN)

Kreyenbuhl J, Buchanan RW, Dickerson FB, Dixon LB (2010) The schizophrenia patient outcomes research team (PORT): updated treatment recommendations 2009. Schizophr Bull 36:94–103

Lehman AF, Lieberman JA, Dixon LB, McGlashan TH, Miller AL, Perkins DO, Kreyenbuhl J, American Psychiatric Association; Steering Committee on Practice Guidelines (2004) Practice guideline for the treatment of patients with schizophrenia, second edition. Am J Psychiatry 161:1–56

Leucht S, Cipriani A, Spineli L, Mavridis D, Örey D, Richter F, Samara M, Barbui C, Engel RR, Geddes JR, Kissling W, Stapf MP, Lässig B, Salanti G, Davis JM (2013) Comparative efficacy and tolerability of 15 antipsychotic drugs in schizophrenia: a multiple-treatments meta-analysis. Lancet 382:951–962

Leucht S, Kissling W, Davis J (2009) Second-generation antipsychotics for schizophrenia: can we resolve the conflict? Psychol Med 39:1591–1602

Lysaker PH, Lancaster RS, Nees MA, Davis LW (2004) Patterns of obsessive-compulsive symptoms and social function in schizophrenia. Psychiatry Res 125:139–146

Lysaker PH, Whitney KA (2006) Clinical and psychosocial correlates of obsessive compulsive symptoms in schizophrenia. In: Columbus A (ed) Advances in psychology research, vol 43. Nova Science Publishers, Hauppauge, New York, pp 1–22

Lysaker PH, Whitney KA (2009) Obsessive-compulsive symptoms in schizophrenia: prevalence, correlates and treatment. Expert Rev Neurother 9:99–107

MacCabe JH, Marks IM, Murray RM (2002) Behavior therapy attenuates clozapine-induced obsessions and compulsions. J Clin Psychiatry 63:1179–1180

Margetic B, Aukst-Margetic B, Jakovljevic M (2008) Aggravation of schizophrenia by clomipramine in a patient with comorbid obsessive-compulsive disorder. Psychopharmacol Bull 41:9–11

Moritz S, Peters MJ, Laroi F, Lincoln TM (2010) Metacognitive beliefs in obsessive-compulsive patients: a comparison with healthy and schizophrenia participants. Cogn Neuropsychiatry 15:531–548

Mukhopadhaya K, Krishnaiah R, Taye T, Nigam A, Bailey AJ, Sivakumaran T, Fineberg NA (2009) Obsessive-compulsive disorder in UK clozapine-treated schizophrenia and schizoaffective disorder: a cause for clinical concern. J Psychopharmacol 23:6–13

Öngür D, Goff DC (2005) Obsessive-compulsive symptoms in schizophrenia: associated clinical features, cognitive function and medication status. Schizophr Res 75:349–362

Pallanti S, Grassi G, Cantisani A, Sarrecchia E, Pellegrini M (2011) Obsessive-compulsive disorder comorbidity: clinical assessment and therapeutic implications. Front Psychiatry 2

Pallanti S, Quercioli L (2006) Treatment-refractory obsessive-compulsive disorder: methodological issues, operational definitions and therapeutic lines. Prog Neuropsychopharmacol Biol Psychiatry 30:400–412

Patel DD, Laws KR, Padhi A, Farrow JM, Mukhopadhaya K, Krishnaiah R, Fineberg NA (2010) The neuropsychology of the schizo-obsessive subtype of schizophrenia: a new analysis. Psychol Med 40:921–933

Peasley-Miklus C, Massie E, Baslett G, Carmin C (2005) Treating obsessive-compulsive disorder and schizophrenia: the case of Sam. Cogn Behav Pract 12:379–383

Rodriguez CI, Corcoran C, Simpson HB (2010) Diagnosis and treatment of a patient with both psychotic and obsessive-compulsive symptoms. Am J Psychiatry 167:754–761

Romanelli RJ, Wu FM, Gamba R, Mojtabai R, Segal JB (2014) Behavioral therapy and serotonin reuptake inhibitor pharmacotherapy in the treatment of obsessive-compulsive disorder: a systematic review and meta-analysis of head-to-head randomized controlled trials. Depression and Anxiety 31:641–652

Rosa-Alcazar AI, Sanchez-Meca J, Gomez-Conesa A, Marin-Martinez F (2008) Psychological treatment of obsessive-compulsive disorder: a meta-analysis. Clin Psychol Rev 28: 1310–1325

Rosen I (1957) The clinical significance of obsessions in schizophrenia. J Ment Sci 103:773–785

Rufer M, Hand I, Alsleben H, Braatz A, Ortmann J, Katenkamp B, Fricke S, Peter H (2005) Long–term course and outcome of obsessive–compulsive patients after cognitive-behavioral therapy in combination with either fluvoxamine or placebo. Eur Arch Psychiatry Clin Neurosci 255:121–128

Rufer M, Watzke B (2006) Ambulante Verhaltenstherapie mit intensiver Exposition einer Patientin mit Zwangsstörung und früherer Psychose. In: Fricke S, Rufer M, Hand I (ed) Verhaltenstherapie bei Zwangsstörungen, Fallbasierte Therapiekonzepte, pp 147–164. München: Urban & Fischer.

Salkovskis PM (2007) Psychological treatment of obsessive-compulsive disorder. Psychiatry 6:229–233

Sarin F, Wallin L, Widerloev B (2011) Cognitive behavior therapy for schizophrenia: a meta-analytical review of randomized controlled trials. Nord J Psychiatry 65:162–174

Schirmbeck F, Boyette L-L, Valk Rvd, Meijer C, Dingemans P, Van R, de Haan L, Kahn RS, de Haan L, van OsJ, Wiersma D, Bruggeman R, Cahn W, Meijer C, Myin-Germeys I (2014) Relevance of Five-Factor Model personality traits for obsessive–compulsive symptoms in patients with psychotic disorders and their un-affected siblings. Psychiatry Research doi: org/10.1016/j.psychres.2014.11.066

Schirmbeck F, Zink M (2012) Obsessive-compulsive syndromes in schizophrenia: a case for polypharmacy? In: Ritsner M (ed) Polypharmacy in psychiatric practice. Springer, Dordrecht. ISBN 978-94-007-5798-1

Schirmbeck F, Zink M (2013a) Cognitive behavioural therapy for obsessive-compulsive symptoms in schizophrenia. Cogn Behav Ther 6:1–13

Schirmbeck F, Zink M (2013b) Comorbid obsessive-compulsive symptoms in schizophrenia: contributions of pharmacological and genetic factors. Front Pharmacol 4:99

Schirmbeck F, Esslinger C, Rausch F, Englisch S, Meyer-Lindenberg A, Zink M (2011) Antiserotonergic antipsychotics are associated with obsessive-compulsive symptoms in schizophrenia. Psychol Med 41:2361–2374

Schirmbeck F, Rausch F, Englisch S, Eifler S, Esslinger C, Meyer-Lindenberg A, Zink M (2012) Stable cognitive deficits in schizophrenia patients with comorbid obsessive-compulsive symptoms: a 12-month longitudinal study. Schizophr Bull. doi:10.1093/schbul/sbs123

Schirmbeck F, Rausch F, Englisch S, Eifler S, Esslinger C, Meyer-Lindenberg A, Zink M (2013) Differential effects of antipsychotic agents on obsessive-compulsive symptoms in schizophrenia: a longitudinal study. J Psychopharmacol 27:349–357

Sevincok L, Akoglu A, Kokcu F (2007) Suicidality in schizophrenic patients with and without obsessive-compulsive disorder. Schizophr Res 90:198–202

Simpson H, Foa EB, Liebowitz MR et al (2013) Cognitive-behavioral therapy vs risperidone for augmenting serotonin reuptake inhibitors in obsessive-compulsive disorder: a randomized clinical trial. JAMA Psychiatry 70:1190–1199

Stengel E (1945) A study on some clinical aspects of the relationship between obsessional neurosis and psychotic reaction types. J Ment Sci 91:166–187

Tundo A, Salvati L, Busto G, Di Spigno D, Falcini R (2007) Addition of cognitive-behavioral therapy for nonresponders to medication for obsessive-compulsive disorder: a naturalistic study. J Clin Psychiatry 68:1552–1556

Tundo A, Salvati L, Di Spigno D, Cieri L, Parena A, Necci R, Sciortino S (2012) Cognitive-behavioral therapy for obsessive-compulsive disorder as a comorbidity with schizophrenia or schizoaffective disorder. Psychother Psychosom 81:58–60

Tundo A, Salvati L, Cieri M, Daniele M, Di Spigno D, Necci R, Parena A (2014) Effectiveness and outcome predictors of cognitive-behavioural therapy for obsessive-compulsive disorder co-occurring with psychosis. J Psychopathol 20:127–133

van den Berg DPG, van der Gaag M (2012) Treating trauma in psychosis with EMDR: a pilot study. J Behav Ther Exp Psychiatry 43:664–671

van Oppen P, van Balkom AJ, de Haan E, van Dyck R (2005) Cognitive therapy and exposure in vivo alone and in combination with fluvoxamine in obsessive-compulsive disorder: a 5-year follow-up. J Clin Psychiatry 66:1415–1422

Veale D (2007a) Cognitive-behavioural therapy for obsessive-compulsive disorder. Adv Psychiatr Treat 13:438–446

Veale D (2007b) Treating obsessive-compulsive disorder in people with poor insight and overvalued ideation. In: Antony MM, Summerfeldt LJ (eds) Psychological treatment of obsessive-compulsive disorder: fundamentals and beyond. American Psychological Association, Washington, DC, pp 267–280

Wykes T, Steel C, Everitt B, Tarrier N (2008) Cognitive behavior therapy for schizophrenia: effect sizes, clinical models, and methodological rigor. Schizophr Bull 34:523–537

Ziedonis D, Smelson D, Rosenthal RN, Batki SL, Green AI, Henry RJ, Montoya I, Parks J, Weiss RD (2005) Improving the care of individuals with schizophrenia and substance use disorders: consensus recommendations. J Psychiatr Pract 11:315–339

Conclusions and Future Directions of Research

Clinical Significance of OCS in Schizophrenia

The wealth of data in this book regarding prevalence rates, clinical importance, insight into phenomenological heterogeneity and multiple etiological mechanisms highlights the significance of co-morbid obsessive-compulsive symptoms (OCS) in patients with schizophrenia and other psychotic disorders.

To summarize former chapters, one can conclude that OCS occur relatively common, affecting almost one third of patients with a psychotic disorder and result in poorer subjective well-being, additional functional impairment and are often associated with more psychotic and depressive symptoms. Hence, the effective treatment of co-morbid OCS will be of significant importance for the overall treatment success.

In clinical practice, the attribution of distressing cognitions, ruminations, repetitive or stereotypic behavior to either OCS or the psychotic syndrome is often a challenge due to the dimensional overlap of symptoms. This book provides evidence-based guidelines and detailed descriptions of clinical aspects, which help to differentiate between OCS and psychotic symptoms and provides comprehensive knowledge on the co-occurrence of OCS and schizotypal personality disorder. The detailed description of clinical symptoms and comorbid constellations must be accompanied by increased insight into relevant genetic risk factors, neuroimaging findings and other biological markers. In perspective, these steps will elucidate the pathogenesis of comorbid OCS in schizophrenia.

In addition, several well described case studies and small therapeutic trials inform treatment guidelines for OCS in schizophrenia. Based on their findings we are able to provide preliminary advice regarding risk prediction, early recognition and pharmacological and psychotherapeutical treatment.

Taken together, the findings underscore the substantial clinical relevance to diagnose OCS in schizophrenia and indicate treatment options.

L. De Haan et al. (eds.), *Obsessive-Compulsive Symptoms in Schizophrenia*,
DOI 10.1007/978-3-319-12952-5

Unmet Needs: Major Aims of Forthcoming Research

To date, our pathogenic understanding is certainly limited and we do not sufficiently understand which and how genetic and environmental risk factors contribute to the clinical manifestation of OCS in schizophrenia, nor how they interact with each other. Moreover we do not sufficiently understand the distinctive underlying neurobiological processes involved in the development of comorbid OCS.

Preliminary evidence from prospective investigations suggests diverse courses of OCS over time, with remission, fluctuation or aggravation of symptoms. So far little is known about risk and resilience factors which influence this longitudinal outcome. The diverse clinical presentation certainly suggests multi-causal explanations.

The greatest need concerns sound evidence for clinical interventions. Here several questions remain unanswered. It can be assumed that depending on the severity and persistence of comorbid OCS, specific subgroups of patients will profit from different interventions. Patients with mild symptomatology and a fluctuating course might already profit from psychoeducation or brief CBT interventions, whereas those with ongoing OCS should probably be treated with more extensive CBT, and/or antidepressive medication. Moreover, several findings suggest a causal interrelation between antipsychotic medication and the risk to develop OCS in patients with schizophrenia, most likely as a gene-environment interaction. Hence, there is need for evidence based guidelines for first choice antipsychotic treatment and for augmentation and combination strategies.

Methods and Milestones

To date, several theoretic concepts have been suggested to classify patients with co-occurring psychosis and OCS, for example the introduction of a new diagnostic entity within the psychosis spectrum. The ongoing debate on possible classifications should not distract from the clinical point: to identify the various problems of patients and to deliver effective treatment that ameliorates their condition. For this purpose, researchers should try to define more homogeneous subgroups based on the onset and course of OCS over time. Multimodal research focusing on these subgroups will more likely be successful to uncover the distinctive neurobiological and environmental risk factors, as has been shown for the subgroup of patients who report onset of OCS subsequent to the start of antipsychotic medication. Large scale collaborations are needed to provide studies with enough power to disentangle genetic risk factors. With respect to pharmacological as well as psychotherapeutic interventions, controlled multicenter treatment trials are needed.

Ultimately the goal is to provide individualized treatment adapted to the stage and individual profile of patients, where the co-occurrence of OCS is certainly of clinical relevance.

Here, experience sampling can be a valuable approach. This method captures the course of symptoms on a day-to-day basis and helps to identify contextual triggers, thereby providing important information for individualized interventions.

This change in perspective might also help to overcome the abovementioned conceptual discussions that are often the mere consequence of mixing and comparing heterogeneous conditions.

Concluding Remarks

We thank all the authors for their contribution to this book and are confident that the input provided by many experts in the field will help to identify, to understand and to relieve OCS in patients with schizophrenia. Furthermore, we hope that this book will stimulate research and progress in the near future.

MIX
Papier aus verantwortungsvollen Quellen
Paper from responsible sources
FSC® C105338
FSC
www.fsc.org

If you have any concerns about our products,
you can contact us on
ProductSafety@springernature.com

In case Publisher is established outside the EU,
the EU authorized representative is:
Springer Nature Customer Service Center GmbH
Europaplatz 3, 69115 Heidelberg, Germany

Printed by Libri Plureos GmbH
in Hamburg, Germany